**SORENSEN and LUCKMANN**

## Instructor's Manual To Accompany
# BASIC NURSING
## A Psychophysiologic Approach

### SECOND EDITION

## Brenda S. McMillan
Assistant Professor—Fundamentals Coordinator
California State University—Fresno
Fresno, California

**1986**

W.B. SAUNDERS COMPANY
Philadelphia   London   Toronto   Mexico City   Rio de Janeiro   Sydney   Tokyo   Hong Kong

W. B. Saunders Company: West Washington Square
Philadelphia, PA 19105

Instructor's Manual To Accompany Basic Nursing          ISBN 0-7216-2109-0

678 066 5432

# PREFACE

This Instructor's Manual has been prepared in conjunction with the second edition of the textbook, <u>Basic Nursing: A Psycho-physiologic Approach</u>. It has been designed to promote optimal learning experiences for the student, while providing an invaluable resource to assist the instructor in efficient utilization of the text. Each section includes: General chapter objectives, specific learning outcomes, teaching/learning strategies, and multiple-choice questions to assist in evaluation of chapter content. Chapters 13, 14, and 15 have been grouped into one since they all relate to Nursing Process.

Specific learning outcomes have been closely correlated with the general objectives listed at the beginning of each chapter. These learning outcomes clarify the objectives by outlining in detail, the chapter content that can be used to assist the student in attainment of the objectives.

Numerous teaching/learning strategies have been designed to facilitate achievement of the cognitive, affective, and psycho-motor chapter objectives. The strategies used in the text include: Lecture/Discussion, written exercises, group activities, class activities, guest speakers, panel presentations, values clarification exercises, communication activities, campus laboratory experiences, and clinical laboratory experiences. The specific strategies provided are contingent upon the chapter objective to be achieved. Appropriate strategies for each nursing course will depend upon available resources and facilities, and the instructor's teaching preferences.

> <u>Lecture/Discussion</u>--Suggestions for lecture/discussion correlate directly with chapter content, and in many instances, present conceptual ideas related to the chapter.

> <u>Written exercises</u>--Written exercises are frequently recommended throughout the manual to reinforce the material presented in the chapter. These exercises include such activities as, diaries, detailed outlines, and essays.

<u>Group activities</u>--A wide variety of classroom group activities have been designed to encourage active student participation in the educational process.

<u>Class activities</u>--Numerous class projects (such as visiting a community health agency) have been included to augment knowledge gained from the text.

<u>Guest speakers and panel presentations</u>--Teaching/learning activities frequently encourage the utilization of community resource personnel who demonstrate expertise in the chapter content being covered.

<u>Values clarification exercises</u>--Specific value clarification exercises have been designed to foster the student's attainment of affective learning.

<u>Communication activities</u>--Interview and role playing activities are recommended throughout the manual to assist the student in the development of interpersonal communication skills.

<u>Campus laboratory experiences</u>--Demonstration/return demonstration activities for specific psychomotor nursing skills are suggested when appropriate.

<u>Clinical laboratory experiences</u>--Community, clinic, and hospital learning experiences are frequently recommended to assist students in the application of cognitive, affective, and psychomotor chapter content.


Multiple-choice questions have been formulated to ensure representative coverage of chapter content. Appropriate rationale statements are included for each question.

# 1

# MEETING HUMAN NEEDS THROUGH THE NURSING PROCESS

## OBJECTIVES

1.0 Discuss nursing as both a science and an art.

    1.1 Compare and contrast the definitions of a science and an art as defined in this chapter. (p. 3)

    1.2 Identify the relationship of "science" and "art" in the profession of nursing. (p. 3)

    1.3 Describe the concept of holistic nursing. (p. 4)

2.0 Discuss what a system is and why people are natural systems utilizing input, output, transformation, and feedback.

    2.1 Outline the major components of General System's Theory as developed by Ludwig Von Bertalanffy. (p. 4)

    2.2 Define the term system. (p. 4)

    2.3 Explain the significance of goal setting within a system. (p. 4)

    2.4 Identify the general characteristics of an open system and a closed system. (p. 5)

    2.5 Discuss the importance of an internal and external environment as they relate to General System's Theory. (p. 5)

    2.6 Briefly discuss major functions of the internal "milieu" within a living system. (p. 5)

    2.7 Explain the concept of subsystem as it applies to the Nursing System. (p. 5)

    2.8 Identify essential components of effective communication: Input, feedback, and transformation. (p. 5)

3.0 Discuss what is meant by the hierarchy of human needs.

    3.1 Identify basic physiologic/sociocultural needs that must be fulfilled by the individual to maintain homeostasis. (p. 5)

    3.2 State the ultimate goal of nursing. (p. 6)

## TEACHING/LEARNING STRATEGIES

### Written Exercise

Ask each student to write their own personal definition of a science and an art. When completed, assist students in understanding how nursing fulfills the requirements for both a science and an art.

### Lecture/Discussion

Explain how a general systems approach can be applied in the health care setting.

Using general systems terminology, discuss the concept of adaptation as it relates to man.

Discuss how a human functions as an open system.

### Lecture/Discussion

Review the case record of a selected individual in the clinical area. Afterwards, ask students to identify any potential individual problems and then rank them according to Maslow's hierarchy of needs.

3.3 Outline Maslow's Hierarchy of Human
Needs. Briefly explain the relationship
between the various levels. (p. 7)

4.0 Describe human needs theory as adapted by
nurse theorists.

4.1 Discuss, and give examples of, the
influence human needs theory has had on
the development of theories for
nursing. (p. 7)

4.2 Describe the three categories of human
needs formulated by Dorothea Orem in the
"Self-Care" theory of nursing. (p. 7)

4.3 Identify Yure and Walsh's two basic
categories of human needs and give
examples of each. (p. 8)

5.0 Describe what happens to homeostatic balance
in an individual when even one basic need is
not met.

5.1 Define the concepts of equilibrium and
disequilibrium. (p. 10)

5.2 Identify the relationship between unmet
human needs and problems. (p. 10)

5.3 Identify common obstacles that may
interfere with need satisfaction. (p. 11)

5.4 Discuss the significance of establishing
a state of equilibrium or a homeostatic
balance within a system. (p. 5)

6.0 Define the nursing process and describe each
of the five steps.

6.1 Describe three basic ways the nurse can
help people satisfy unmet needs and
solve problems. (p. 12)

6.2 Define "nursing process." (p. 12)

6.3 Briefly identify and describe the five
basic steps of the "nursing process."
(p. 12)

6.4 Discuss the influence that utilization
of the nursing process can have when
assisting an individual to regain or
maintain homeostatic balance. (p. 12)

## Written Exercise

After discussion of chapter content, instruct
students to write a brief summary of the primary
human needs experienced by a person of their age
and developmental status.

## Lecture/Discussion

Compare and contrast the human needs framework of
a major nursing theory with that of Maslow.

## Lecture/Discussion

Ask students to identify the primary and secondary
needs that they consider essential for the
maintenance of health. How do these needs compare
with Maslow's hierarchy of human needs?

## Lecture/Discussion

Facilitate a discussion of the major differences
that exist between a nursing process approach
based on the general system's theory and the
nursing process approach based on the
problem-solving technique.

---

## MULTIPLE CHOICE QUESTIONS

1. Which of the following statements about
"systems" is incorrect?

A. A system is a set of interrelated parts
which form a unified whole.
B. Systems are constantly in a state of
homeostatic balance.
C. Systems are composed of smaller parts or
subsystems.
D. A system reacts holistically to changes
in any one of its subsystems.

## CORRECT ANSWER AND RATIONALE

B    Responses A, C, and D are correct statements
about "systems." Response B is incorrect
because systems are continuously involved in
a process input, transformation, and
feedback. Therefore, they tend to be in a
state of disorganization and disequilibrium.
(pp. 4-5)

2. After a few days in the hospital Bill is discharged. Evaluation reveals that all immediate health care needs were met. This is an example of system:

   A. Transformation
   B. Homeostasis
   C. Input
   D. Output

D    Output is the end product of a system. The output of a health-care system may be analyzed by evaluating the attainment of health-care goals/needs of those individuals leaving the system. (p. 5)

3. Homeostasis is correctly defined as:

   A. A state of equilibrium or balance
   B. Psychophysiologic equilibrium
   C. A steady state
   D. All of the above

D    All responses are correct statements defining homeostasis. (pp. 5-6)

4. According to Maslow, the most basic level of human needs are:

   A. Esteem needs
   B. Love and belonging needs
   C. Physiologic needs
   D. Safety needs

C    Maslow organized human needs according to the following hierarchy: Physiologic, safety, belonging and love, esteem, and self-actualization needs. (p. 7)

5. Which of the following problems would take priority when caring for a patient?

   A. Inadequate oxygen intake
   B. Inability to retain urine
   C. Difficulty falling asleep
   D. Inadequate food intake

A    According to Maslow, some needs require immediate gratification (e.g., respiratory needs), some needs can be temporarily postponed (e.g., food, sleep, elimination), and still other needs can be postponed indefinitely (e.g., sexual needs). (p. 7)

6. Achieving or maintaining independence is a human need relating to:

   A. Personal growth and maturity
   B. Self-esteem
   C. Self-actualization
   D. Full development of potential

B    Self-esteem needs include all of the following: Sense of value, usefulness; high evaluation of self; adequacy, self-reliance; goal attainment; mastery and competency in skills; independence; and endurance. Selections A, C, and D all pertain to human self-actualization needs. (p. 8)

7. The central theme of Dorothea Orem's theory of nursing is:

   A. The concept of self-care
   B. Universal self-care requisites
   C. Basic human needs
   D. Needs arising from illness

A    Dorothea Orem bases her theory of nursing on the concept of self-care. Self-care is defined as those activities that individuals practice to maintain life, health, and well-being. Orem groups human needs into three categories: Universal health-care requisites, developmental self-care requisites, and health-deviation self-care requisites. (p. 7)

8. Unmet human needs result in:

   A. Individual problems
   B. Disequilibrium
   C. Illness
   D. All of the above

D    When human needs go unmet, disequilibrium and eventual illness results. In nursing terminology, the unmet human need develops into an individual problem. (p. 10)

9. The nurse administers medication to control Mr. Black's postoperative pain. This nursing activity would assist the individual to meet which kind of human need?

   A. Belonging
   B. Physiological
   C. Safety
   D. Universal

C    According to Maslow, achieving freedom from pain is a safety need. (p. 8)

10. Which of Maslow's basic human needs cate-
    gories contains both physiological and
    psychosocial needs?

    A. Belonging
    B. Physiologic
    C. Safety
    D. Self-esteem

C   An analysis of the subcategories outlined on
    page 8 of the text reveals that both
    physiologic and psychologic needs are indexed
    only under safety needs. The most basic
    level, physiological needs, deals with
    physical human needs; all other levels (with
    the exception of safety) deal with
    psychological human needs. (p. 8)

11. Mr. Jackson has just expired. According to
    Orem, his significant others may be
    experiencing a human need associated with:

    A. Developmental self-care requisites
    B. Human developmental processes
    C. Conditions or events that occur during
       the normal life cycle
    D. All of the above

D   Developmental self-care requisites are
    associated with human developmental processes
    and with conditions and events occurring
    during various stages of the life cycle and
    events that can adversely affect development,
    such as, the loss of a significant other.
    (p. 8)

12. Nursing intervention to meet a person's
    physiological needs include all of the
    following except:

    A. Allowing the person to choose the foods
       to be consumed
    B. Administering medication for pain control
    C. Measuring the temperature, pulse, and
       respiration
    D. Walking the person in the hallway three
       times a day

A   Although selection A indirectly affects
    physiological needs, it more appropriately
    promotes self-esteem needs by encouraging the
    person to maintain a sense of independence.
    (p. 8)

13. The nurse includes the family in the planning
    phase of the nursing process. This activity
    assists the person with which type of basic
    human needs?

    A. Belongingness
    B. Safety
    C. Security
    D. Self-esteem

A   Including the family when planning care for a
    person promotes the fulfillment of love and
    belonging needs. It provides continued unity
    with loved ones, and promotes mutually
    meaningful relationships. (p. 8)

14. Nursing intervention to prevent the
    development of unmet needs and problems
    should include all of the following except:

    A. Assisting the person to remove or
       diminish obstacles to need satisfaction.
    B. Utilization of the teaching/learning
       process.
    C. Making referrals to other appropriate
       health professionals for further
       education and counseling.
    D. Encouraging individual participation in a
       program for rehabilitation.

D   Selections A, B, and C are measures that can
    be used to prevent the development of needs
    and problems. Selection D is designed to
    assist the person to attain a state of
    optimal independence so they can care for
    themselves as much as possible and meet their
    own needs. (p. 11)

15. Which of the following statements about the
    nursing process is incorrect?

    A. It promotes more effective, meaningful
       nursing care.
    B. It begins with a statement of the
       person's health care problems.
    C. It is designed to meet the needs of
       individuals.
    D. It enables the nurse to deliver holistic
       nursing care.

B   Selection B is the most incorrect statement
    related to the nursing process. The nursing
    process consists of a series of five basic
    steps: Data-gathering, nursing diagnosis,
    the nursing care plan, implementation, and
    evaluation. (p. 12)

# THE NEED TO UNDERSTAND THE SELF

OBJECTIVES

1.0 Discuss components of the "healthy self."

   1.1 Identify 11 basic generalizations or characteristics of the "self." (p. 17)

   1.2 Briefly describe the impact that health and illness may have on each of the 11 characteristics of the "self." (p. 17)

   1.3 Interpret the meaning of the phrase, "The healthy self has a sense of personal integration or coherent wholeness." (p. 17)

   1.4 Explore the positive and negative effects of introspection on the "self." (p. 17)

   1.5 Interpret the meaning of the phrase, "The healthy self strives to maintain some autonomy; i.e., a sense of uniqueness." (p. 17)

   1.6 Discuss the meaning of the phrase, "The self is largely determined and recognized by the values it assumes." (p. 18)

   1.7 Interpret the meaning of the phrase, "The healthy self is characterized by energy directed toward self-actualization." (p. 18)

   1.8 Discuss the significance of the statement, "The self is capable of introspection and is aware of time." (p. 18)

   1.9 Explain the meaning of the statement, "The healthy self is not entirely free from emotional conflicts or symptoms of illness." (p. 19)

   1.10 Translate the meaning of the phrase, "Even though individual 'selves' are separate from one another, it is possible to form bonds with others." (p. 19)

   1.11 Discuss the statement: "Self-concept is founded on perceptions of oneself. At times we perceive ourselves differently from the way others perceive us." (p. 19)

   1.12 Interpret the significance of the statement, "Beyond concepts of the 'individual self' are broader, deeper concepts of the 'universal self'". p. 17)

TEACHING/LEARNING STRATEGIES

**Lecture/Discussion**

Ask students to identify factors that influence their own health behavior.

**Group Activity**

Instruct to describe characteristics of a totally healthy person at each stage in the life span. Divide students into small groups and ask them to compare the similarities and differences in the characteristics they have written.

2.0 Incorporate understandings of the self into planning nursing care for ill people.

   2.1 Explore ways in which the nurses' appreciation of the uniqueness and individuality of each person can contribute to the quality of nursing care rendered. (p. 21)

   2.2 Identify measures the nurse can utilize to promote and reinforce a person's sense of autonomy during illness. (p. 21)

   2.3 Briefly discuss the influence of illness-related stress and change on an individual's drive for self-actualization. (p. 21)

   2.4 Identify special needs of the ill individual with relation to the concepts of introspection and time. (p. 21)

   2.5 Discuss the importance of understanding conflict and illness as a normal life experience. (p. 22)

   2.6 Discuss the value of using therapeutic communication in interactions with individuals experiencing illness. (p. 26)

   2.7 List actions the nurse might take to help reduce differences between the public and private self in individuals requiring nursing care. (p. 22)

   2.8 Discuss ways in which personal self-concept can influence the nurse's perception of others. (p. 23)

3.0 Discuss the concept of the "universal self."

   3.1 Recognize the importance of nonjudgmental support for individuals contemplating the relationship between their "individual self" and the "universal self." (p. 23)

   3.2 Understand the impact that interactions with "significant others" has in the development of an individual's personality and self-concept. (p. 23)

   3.3 Define the terms: Significant other, family, nuclear family, and extended family. (p. 23)

## Lecture/Discussion

Ask students to identify psychological coping mechanisms that are effective in assisting an individual to cope with the challenges created by illness.

## Written Exercise

Ask students to keep a daily journal of the activities that influence their own wellness level. Have them identify practices that are beneficial, as well as those activities that are hazardous to the maintenance of high level wellness.

## Values Clarification

Encourage students to explore the following questions: "Why do I want to be a nurse?" "Which of my own needs will be met by being a nurse?" "What caused me to feel good during my last clinical experience?"

Ask students to keep a diary of the feelings elicited each day in the clinical setting.

## Values Clarification

Ask students to identify the time in their life when they were most happy. Encourage them to explore reasons for their happiness during that period of time.

Ask students to describe a person that they feel is "self-actualized." Have them discuss reasons for their choice.

---

## MULTIPLE CHOICE QUESTIONS

1. All of the following are characteristics of the "healthy self" except:

   A. Has a sense of personal integration and coherent wholeness.
   B. Is capable of introspection and is aware of time.
   C. Is entirely free from emotional conflicts or symptoms of illness.
   D. Is able to cope with difficulties of life and continue to pursue self-actualization.

## CORRECT ANSWER AND RATIONALE

C  Statements A, B, and D are characteristics of the "healthy self." The "healthy self" is not entirely free from emotional conflicts or symptoms of illness. A certain amount of imbalance, conflict, or illness is a natural part of life. (p. 19)

2.  The process of getting to know oneself is called:

    A.  Introversion
    B.  Introsusception
    C.  Intubation
    D.  Introspection

D   Introspection is correctly defined as the process of getting to know oneself. (p. 17)

3.  The individuality and uniqueness of an individual are influenced by:

    A.  Genetic background
    B.  Age and developmental status
    C.  Experiential forces
    D.  All of the above

D   Individual uniqueness is influenced by the interaction of a number of variables. The three most important variables are: Time (age and developmental status), heredity (genetic background), and environment (experiential forces). (p. 18)

4.  Mr. Bender refuses his breakfast. He tells the nurse that he cannot eat the food that has been served because he is Jewish and consumes only kosher foods. Mr. Bender's action reflects a personal:

    A.  Belief
    B.  Opinion
    C.  Value
    D.  Custom

C   Mr. Bender's action reflects a personal value. The values a person embraces are strongly influenced by beliefs and customs, but are not values unless they are the basis for action. (p. 21)

5.  Healthy individuals attempt to maintain a sense of autonomy. This means that the individual:

    A.  Seeks involvement in social affairs
    B.  Strives to develop their fullest potential
    C.  Learns to like and accept himself
    D.  Achieves a sense of uniqueness

D   The autonomous person achieves a sense of individuality or uniqueness, and is able to function independently. (p. 18)

6.  Mr. Jones refuses to take a morning bath, stating that he always takes a shower at bedtime. The best way to deal with this situation would be to:

    A.  Tell Mr. Jones that all baths must be taken in the morning.
    B.  Allow Mr. Jones to take his bath in the evening.
    C.  Remind Mr. Jones of general hospital routines.
    D.  Offer Mr. Jones a bath later in the afternoon.

B   The nurse could best assist Mr. Jones to maintain a sense of autonomy by allowing him to take a bath in the evening as requested. (p. 21)

7.  The nurse can assist an ill individual to maintain a sense of integration or wholeness by:

    A.  Allowing the person to participate in the decision making process.
    B.  Notifying the individual of any changes that occur.
    C.  Discussing the general hospital routines upon admission.
    D.  All of the above.

D   The nurse can assist a hospitalized individual to maintain a sense of order and personal integration by implementing all of the above activities. (p. 21)

8.  The process of self-actualization:

    A.  Is strongly influenced by culture and personal life goals
    B.  Is the need to develop one's potential as a human being
    C.  Can be attained by all who seek it
    D.  All of the above

B   Self-actualization is the need to become what one can become, to develop one's full potential. People strive for self-actualization, regardless of cultural diversity and personal life goals. The self-actualized person has developed a sense of self-awareness, something that is not possible for everyone to attain. (p. 18)

9.  Interaction with significant others is very
    important in the development of one's
    self-concept.  Significant others are <u>best</u>
    described as:

    A.  Members of the nuclear family
    B.  Both nuclear and extended family members
    C.  Anyone who is personally important to
        the individual
    D.  Friends, peers, and teachers

C   The term "significant others" refers to
    anyone who is personally significant in the
    life of the individual.  Significant others
    may include not only one's family, but also
    other people, such as, friends, peers, and
    teachers.  (p. 23)

10. An individual's self-concept:

    A.  Influences the way in which he reacts to
        others
    B.  Is primarily subjective in nature
    C.  Develops and changes throughout the
        lifespan
    D.  All of the above

D   Self-concept is founded on perceptions of
    oneself.  It greatly influences the way an
    individual acts toward others and how others
    act to him.  Since it is based on one's
    feeling about himself, it is primarily
    subjective in nature.  (p. 23)

# THE NEED TO ADAPT TO STRESS

| OBJECTIVES | TEACHING/LEARNING STRATEGIES |
|---|---|
| | **Class Activity** |
| 1.0 Discuss theories of stress. | Ask students to complete the Holmes-Rahe Social |
| | Readjustment scale. Ask them how their present |
| 1.1 Discuss the historical development of stress theory. (p. 26) | level of wellness correlates with the scores obtained on the scale. |
| 1.2 Briefly summarize three models of stress: Selye's General Theory of Stress; Holmes and Rahe's Model of Adaptation to Life Change and Subsequent Onset of Illness; and the Lazarus Model of Stress and Coping. (p. 28) | |
| 2.0 Distinguish between stressors and stress responses. | **Lecture/Discussion** |
| 2.1 Identify common difficulties related to the process of defining stress. (p. 26) | Help students to understand the relationship between stress and illness. |
| 2.2 Define the terms: stressor and stress response. (p. 26) | |
| 2.3 Give examples of "stressors" that may challenge the adaptive capabilities of an organism or person. (p. 26) | |
| 2.4 Identify two general "stress response" categories, and gives examples of each. (p. 26) | |
| 2.5 Discuss general conclusions drawn from past research studies related to stressors and stress reactions. (p. 27) | |
| 2.6 Discuss the physiologic impact of stress as formulated by Selye. (p. 28) | |
| 3.0 Describe coping responses and defense mechanisms. | **Lecture/Discussion** |
| 3.1 Briefly describe Selye's general and local adaptation syndromes. Include in this description, a comparison of the syndrome's similarities and differences. (p. 29) | Discuss criteria used to differentiate between pathologic and nonpathologic use of defense mechanisms. |
| 3.2 Describe Selye's concept of "faulty adaptation." (p. 29) | |
| 3.3 Identify common health problems that may occur as a result of "faulty adaptation." (p. 29) | |
| 3.4 Discuss the relationship between change and illness as formulated by Holmes and Rahe. (p. 29) | |

3.5 Explain the role that major life changes may play in the development of an illness. (p. 30)

3.6 Give examples of major life events that may produce significant life changes. (p. 30)

3.7 Discuss major elements included in Lazarus's stress and copying paradigm: demands, primary appraisal of demands, secondary appraisal, stress, coping, emotion, and reappraisal. (p. 30)

3.8 Describe three major types of coping responses as stated by Pearlin. (p. 33)

3.9 Describe five major types of coping responses as stated by Lazarus. (p. 33)

3.10 Define "defense mechanisms." (p. 33)

4.0 Describe physiologic responses to stressors.

4.1 Identify physiologic and psychologic forces that initially influence our response to internal and external stressors. (p. 33)

4.2 Explain the relationship of defense mechanisms to self-concept and healthy adaptation. (p. 33)

4.3 Name and define the most common types of defense mechanisms and give nursing care examples of each. (p. 34)

4.4 Identify the three most commonly used mechanisms of defense. (p. 34)

4.5 List the major physiologic responses of the body to stressors. (p. 34)

4.6 Identify the major psychologic response of the body to stressors. (p. 36)

5.0 Discuss the causes of anxiety, how it is communicated and assessed.

5.1 Define the term anxiety. (p. 37)

5.2 Compare and contrast the terms, anxiety and fear. (p. 37)

5.3 Explore ways in which perception of anxiety may influence an individual's psychologic response to stressors. (p. 37)

5.4 Identify life events/situations that may provoke or produce anxiety. (p. 37)

5.5 Identify essential sources of data to be obtained when assessing anxiety. (p. 37)

5.6 Describe indices used to assess the intensity of anxiety: ataraxia, well-being, mild anxiety, moderate anxiety, severe anxiety, and panic. (p. 37)

**Class Activity**

Ask students to identify the most stressful experience they ever encountered. Have them share their feelings elicited by the experience, the coping styles used, and the outcome of the situation.

**Lecture/Discussion**

Ask students to describe the behavior displayed by an individual experiencing the various levels of anxiety; Ataraxia, well-being, mild anxiety; moderate anxiety, severe anxiety, and panic. (p. 38)

Have students identify data that should be gathered when assessing a person in a state of anxiety. (p. 38)

5.7 Outline, in ascending order, the three major lines of defense used by an individual in response to agents or factors that challenge personal adaptive capacities. (p. 50)

6.0 Describe the four methods for dealing with stressful demands and begin to use these methods in your own life.

6.1 State the ultimate nursing goal of stress management. (p. 31)

6.2 Identify data required to assess an individual's perceptions or vulnerability to stressors, responses to stressors, and coping resources. (p. 31).

6.3 Describe basic nursing intervention useful in assisting persons to cope with stress responses and stress-related illnesses. (p. 31)

6.4 Identify four essential self-help measures that can be used by the individual to counter and control stress reactions. (p. 38)

6.5 List questions to be asked when attempting to identify the source of a stressor. (p. 39)

6.6 Identify actions an individual might take to deal with an identified stressor. (p. 39)

6.7 List essential data to be obtained when assessing the "feelings" associated with stressful situations. (p. 39)

6.8 Briefly discuss the importance of acknowledging the feelings that often accompany stressful situations. (p. 39)

6.9 Identify sources of professional health care that can be utilized as a line of defense against stressors. (p. 40)

6.10 Discuss the impact that a supportive network of significant others can have on an individual encountering stressful situations. (p. 39)

7.0 Elaborate on the role of stress responses in disease causation.

7.1 Summarize the relationship between physical condition and response to stressors. (p. 40)

7.2 Identify four factors that may be influential in the development of stress-related physical or mental disorders. (p. 40)

7.3 Identify manifestations of and factors contributing to the development of chronic disease. (p. 41)

### Lecture/Discussion

Instruct students to identify the activities they engage in to promote relaxation. Ask them to discuss the activities that they find most useful.

### Lecture/Discussion

Ask students to outline the stress-producing factors they feel influence a person's homeostatic balance at each stage in the life cycle.

7.4 Give examples of successful and unsuccessful stress management. (p. 41)

8.0 Describe levels of adaptation.

   8.1 Explain the meaning of the term adaptation. (p. 41)

   8.2 List and briefly describe four levels of human adaptation. (p. 42)

### Lecture/Discussion

Ask students to summarize the characteristics of the four levels of human adaptation: Physiologic, psychologic, sociocultural, and technologic. (p. 42)

Ask students to compare and contrast the various levels of human adaptation: Physiologic, psychologic, sociocultural, and technologic.

9.0 List and give examples of the characteristics of adaptation.

   9.1 Identify ten common characteristics of human adaptive mechanisms. (p. 43)

   9.2 Briefly summarize the role of the nursing process in assisting others to adapt successfully to stressors. (p. 45)

### Lecture/Discussion

Facilitate a discussion of the similarities and differences between Selye's general and local adaptation syndromes.

10.0 Describe the characteristics of life crises.

   10.1 Outline Caplan's four developmental phases of crisis. (p. 45)

   10.2 Briefly discuss the "crisis continuum." (p. 45)

   10.3 State the definition of the "crisis" and give examples of situations that may produce crises. (p. 45)

   10.4 Cite common characteristics of life crises. (p. 45)

### Lecture/Discussion

Encourage a discussion of the following: Has entry into nursing school caused an increase or decrease in their stress level? Have they used their time more efficiently or less efficiently?

Ask students to share the thoughts, feelings and behaviors they displayed when a crisis situation was encountered.

### Written Exercise

Ask each student to write their definition of a crisis. Allow volunteers to read their definitions in class.

11.0 Discuss how potential crises may be averted and how actual crises can be treated.

   11.1 Analyze typical psychologic and physiologic reactions of people in crisis. (p. 46)

   11.2 Identify factors that may have an influence on the development of a problem into a crisis situation. (p. 46)

   11.3 Describe basic nursing intervention useful is assisting persons who are confronted with actual crises. (p. 46)

12.0 Appreciate the stress of hospitalization and be aware of ways you can help people adjust to their stressful environment.

   12.1 Explore the interrelationships of stressors, illness, and hospitalization. (p. 47)

   12.2 Outline five major tasks of individuals attempting to cope with illness and hospitalization, and nursing implications for each. (p. 48)

### Lecture/Discussion

Ask students to identify ways in which the nurse-individual, relationship can be used effectively to reduce a person's anxiety.

### Written Exercise

Have students outline specific techniques that can be used to help a person cope effectively with stress.

3-4

12.3 Identify basic hospital stress factors and give examples of each. (p. 49)

13.0 Understand that nurses are also under stress and be aware of ways to deal with stressors in your life and potential burnout.

    13.1 Explore causes for professional "burnout" in nursing. (p. 50)

    13.2 Identify behavioral indicators, physical signs, and emotional indicators of professional burnout. (p. 50)

    13.3 Outline guidelines the nurse may enact to prevent or intervene in the development of professional burnout. (p. 50)

14.0 Appreciate the interrelatedness of body, mind, and life experience in reacting to stressors.

## Clinical Laboratory Experience

Have students incorporate stress management techniques into actual individual situations.

---

## MULTIPLE CHOICE QUESTIONS

1. Stressors are:

   A. Agents or factors that pose a real threat to the individual.
   B. External factors that challenge the adaptive capacities of a person.
   C. Physiologic and psychologic responses to stress.
   D. Forces that place a strain upon the person, resulting in a stress response.

2. All of the following are examples of physical stressors, except:

   A. Inadequate sleep
   B. Lack of food
   C. Unmet sexual needs
   D. Pregnancy

3. The nurse needs to be aware that an individual's response to stress is influenced by:

   A. Perception of the stressor.
   B. Number of stressors to be coped with.
   C. Past experience with a comparable stressor.
   D. All of the above.

4. The three stages of the General Adaptation Syndrome are:

   A. Alarm, resistance, and exhaustion.
   B. Alarm, resistance, and fatigue.
   C. Alarm, reaction, and exhaustion.
   D. Alarm, reaction, and fatigue.

## CORRECT ANSWER AND RATIONALE

D   Stressors are agents or factors that challenge the adaptive capacities of an organism or person. They arise from both internal and external stimuli, that pose a real or perceived threat to the individual.

    Response to stress may be categorized as physiologic or psychologic. (p. 27)

C   Selections A, B, and D are all examples of physical stressors. Unmet sexual desires is a psychological stressor. (p. 27)

D   Individual responses to stressors are mediated by personality, perception of the stressor, and resources for coping. Stress responses generally result from many stressors. (p. 27)

A   Selye suggested that the GAS developed in three distinct stages: (1) alarm, (2) resistance, and (3) exhaustion. (p. 29)

5. Holmes and Rahe developed the Social Readjustment Rating Scale. This is best described as:

   A. A ranking of physiological and psychological responses to stress.
   B. A ranking of major life events to life change units.
   C. A ranking of the common reactions to stressful events.
   D. A schedule or list of major life events.

B. The SRRS is best described as a ranking of major life events according to life change units. Major life changes are assigned numerical values on the basis of their significance to the person. (p. 29)

6. According to Holmes and Rahe, which of the following life change events ranks highest as a stressor:

   A. Death of close family member
   B. Death of a spouse
   C. Retirement
   D. Divorce

B. Death of a spouse ranks highest as a stressor. (p. 30)

7. Mrs. Carter has just received news that her husband has expired. Physiological responses to this stressful situation may include all of the following except:

   A. Increased heart rate
   B. Increased blood pressure
   C. Reduced oxygen intake
   D. Increased blood sugar

C. Physiologic stress response indicators include all of the following: Increased heart rate; increased blood pressure; increased oxygen intake; increased serum glucose levels; decreased inflammatory and immune responses; pupil dilation; reduced peristaltic action; and increased alertness. Generally, the cardiovascular system is stimulated and the gastrointestinal system is inhibited during stress response. (p. 32)

8. Which of the following statements are correct?

   A. The most commonly used defense mechanisms are denial, selective inattention, and rationalization.
   B. Defense mechanisms change the way in which a person thinks about whatever is disturbing him.
   C. A defense mechanism is a conscious process that is used to protect the individual from anxiety.
   D. Defense mechanisms can be used to solve problems and alter the conditions of the anxiety itself.

B. Defense mechanisms are largely unconscious mental processes and behaviors that protect and enhance our self-esteem and self-concept. These adaptive mental mechanisms protect us from anxiety reactions by distorting perception, memory, action, motivation, and thinking. (p. 34)

9. The individual who involuntarily forgets about unacceptable ideas, impulses, or events is using which defense mechanism?

   A. Denial
   B. Rationalization
   C. Repression
   D. Suppression

C. Repression is an unconscious process that is used to put stress-provoking thoughts out of awareness. Once the idea has been repressed, the material cannot be voluntarily recalled to memory. (p. 34)

10. After being told that she will never be able to conceive a child, Sally focuses all energy on her professional career development. Which of the following defense mechanisms is she using?

    A. Compensation
    B. Displacement
    C. Sublimation
    D. Suppression

C. Sublimation involves the unconscious diversion of energy from an unattainable goal to a more acceptable endeavor or socially acceptable behavior. (p. 35)

11. Mr. Carr has failed to adhere to his prescribed medical regime. He explains that his daughter was supposed to remind him to perform the prescribed activities, but forgot to do so. Which defense mechanism is being used?

    A. Displacement
    B. Intellectualization
    C. Projection
    D. Rationalization

C    Projection is the process by which a person attributes to others exaggerated amounts of undesirable qualities that they have but do not wish to recognize in themselves. (p. 34)

SITUATION: Kaye, a first semester nursing student, is seen in school health clinic with complaints of nausea, loss of appetite, and diarrhea. She appears tense and apprehensive. A complete physical examination reveals no physiologic reason for Kaye's complaints. Questions 12 to 15 apply to this situation.

12. It is determined that Kaye is suffering from anxiety. Which of the following statements about anxiety is correct?

    A. Anxiety is primarily an objective experience.
    B. Anxiety is more difficult to handle than fear.
    C. Anxiety is communicated nonverbally.
    D. Anxiety first appears during adolescence.

B    Anxiety is related to an unidentifiable source of anticipated danger, and is therefore more difficult to manage than fear, where the source of danger is recognized and can be identified. Anxiety is primarily a subjective experience that is communicated both verbally and nonverbally. It first appears during infancy, at the age of 7 to 8 months. (p. 37)

13. The nurse caring for Kaye is aware that the complaints of nausea, loss of appetite, and diarrhea:

    A. Are somatic symptoms generated by her anxiety
    B. Can eventually cause disease by keeping Kaye's body in an abnormal state
    C. Are physiologic effects of Kaye's anxiety
    D. All of the above

D    Anxiety often generates somatic symptoms. Some of the physiologic effects of anxiety are anorexia, nausea, vomiting, abdominal cramps, and diarrhea. Each individual experiences different somatic responses to anxiety. If the anxiety is short-lived, these effects do no harm. However, sustained or chronic anxiety eventually causes disease by keeping the body in an abnormal state. (p. 38)

14. Initially the nurse could best assist Kaye to identify the source of her anxiety by:

    A. Reviewing her past healthy clinic records
    B. Interviewing her significant others at school
    C. Encouraging self-assessment
    D. All of the above

C    It is not always easy for an individual to identify the source of anxiety. Initial nursing intervention to assist in identification of the stressor should be directed toward self-assessment of feelings that are being experienced and their possible sources. (p. 39)

15. Kaye realizes that her anxiety experience began shortly after her failure on two nursing examinations. She states that her home and work responsibilities often left little time for study. In order to deal with the identified stressors, Kaye should be encouraged to do all of the following except:

    A. Reduce her required work time by obtaining financial assistance
    B. Delegate household tasks to others living in her home
    C. Quit school and resume her education at a less stressful time
    D. Develop a reasonable time management schedule

C    Once the source of a problem has been identified, the person should be encouraged to deal with the stressor by changing the situation, or the perception and response to the situation. Terminating her education would be the least appropriate way for Kaye to deal with this situation. She should first attempt to change her perception and response to the situation. (p. 39)

16. Nursing intervention for an extremely anxious person should include all of the following except:

   A. Keep communication clear and brief
   B. Use nonverbal communication to clarify communication
   C. Give clear, detailed explanations
   D. Encourage discussion of feelings

C   The extremely anxious person easily misunderstands what is said, so keep communication clear and brief. Repeat statements as necessary. Nonverbal communication should be utilized to aid in clarifying the communication. Also remember that the anxious person needs an opportunity to discuss feelings with a calm, nonjudgmental person. (p. 38)

17. Which of the following general statements about adaptation is incorrect?

   A. Adaptability varies from individual to individual.
   B. Adaptive responses are more limited in number and scope at the psychologic level.
   C. All adaptive mechanisms attempt to maintain homeostasis.
   D. Adaptive responses may be inadequate, excessive, or inappropriate.

B   Responses A, C, and D are all characteristics of adaptation. Response B is incorrect: adaptive responses are much more limited in number and scope at the physiologic level than they are at the social and psychologic level. (p. 44)

18. Mr. Smith is experiencing severe financial problems as a result of prolonged hospitalization for a serious illness. A crisis could develop if:

   A. Mr. Smith is unable to view the situation realistically
   B. Mr. Smith's previously learned coping mechanisms fail
   C. Mr. Smith has inadequate support from significant others
   D. All of the above

D   According to Aguilera, whether a problem develops into a crisis depends upon three factors: (1) the individual's perception of the problem or event, (2) available situational supports, and (3) coping mechanisms. If one of more of these factors are missing, the problem may not be resolved, and a crisis could develop. (p. 46)

19. The nurse providing crisis intervention for a person should be aware that:

   A. Most crises develop in an unpredictable fashion
   B. Crises tend to occur in cycles, with one crisis following another
   C. Individuals experiencing crises are often resistant to crisis intervention measures
   D. Most crises are resolved successfully in four to six months

B   Crisis intervention theory is based on the following assumptions:
   (1) Crisis is a universal experience; (2) Crisis is usually time limited, with resolution within four to six weeks; (3) Crisis exists on a continuum; (4) Crises tend to occur in cycles; and (5) People undergoing crises are highly responsive to crisis intervention. (p. 45)

20. As a nurse you are aware that the initial step in crisis intervention is:

   A. Exploring individual coping mechanisms
   B. Assessment of the crisis situation
   C. Explaining the crisis situation or event
   D. Exploring individual feelings evoked by the event

B   Crisis intervention begins with an initial assessment of the individual and the circumstances that led to the crisis. (p. 46)

21. Which of the following nurses is most likely to be at risk for burnout?

   A. Sally, a recent graduate, who has learned to effectively cope with stressful situations
   B. Joy, who skips lunch each day to meet individual demands
   C. Jack, who occasionally volunteers to work his days off
   D. Sue, who requests additional help when there is insufficient nursing staff to meet needs

B   Joy is not using effective stress management measures. When work loads are too heavy, demands are too great, and nursing care suffers. Her ideals may clash head-on with reality. The resulting disappointment and failed personal expectations are a breeding ground for burnout. (p. 50)

# 4

# THE NEED TO MAINTAIN A STATE OF BALANCE

## OBJECTIVES

1.0 Describe the major physiologic homeostatic regulators and their role in the maintenance of homeostasis.

   1.1 Discuss Hippocrates' definition of health. (p. 53)

   1.2 Explain the theory of homeostasis as developed by Cannon. (p. 53)

   1.3 Identify internal physiological processes that regulate the homeostasis of biological organisms. (p. 53)

   1.4 Briefly define the concepts of cybernetics and feedback. (p. 54)

   1.5 Compare the differences in historical views of homeostasis with current views of homeostasis. (p. 54)

   1.6 Explain the meaning of automaticity and rhythmicity as they relate to the homeostatic process. (p. 54)

   1.7 Summarize changes in physiologic homeostasis in health and illness. (p. 54)

   1.8 Discuss the impact that homeostatic imbalance can have on the individual. (p. 54)

   1.9 State the goal of all nursing care in relation to the concept of homeostasis. (p. 54)

   1.10 Identify two major homeostatic regulators functioning within the body. (p. 54)

   1.11 Identify three major functions of the autonomic nervous system. (p. 54)

   1.12 Outline the anatomical components of the endocrine system and briefly describe their role in the homeostatic process. (p. 54)

   1.13 Outline general functions of hormones in the body. (p.54)

   1.14 State three common characteristics of all endocrine glands. (p.56)

   1.15 Discuss the role of other body systems in maintaining an individual's homeostasis: GI system, respiratory system, cardiovascular system, kidneys, and the liver and pancreas. (p.56)

## TEACHING/LEARNING STRATEGIES

### Lecture/Discussion

Ask students to briefly discuss the role of other major body systems in the maintenance of physiologic homeostasis: GI system, biliary system, respiratory system, cardiovascular system, and the renal system.

Have students discuss the role of the autonomic nervous and the endocrine system in the maintenance of physiologic homeostasis.

1.16 Explore the impact the external environment can have on the homeostasis of the body's internal environment. (p.56)

1.17 Identify nine characteristics that indicate an emotionally balanced person. (p.56)

1.18 Identify major factors influencing the development of an emotional disequilibrium. (p.57)

1.19 Describe the role emotional equilibrium plays in the maintenance of an individual's homeostasis. (p. 56)

2.0 Discuss the basic characteristics of homeostatic mechanisms.

   2.1 Explain the compensatory nature of homeostatic devices. (p. 57)

   2.2 Discuss the self-regulatory nature of homeostatic mechanisms. (p. 58)

   2.3 State the main objective of a homeostatic mechanism. (p. 58)

**Lecture/Discussion**

Discuss the self-regulatory nature of homeostatic devices.

Discuss the compensatory nature of homeostatic devices.

3.0 List physiologic and psychosocial elements that must be present in our environment if homeostasis is to be maintained.

   3.1 List essential requirements of the body that are necessary in the maintenance of homeostasis. (p. 57)

**Lecture/Discussion**

Ask students to identify an example of a physiological body process that is under the control of several homeostatic mechanisms.

**Written Exercise**

Ask students to list the prerequisites that must be fulfilled for the maintenance of homeostasis.

Ask students to list the characteristics of a person who is in a state of psychologic homeostatic balance.

4.0 Compare a thermostat-regulated furnace with regulation of body temperature.

   4.1 Identify and briefly describe two examples of compensatory mechanisms at work in the body. (p. 57)

   4.2 Identify two features of a thermostatic negative feedback system. (p. 58)

5.0 Differentiate between positive and negative feedback.

   5.1 Describe the operation of negative feedback within the body. (p. 58)

**Lecture/Discussion**

Have students identify the difference in negative feedback and positive feedback.

6.0 Describe how negative feedback works in maintaining physiologic homeostasis and give examples.

   6.1 Discuss, using examples, the effect of positive and negative feedback on homeostatic balance. (p. 58)

**Lecture/Discussion**

Discuss factors that influence a homeostatic mechanism's ability to correct the errors it commits.

Help students to understand the way in which negative feedback is used to maintain homeostasis.

6.2 Give examples of the use of negative feedback to maintain homeostasis. (p. 59)

6.3 Understand that a single physiologic process may be under the control of several homeostatic mechanisms. (p. 61)

6.4 Give examples of single physiologic processes that are under the control of several homeostatic mechanisms. (p. 61)

6.5 Identify situations in which biologic organisms tolerate limited positive feedback. (p. 61)

7.0 List the major types of physiologic homeostatic disruptions that can occur and give examples of each.

7.1 Identify six reasons some degree of deviation of error exists in all homeostatic systems. (p. 61)

7.2 State an example of oscillations occurring in a negative feedback system, and describe the impact on body systems if these oscillations become too great. (p. 62)

7.3 Briefly describe limitations common to all homeostatic mechanisms. (p. 62)

7.4 Discuss the result an overdriven system may have on homeostatic balance. (p. 62)

7.5 Explore the effect disease processes may have on homeostatic mechanisms. (p. 62)

7.6 Discuss, using an example, the effects of rapid and complete breakdown of the homeostatic process. (p. 63)

7.7 Identify two new areas of research in the field of homeostasis and feedback. (p. 63)

### Lecture/Discussion

Give clinical examples of disruptions that occur in homeostatic mechanisms.

Ask students to identify the common limitations of homeostatic mechanisms.

8.0 Apply the concept of homeostasis to nursing care.

8.1 Briefly explain ways in which knowledge of the homeostatic process can be used when assessing and planning nursing intervention for individuals. (p. 66)

### Lecture/Discussion

Ask students to discuss ways in which homeostatic principles could assist them when planning nursing care.

9.0 Describe circadian rhythms in human beings and discuss their relevancy to illness and health.

9.1 Define basic terms used to describe biologic rhythms: Cycle, period, frequency, and amplitude. (p. 63)

9.2 Identify natural body cycles that influence homeostatic balance. (p. 63)

9.3 List and briefly describe six examples of circadian rhythms functioning within humans. (p. 64)

### Lecture/Discussion

Discuss the effects of environmental and social factors on a person's internal circadian rhythms.

Discuss the influence of biologic rhythms on maintenance of body homeostasis.

Ask students to differentiate between circadian, ultradian, and infradian rhythms. Have them give an example of each.

Ask students to identify the major circadian rhythms regulating physiologic processes within the body.

9.4 Briefly describe two factors that help synchronize an individual's internal circadian rhythm. (p. 64)

9.5 Identify specific physiologic and emotional changes that can lead to a disruption of biologic rhythms. (p. 65)

9.6 Discuss, using examples, the impact time changes can have on the circadian rhythm. (p. 65)

Class Activity

Ask students to identify the "highs" and "lows" they feel during a normal day. Have them identify ways in which their feelings may have been affected by biologic rhythms.

10.0 Discuss how our growing knowledge concerning circadian rhythms will affect nursing care in the future.

10.1 Explore ways in which chronobiologic principles may be applied to health care. (p. 65)

Lecture/Discussion

Ask students to identify specific emotional and physiological changes that can disrupt the functioning of circadian rhythms.

11.0 Discuss the basic concepts of biofeedback.

11.1 Define the principle of biofeedback. (p. 65)

11.2 Identify recent changes in the belief of a rigid dicotomy between the voluntary and involuntary physiologic functions of the body. (p. 66)

11.3 Discuss clinical applications of biofeedback training. (p. 66)

Lecture/Discussion

Summarize ways in which the application of basic chronobiologic principles may benefit health care.

12.0 Describe the technique of biofeedback.

12.1 Describe the process of biofeedback training. (p. 66)

Lecture/Discussion

Discuss the technique of biofeedback training. Identify specific clinical disorders treated by biofeedback techniques.

---

## MULTIPLE CHOICE QUESTIONS

1. The two major homeostatic regulators of the body are:

   A. Autonomic Nervous System and Exocrine System
   B. Autonomic Nervous System and Endocrine System
   C. Autonomic Nervous System and Neuroendocrine System
   D. Voluntary Nervous System and Endocrine System

2. Which of the following statements about the autonomic nervous system is incorrect?

   A. Operates automatically or without conscious control
   B. Is composed of the thoracolumbar system and the craniosacral system
   C. Exerts its major influence when exposed to stressful situations
   D. Regulates visceral activities

## CORRECT ANSWER AND RATIONALE

B  The major homeostatic regulators are the autonomic nervous system and the endocrine system. Because the nervous system and endocrine system complement one another in promoting homeostasis, the two systems are often linked and called the neuroendocrine system. The autonomic nervous system is largely involuntary. (p. 54)

C  The autonomic nervous system is composed of two major divisions: the sympathetic (thoracolumbar) and parasympathetic (craniosacral) systems, which usually affect them both in opposite ways. The sympathetic nervous system is initiated during stressful conditions; the parasympathetic nervous system exerts its major influence during periods of rest. (p. 54)

3.  The body's ability to maintain homeostasis is influenced by:

    A.  Fulfillment of basic physiologic needs
    B.  Socioeconomic factors
    C.  Physical integrity
    D.  All of the above

    D   To maintain homeostasis, the body must meet basic physiologic requirements for oxygen, water, nutrients, and tissue-building materials. Homeostasis also depends upon the maintenance of physical integrity and socio-cultural factors. (p. 57)

4.  Circadian rhythm refers to:

    A.  A biologic cycle shorter than 24 hours
    B.  A biologic rhythm of approximately 24 hours
    C.  The 28-day monthly cycle
    D.  A biologic cycle longer than 24 hours

    B   A circadian rhythm is a cycle that occurs at intervals of approximately 24 hours. (p. 63)

5.  Mrs. Grey has recently had her right breast surgically removed. The degree of threat this loss poses to her self-concept and psychological equilibrium depends upon:

    A.  Mrs. Grey's ability to successfully cope with the stress induced by the loss.
    B.  The value Mrs. Grey placed on her breasts.
    C.  Support received from significant others.
    D.  All of the above

    D   Emotional imbalance can develop when one's self-image is threatened. Resolution of the related crisis and a return to emotional balance depend upon support from significant others, good nursing and medical care, professional counseling, and the person's learned coping skills. (p. 57)

6.  Which of the following statements about homeostatic feedback systems is correct?

    A.  Positive feedback systems inhibit change, whereas negative feedback systems stimulate change.
    B.  Almost all biologic systems are controlled by negative feedback.
    C.  A positive feedback system leads the organism back to the status quo.
    D.  Positive feedback systems tend to be disruptive for biologic systems.

    D   Homeostatic devices use negative feedback to inhibit change, and positive feedback to encourage or stimulate change. Almost all biologic systems are controlled by negative rather than positive feedback. Positive feedback systems lead an organism away from the status quo and, therefore, tend to be disruptive for biologic systems. (p. 58)

7.  An event that repeats itself at predictable intervals is called a:

    A.  Cycle
    B.  Period
    C.  Rhythm
    D.  Revolution

    A   A cycle is an event that repeats itself at predictable intervals, e.g., the menstrual cycle. (p. 63)

8.  The 28 day female menstrual cycle is an example of which type of biologic rhythm?

    A.  Circadian
    B.  Infradian
    C.  Hormonal
    D.  Ultraradian

    B   The menstrual cycle, which occurs in women every 28 days or so, is an example of a infradian rhythm. Infradian rhythms occur at intervals longer than 24 hours. (p. 63)

9.  Mr. Simmons must be awakened frequently during his normal sleeping hours to take medication. The nurse caring for Mr. Simmons should be aware that this disruption in his established sleep-wakefulness rhythm can:

    A.  Have a more detrimental effect than a decrease in the total number of sleeping hours.
    B.  Cause alterations in mood.
    C.  Cause a deterioration in psychomotor performance.
    D.  All of the above

    D   When sleep-wakefulness rhythms are disrupted, as is often the case when a person is hospitalized, the mood of the individual suffers, and psychomotor performance deteriorates. Disruption of the sleep-wakefulness rhythm has a more detrimental effect than does a decrease in the total hours of sleep. (p. 64)

10. Which of the following statements is _incorrect_?

   A. Almost all organs and tissues of the body perform functions to assist in the maintenance of homeostasis.
   B. A biologic organism will continue to live and function properly as long as normal conditions are maintained within the internal environment.
   C. Essentially all homeostatic mechanisms operate by the process of positive feedback.
   D. Homeostasis is the tendency of biologic organisms to maintain static, or constant condition within the internal environment.

C   Homeostatic mechanisms tend to be negative feedback systems. Almost all biologic systems are controlled by negative rather than positive feedback. (p. 58)

11. An individual's gastrointestinal motility, body temperature, and urinary output are controlled almost entirely by:

   A. Autonomic nervous system
   B. Circadian rhythms
   C. Parasympathetic nervous system
   D. Sympathetic nervous system

A   The autonomic nervous system regulates visceral activities, such as the activities of smooth muscle, cardiac muscle, and glands. It is composed of two major divisions: The sympathetic and the parasympathetic, which usually affect body functions in opposite ways. The impact of circadian rhythm has been shown to affect these functions and, therefore, are worthy of consideration. (pp. 54, 63)

# 5

# THERAPEUTIC INTERACTION

OBJECTIVES

1.0 Understand the basic characteristics common to all helping professionals.

   1.1 Summarize the meaning of the term "help." (p. 72)

   1.2 Identify the role of the nurse as a "helper." (p. 72)

   1.3 Discuss the importance of interpersonal relationships as they relate to nursing. (p. 72)

   1.4 Discuss the significance of interpersonal relationships within the nursing process. (p. 72)

   1.5 Outline factors that influence the development of a therapeutic relationship within the helpee and helper systems of health care. (p. 73)

2.0 Give attention to your own personal growth in physical, emotional, and intellectual realms.

   2.1 Explain, using examples, how interpersonal behavior may influence the nurse-individual relationship. (p. 73)

   2.2 Identify characteristics of the "helpful" nurse. (p. 73)

   2.3 Discuss the influence of personal experiences, specific health-oriented experiences, and general life experiences on the development of a therapeutic relationship. (p. 73)

   2.4 Discuss reasons the nurse is personally obligated to maintain health in physical, emotional, and intellectual realms. (p. 75)

3.0 Understand the concepts of genuineness, non-possessive warmth, accurate empathy, concreteness in communication, immediacy in communication, and sensitive confrontation.

   3.1 Compare and contrast the role of the nurse in interpersonal and therapeutic relationships. (p. 73)

   3.2 Identify two categories of skills that the nurse brings to the therapeutic relationship. (p. 74)

TEACHING/LEARNING STRATEGIES

Lecture/Discussion

Ask students to identify the factors they feel facilitate the development of a "therapeutic" nurse-individual relationship.

Lecture/Discussion

Review the elements of the communication process.

Discuss the significance of effective communication skills in the nursing process.

Written Exercise

Have students list the characteristics they feel are necessary to promote a "helping" relationship. Allow time for discussion in class.

3.3 Identify and briefly describe three phases of the therapeutic relationship. (p. 74)

3.4 Describe the function of the nurse as a professional helper. (p. 74)

3.5 Identify and briefly describe two major characteristics of a helpful person. (p. 78)

3.6 List and briefly describe facilitative characteristics that may be used by the nurse to enhance the therapeutic relationship. (p. 78)

3.7 List and briefly describe action-oriented characteristics of the nurse that may be used to enhance the therapeutic relationship. (p. 78)

3.8 List factors influencing the development of a therapeutic environment. (p. 77)

4.0 Assess your own behavior within therapeutic relationships for genuineness, nonpossessive warmth, accurate empathy, concreteness in communication, and sensitive confrontation.

4.1 Describe the concept of appropriate confidentiality as it relates to the therapeutic relationship. (p. 81)

4.2 Explore ways in which the nurse can utilize knowledge of personal and environmental factors distorting communication to facilitate therapeutic communication. (p. 82)

4.3 Identify five levels of communication as formulated by Powell. (p. 84)

4.4 Describe the five levels of communication and discuss the influence each can have on the therapeutic relationship. (p. 84)

4.5 Identify and briefly discuss five major categories of responses that may block effective communication. (p. 85)

4.6 Briefly describe four problem-solving communication skills that may be used by the nurse to enhance the therapeutic relationship. Give specific examples of each. (p. 88)

4.7 Summarize ways in which the nurse can use self-disclosure to facilitate a therapeutic interaction. (p. 89)

4.8 Identify four ways silence can be used during the interview process to facilitate the therapeutic interaction. (p. 89)

4.9 Discuss the role touch can play in the communication process. (p. 90)

## Lecture/Discussion

Provide examples of communication techniques that can be used to facilitate therapeutic communication.

Provide examples of communication techniques that can block effective communication.

## Communication Activity

Request two students to participate in a role-playing exercise. Ask one student to assume the role of a newly hospitalized person and the other student the role of the nurse. Ask the nurse to conduct an introductory interview with the newly hospitalized person. Have other students critique the communication occurring between these two individuals.

4.10 Identify ways touch can be used as a
powerful communication tool. (p. 90)

4.11 State five basic Neuro Linguistic
Programming processes that may be used
in nursing communication situations.
(p. 90)

4.12 Explain the purpose of using structured
interview sessions within therapeutic
relationships. (p. 90)

5.0 Use listening skills effectively.

5.1 List guidelines that can be used by the
nurse to promote effective listening
techniques. (p. 86)

5.2 Briefly describe three categories of
listening skills that may be used by the
nurse to enhance the therapeutic relationship: Attending, perception checking, and reflecting. Give specific
examples of each. (p. 87)

6.0 Make careful nursing assessment using
interviewing skills.

6.1 Identify four distinct phases of the
interviewing process. (p. 91)

6.2 Discuss measures the nurse can take to
prepare for the interview process.
(p. 91)

6.3 Identify nursing measures used to
prepare a person for the interview
process. (p. 91)

6.4 Identify specific techniques that can be
used by the nurse to open the interview
process. (p. 92)

6.5 Identify six ways the nurse can use
interviews within the context of professional therapeutic relationships.
(p. 91)

6.6 Describe two basic types of interviews
and discuss the role of the nurse in
each. (p. 91)

6.7 Briefly describe the process of communication. (p. 81)

6.8 Outline and give examples of personal
and environmental factors that may contribute to the distortion of variables
in the communication process. (p. 82)

6.9 Briefly describe the concepts of verbal
and nonverbal communication. (p. 83)

6.10 Briefly describe and give examples of
verbal and nonverbal techniques of
communication. (p. 83)

## Communication Activity

Ask students to conduct a 10 minute interview with
an individual in the clinical setting. After the
interview, ask students to record the verbal and
nonverbal communication that occurred. Have them
identify the therapeutic and nontherapeutic
communication they used during the interview.

6.11 Identify seven general types of non-
    verbal communication. Give examples of
    each, and the general message they
    convey to others. (p. 84)

6.12 Briefly describe the three elements that
    characterize interview interactions:
    Questions, responses, and nonverbal
    communication patterns. (p. 92)

6.13 Discuss the importance of using knowl-
    edge related to questions, responses,
    and nonverbal communication patterns to
    facilitate completion of the objectives
    of the interview. (p. 92)

6.14 Outline nine techniques used by the
    nurse to assist in the effective wording
    of questions. (p. 92)

6.15 Enumerate the strengths and weaknesses
    of the various types of questions:
    Open, closed, direct, indirect, primary,
    and secondary. (p. 93)

6.16 Identify techniques that may be used by
    the nurse to successfully close the
    interview process. (p. 93)

6.17 Identify data indicative of concealed
    messages. (p. 94)

6.18 Give examples of responses the nurse can
    make when concealed issues are
    suspected. (p. 94)


7.0 Communicate successfully in situations
    involving anger, violence, crying, depres-
    sion, language barriers, serious physical
    illness, hearing impairment, visual impair-
    ment, dysphagia, conditions of the larynx.

    7.1 Identify measures the nurse can utilize
        in dealing with special circumstances
        that may impede the communication
        process: Anger, violence, crying,
        depression, language barrier, serious
        physical illness, hearing impairment,
        visual impairment, dysphagia, and
        laryngeal disorders. (p. 94)


8.0 Reevaluate your professional practice within
    therapeutic relationships.

    8.1 Explore ways in which the nurse can
        utilize genuineness, non-possessive
        warmth, accurate empathy, concreteness
        in communication, immediacy in communi-
        cation, and sensitive confrontation to
        evaluate the therapeutic relationship.
        (p. 96)

**Lecture/Discussion**

Ask students to identify ways in which
communication can be affected by illness.

**Lecture/Discussion**

Ask students to identify the reasons why
communication is important among health team
members.

Alert students to the difference between assertive
and aggressive behavior.

Impress upon students the importance of
"appropriate" confidentiality.

9.0 Identify significant characteristics of groups.

    9.1 State the definition of a group. (p. 97)

    9.2 Briefly describe two basic types of groups: Primary and secondary groups. (p. 97)

    9.3 Summarize major differences in formal and informal groups. (p. 97)

    9.4 Define the term group process. (p. 97)

    9.5 Describe the use of sociograms to illustrate group interactions. (p. 97)

    9.6 List and briefly describe three leadership styles that are used by groups. (p. 97)

    9.7 State two major decision-making methods that are used in groups. (p. 97)

    9.8 Briefly discuss variables that occur within groups: Autonomy, cohesiveness, control, dependence, flexibility, general tone, historicity, homogeneity, membership, mores, norms, participation, permeability, position, potency, role, size, and stability. (p. 98)

    9.9 Summarize the roles that are assigned or assumed by group members: Task-oriented roles, group maintenance roles, and self-oriented roles. (p. 98)

    9.10 Discuss practical hints the nurse can use for leading group discussions. (p. 99)

    9.11 Describe typical characteristics of leadership styles and identify situations in which each would be appropriate. (p. 99)

## Group Activity

Ask students to evaluate the group dynamics of their clinical discussion group. Have them determine the leadership style used and whether or not they think the group communicates effectively.

Have students identify the productive and nonproductive conflict that occurs in their clinical discussion group. Ask them how the group generally resolves conflict.

## Class Activity

Ask students to identify groups to which they belong. Have them evaluate one of the groups in terms of its major characteristics/variables, roles of the members within the group, and the leadership style operating within the group.

---

## MULTIPLE CHOICE QUESTIONS

1. Which of the following statements about the therapeutic nursing relationship is _incorrect_?

    A. The nurse is usually in the "power" position in the relationship.
    B. The needs of all participants in the relationship are equally important.
    C. The relationship is purposeful and goal directed.
    D. The relationship is time-limited; it will end when the the goal has been reached.

2. Which of the following is not an instrumental role of the nurse?

    A. Giving medications
    B. Interviewing
    C. Providing wound care
    D. Performing a complete bedbath

## CORRECT ANSWER AND RATIONALE

B  A therapeutic nursing relationship is established purposefully, maintained deliberately, and ended carefully in relation to the particular health care needs of the individuals needing help. The relationship focuses on the needs of the individual requiring care. (p. 73)

B  The professional nurse assumes expressive and instrumental roles within the therapeutic relationship. In the instrumental role the nurse provides direct-care skills, and in the expressive role the nurse is concerned with the activities of communication. (p. 74)

3. When initiating a therapeutic relationship, the nurse should focus primarily on:

   A. Clarification of the nursing role
   B. Establishment of trust
   C. Gathering assessment data
   D. Identification of health care goals

B. The most important task of the initiation phase is to build trust. The working phase cannot begin until trust has been established. (p. 74)

4. To facilitate communication, the nurse should convey:

   A. Accurate empathy
   B. Authenticity
   C. Unconditional positive regard
   D. All of the above

D  The nurse uses facilitative characteristics to create an emotional environment in which a person feels comfortable and safe in communicating. The facilitative characteristics used by the nurse are: Genuineness (authenticity), nonpossessive warmth (unconditional positive regard), and accurate empathy (empathetic understanding). (p. 78)

5. The nurse continually strives to understand exactly what the other person is feeling and experiencing. This conveys:

   A. Accurate empathy
   B. Immediacy in communication
   C. Genuineness
   D. Congruence

A  The nurse conveys accurate empathy by continually seeking to understand exactly what the other person is feeling and experiencing. Other terms used for accurate empathy are: Empathetic understanding, active listening, and creative listening. (p. 80)

6. Choose the statement that best describes the concept of communication:

   A. An Exchange of information, thoughts, and feelings from one person to another.
   B. An interchange of information.
   C. Verbal and nonverbal exchange of information, thoughts, and feelings from one person to another.
   D. Process of sending a verbal/nonverbal message.

C  Option C is the most accurate and complete statement about communication. It includes components discussed in options A, B, and D. (p. 81)

7. The nurse facilitates communication by:

   A. Frequently changing the focus of the conversation.
   B. Offering immediate solutions to a person's concerns.
   C. Sharing personal opinions related to the situation.
   D. Restating in a summary fashion what a person has said.

D  Options A, B, and C are all blocks to effective communication. The nurse demonstrates therapeutic communication when he/she summarizes or restates what a person has said; this is another way of perception checking. (p. 87)

8. A communication technique that involves restating a person's message in different words is:

   A. Clarifying
   B. Paraphrasing
   C. Restatement
   D. Summarizing

B  Paraphrasing means to restate a person's message in different words. (p. 87)

9. During conversation, the nurse tells the person, "I'm not sure I understand what you are trying to tell me about . . ." This is an example of which therapeutic communication technique?

   A. Clarifying
   B. Exploring
   C. Focusing
   D. Validating.

A  The nurse attempts to find or understand the meaning of a communicated message by using clarification. (p. 87)

10. All of the following represent general inter-
    pretations of nonverbal messages.  Which
    association is <u>incorrect</u>?

    A. Direct eye contact - interest, confidence,
       honesty
    B. Pursed lips - Anger
    C. Averted gaze - Secure
    D. Faked smile - Manipulative, placating

11. The person states, "I don't think I'm ever
    going to go home."  The nurse's <u>best</u> response
    would be:

    A. "You shouldn't think like that."
    B. "You'll be fine."
    C. "Why do you feel that way?"
    D. "You feel as if you're never going to go
       home."

12. A person states, "I'm really scared!"  The
    nurse responds, "You're really scared."  The
    communication technique used by the nurse is:

    A. Attending
    B. Paraphrasing
    C. Restating
    D. Validating

13. The use of silence during an interview is
    therapeutic if:

    A. The person is overcome with emotion.
    B. The person appears uncomfortable with the
       topic being discussed.
    C. The nurse is uncomfortable with the
       current discussion.
    D. The nurse wishes to terminate the
       communication session.

14. All of the following nurses have violated a
    person's right to privacy and confidentiality
    <u>except</u>:

    A. Sue, who shares information about the
       person with her nursing instructor.
    B. John, who shares private information with
       the person's significant others.
    C. Sarah, who shares information with an
       interested nurse from another floor.
    D. Carey, who discusses the person's case
       over lunch in the hospital cafeteria.

15. The nurse asks, "How are your feeling this
    evening?"  This is an example of which type of
    question?

    A. Direct
    B. Open
    C. Primary
    D. Secondary

16. Which of the following groups contains an
    example of verbal communication?

    A. Direct eye contact, broad smile, excessive
       gesturing
    B. Disheveled, crying, flared nostrils
    C. Gasping, high tone of voice, standing erect
    D. Well-groomed, eyes open wide, singing

C. An averted gaze generally communicates that
   the person is submissive, untruthful, or
   lacking in confidence. (p. 84)

D. Option D is the only therapeutic response.
   Options A, B, and C block effective communication.  Option A rejects the person, option B
   offers false reassurance; and option C demands
   an explanation. (p. 87)

C  Restatement means to restate or repeat a
   person's words or phrases.  By echoing a
   person's words, the nurse can help a person to
   examine or explore the topic more fully.
   (p. 87)

A  Silence is used during the interview to:  (1)
   allow the person to collect thoughts and
   recall needed information, (2) give a person
   the sense of truly being listened to, (3) give
   the nurse time to organize thoughts in terms
   of further questions and to record data, and
   (4) give the nurse time to note how the person
   communicates nonverbally.  It is essential for
   the nurse to remain silent whenever a person
   is overcome by emotion. (p. 89)

A  Confidential person information should be used
   to improve the quality of a person's care.
   Information that is irrelevant to the health
   care situation should never be discussed.
   Information should be shared only with those
   involved in the individual's professional
   care. (p. 81)

B  The nurse's statement represents an open type
   question.  This broad, unstructured question
   allows the person to state opinions, views,
   and feelings. (p. 93)

D  Singing exchanges information in the form of
   words, and is therefore verbal in
   orientation. (p. 84)

SITUATION: The nurse has just informed Mr. Sleigh that his diagnostic tests have been canceled for the second day in a row. Mr. Sleigh clenches his fist at the nurse as she prepared to leave the room. His lips are pursed and his nostrils flaring. Questions 17 and 18 apply to this situation.

17. Mr. Sleigh's nonverbal behavior indicates:

A. Anger
B. A concealed message
C. Fear
D. Depression

A. Mr. Sleigh's behavior is appropriately labeled as anger. Anger is almost always a sign of fear, anxiety, or helplessness. In this case, Mr. Sleigh's anger is probably a sign that he is anxious about the outcome of the canceled tests. A clenched fist, pursed lips, and flaring nostrils are nonverbal signs indicating anger. (p. 94)

18. The nurse's best response to Mr. Sleigh at this time would be:

A. "Everything is going to be all right Mr. Sleigh, you'll see."
B. "I don't know what you're so upset about."
C. "You seem to be upset. Tell me about it."
D. Silence

C If a person becomes angry, the nurse should: Verify the person's observations, acknowledge and accept the anger, help the person pinpoint the cause of the anger, and encourage physical activity, if possible. (p. 94)

19. When communicating with an individual who has a hearing impairment, the nurse should:

A. Talk directly to the person while facing him.
B. Use nonverbal cues to demonstrate ideas when appropriate.
C. Avoid chewing gum, eating, or covering the mouth when talking to the person.
D. All of the above

D All of the listed options should be utilized to facilitate communication with the hearing impaired individual. (p. 96)

20. All of the following enhance communication with a visually impaired individual except:

A. Raising the voice slightly
B. Always speaking when entering the room
C. Orienting the person to sounds in the environment
D. Always giving the reason for touching the person before doing so

A It is not necessary to raise the voice when engaging in communication with the visually impaired person. The nurse should speak in a normal tone and pitch of voice. Options B, C, and D will facilitate communication with a person who is visually impaired. (p. 96)

21. The expected behaviors of members within a group are called:

A. Mores
B. Norms
C. Values
D. Roles

B Norms are the expected behaviors of members within a group. Norms are maintained by sanctions or consent. (p. 98)

22. All of the following are characteristics of the effective group except:

A. Atmosphere is informal, comfortable, and relaxed.
B. Decision making is done by the highest authority in the group.
C. Goals, tasks and objectives of the group are clearly understood by all members.
D. Ideas and feelings of group members are encouraged.

B Options A, C, and D are characteristics of an effective group. Decisions in the effective group are usually done by consensus. (p. 100)

# UNDERSTANDING THE EXISTENCE
# OF THE ILL

OBJECTIVES

1.0 Draw nursing insights from consideration of your own experiences with illness.

    1.1 Briefly describe the impact that moods and feelings can have on individuals coping with the changes of illness. (p. 105)

    1.2 Appreciate the impact moods and feelings, medications, and sense of awareness have had in your own personal encounters with illness. (p. 104)

    1.3 Identify nursing insights that can be gained from an understanding of moods and feelings commonly experienced by the individual coping with illness. (p. 104)

    1.4 Identify nursing insights that can be gained from an awareness of the effects of medications taken by ill individuals. (p. 105)

    1.5 Briefly outline the nursing insights that can be gained from an understanding of the sense of awareness in individuals coping with illness. (p. 106)

    1.6 Describe the functions of the nurse advocate in the provision of health care. (p. 107)

2.0 Appreciate the uniqueness of each person's experiences with illness.

    2.1 Identify and briefly describe variables that influence the way in which people deal with the symptoms of illness. (p. 107)

3.0 Discuss some common experiences of ill people.

    3.1 Explore ways in which the nurse's understanding of the subjective experiences of illness can affect the nursing care given. (p. 104)

4.0 Describe the experience of illness in terms of stages.

TEACHING/LEARNING STRATEGIES

Written Exercise

Have students write a brief summary of how illness responses are influenced by a person's stage in the life cycle.

Values Clarification

Ask students to review the period in their life in which they experienced their most severe illness. Have them examine their thoughts, feelings, and behaviors during this time.

Class Activity

Have students write their own personal definitions of health and illness, and identify the factors that influence their definitions. Afterwards, ask them to share their definitions in class.

Lecture/Discussion

Ask students to briefly describe the stages of the experience of illness: Transition, acceptance, and convalescence.

Ask students to explain the relationship of physical functioning to psychosocial functioning through the stages of illness.

5.0 List typical behavioral responses of illness.

    5.1 Outline behavioral responses of the individual experiencing signs and symptoms of illness. (p. 107)

    5.2 Briefly describe factors that affect a person's reaction to illness. (p. 108)

**Lecture/Discussion**

Facilitate a discussion of the major factors influencing a person's response to illness.

**Communication Activity**

Have students interview the family member of a person who is experiencing a severe illness regarding the behavior changes that might have occurred since the onset of the illness.

6.0 Discuss various ways people deal with symptoms of illness.

7.0 Identify some of the factors involved in hypochondriasis.

    7.1 Give examples of individuals who seek health care more often than their condition warrants. (p. 108)

**Lecture/Discussion**

Have students explore ways in which the nursing care of a person with an actual illness might differ from that of a person experiencing a "hypochondria."

8.0 Recognize typical reactions to the confirmation of illness.

    8.1 Briefly describe common reactions experienced by individuals upon the confirmation of illness: Anxiety, shock, denial, suspicion, questioning, shame and guilt, insignificance and loneliness, regression and dependency, rejection, fear, and withdrawal and depression. (p. 109)

**Lecture/Discussion**

Ask students to share the reactions of a close significant other upon confirmation of a serious life-threatening illness.

9.0 Describe the general components of the sick role and impaired role.

    9.1 Outline four general aspects of the sick role that characterize the individual experiencing illness. (p. 111)

    9.2 Identify criteria that must be fulfilled for an individual to qualify for the sick role. (p. 111)

    9.3 Give examples of people exhibiting a "deviant sick role." (p. 111)

    9.4 Identify situations in which individuals are assigned an impaired role during illness. (p. 111)

**Lecture/Discussion**

Ask students to describe the various roles assumed by the ill individual. Sick role, deviant-sick role, and the impaired role. Have them give examples of each.

Ask students to discuss the effects of hospitalization that they have observed in their assigned individuals in clinical.

10.0 Identify some of the problems of chronically ill people.

    10.1 Define chronic illness. (p. 111)

    10.2 Identify essential information chronically ill people and their significant others need to know in order to prevent and manage medical crises. (p. 112)

    10.3 Summarize factors that may influence a chronically ill individual's management of prescribed regimes. (p. 112)

**Communication Activity**

Ask students to interview an individual in the community with a chronic illness regarding the significant lifestyle changes that have occurred as a result of their illness.

10.4 Explain the significance symptom control can have on the achievement of a normal life style in chronically ill individuals. (p. 112)

10.5 Explore ways in which chronic illness can promote social isolation. Identify measures to reduce or prevent the occurrence of social isolation. (p. 112)

10.6 Explore situations in which chronically ill individuals may encounter greater difficulty in learning to cope with the changes evoked by their illness. (p. 112)

10.7 Discuss the effects chronic illness can have on time management. (p. 112)

11.0 Describe the significance of change in body image to an individual.

    11.1 Describe the term body image. (p. 112)

    11.2 Discuss factors influencing the development of body image. (p. 113)

    11.3 Give examples of situations that can affect body image. (p. 113)

    11.4 Identify factors that influence a person's reaction to body image changes. (p. 113)

    11.5 Describe common reactions to a change in body image. (p. 113)

    11.6 Give specific examples of situations that may produce changes in body image. (p. 114)

    11.7 Identify indications of maladaptive reactions to body image changes. (p. 115)

    11.8 Identify stages of adaptation to change. (p. 115)

    11.9 Describe nursing intervention strategies effective in the promotion of a positive reaction to body image changes. (p. 115)

## Lecture/Discussion

Ask students to identify situations in which body image integrity may be disturbed.

Ask students to identify individuals in the clinical setting who are more prone to the development of a body image disturbance.

## Values Clarification

Have students write one paragraph summarizing their own physical characteristics. Ask them to identify things they "like" and "dislike" about themselves in relation to these characteristics.

## Clinical Laboratory Experience

Ask students to identify individuals in the clinical agency who may be experiencing a maladaptive reaction to a body image change.

---

## MULTIPLE CHOICE QUESTIONS

1. All of the following are behavior changes that may be associated with illness except:

   A. Narrowed interests
   B. Mood swings
   C. Egocentricity
   D. Decreased sensory awareness

## CORRECT ANSWER AND RATIONALE

B    An ill person's senses are often heightened. Options A, B, and C are common manifestations of illness. (p. 107)

2. When a person experiences symptoms of illness, he may go from one health professional to another seeking someone who will confirm the absence of disease. This behavior indicates that the person:

   A. Seeks provisional validation from others
   B. Is ambivalent about seeking health care
   C. Believes their symptoms are not serious
   D. May be denying the illness

   D   A person who is experiencing some cues of illness may try to prove that the symptoms are not real by increasing activity or denying the illness. They may go from one health professional to another health professional seeking someone who will confirm the absence of disease. This is appropriately labeled counteraction. (p. 107)

3. The psychologic experience of illness can be described in three stages. Arrange the stages in order:

   A. Acceptance, transition, convalescence
   B. Acceptance, transition, recovery
   C. Transition, acceptance, convalescence
   D. Transition, acceptance, recovery

   C   The stages of the psychologic experience of illness are transition, acceptance, and convalescence. (p. 106)

4. Which of the following individuals is most likely to seek health care first?

   A. The person who frequently experiences indigestion.
   B. A person experiencing external bleeding.
   C. A person with concerned significant others.
   D. A person whose symptoms interfere with their normal activities.

   B   People seek health care promptly for frightening or dramatic symptoms. In addition, they are more likely to seek professional help for conspicuous conditions (external bleeding) than for less obvious reasons. (p. 108)

5. Mrs. Black is seen frequently in a local health clinic. She has a tendency to exaggerate the symptoms and severity of her illness. This person is appropriately labeled as a:

   A. Hypochondriac
   B. Malingerer
   C. Neurotic
   D. None of the above

   D   The health professional should avoid the use of labels. It would be more useful to describe Mrs. Black's behavior in nonjudgmental ways, e.g., "shows a high level of concern and preoccupation with body functions;" "seeks medical attention more frequently than appears necessary."

6. Mr. Silver has recently been diagnosed with having tuberculosis, a communicable disease. His behavioral response to this diagnosis will be influenced by:

   A. Number of previous illnesses
   B. Age and socioeconomic status
   C. Attitudes of others toward the disease.
   D. All of the above

   D   Each person's reaction to the confirmation of illness is unique. Factors affecting a person's reaction to illness include: Coping patterns, self-concept, philosophy of life, age, socioeconomic status, general state of personal happiness, number of past illnesses, and the attitudes of others toward the illness. (p. 109)

7. Marsha frequently misses work because she is ill. She does not enjoy her present job, and finds she dislikes her present job and often complains that her work responsibilities are overwhelming. Marsha has assumed a:

   A. Sick role
   B. Deviant sick role
   C. Chronic role
   D. Impaired role

   B   Marsha exemplifies a deviant sick role. Individuals assume deviant sick roles for a variety of reasons: (1) they do not wish to get better and do not comply with treatment, (2) use illness for secondary gains, (3) use illness to avoid responsibilities, and (4) do not care whether they get better or not. (p. 111)

8. A person who appears less mature when ill is in a state of:

   A. Helplessness
   B. Immaturity
   C. Regression
   D. Repression

   C   People often appear less mature when ill. This state of regression is a common reaction to illness; it allows a person to accept the dependency more easily. (p. 110)

9. A person in your care suffers from a chronic illness. You are aware that people with chronic illnesses:

A. Can usually be cured with proper medical management
B. Usually require long-term medical management
C. Were born with the disease
D. Maintain a normal lifestyle

B   Chronic, incurable illnesses are long-term and require palliation or medical management. These illnesses usually cause alterations in the daily lives of the ill person and their significant others. (p. 112)

10. Which of the following individuals would probably find a change in body image most stressful?

A. A man who has all of his teeth extracted in preparation for dentures.
B. An elderly woman experiencing changes due to the normal aging process.
C. An adolescent who suddenly develops severe facial acne.
D. A woman who undergoes revision of an old abdominal surgical scar.

C   The adolescent would probably find their change in body image most stressful because: (1) Body image is particularly important for an adolescent, who is usually very concerned about developing "normally" or attractively; and (2) Changes in the face are particularly significant, since the face is synonymous with the self. (p. 113)

11. The initial stage of adaptation to a body image change is called:

A. Acknowledgment
B. Impact
C. Shock
D. Denial

B   The stages of adaptation to a body image change are, in order: Impact, retreat, acknowledgment, and reconstruction. (p. 115)

# 7

# HUMAN NEEDS DURING ILLNESS

OBJECTIVES

1.0 List the various levels of Maslow's hierarchy of basic human needs.

   1.1 Outline Maslow's hierarchy of human needs. (p. 118)

   1.2 Identify basic survival needs of individuals during health and illness. (p. 118)

   1.3 Explore the impact impaired survival needs may have on the individual. (p. 118)

   1.4 Identify stimulation needs of individuals during health and illness. (p. 119)

   1.5 Identify safety and security needs during health and illness. (p. 119)

   1.6 Identify specific love and belonging needs during health and illness. (p. 120)

   1.7 Identify fundamental self-actualization needs of the individual during health and illness. (p. 121)

2.0 Discuss the ways illness can disrupt normal satisfaction of basic human needs.

   2.1 Discuss ways in which survival needs may be altered by illness. (p. 118)

   2.2 Identify ways in which the sick individual may exhibit unmet stimulation needs during illness. (p. 119)

   2.3 Explore the impact an impaired role may have on the attainment of stimulation needs. (p. 119)

   2.4 Identify data indicative of unmet stimulation needs during illness. (p. 119)

   2.5 Describe the impact that illness can have on an individual's attainment of safety and security needs. (p. 119)

   2.6 Summarize behaviors that indicate unmet safety and security needs during illness. (p. 119)

   2.7 Identify basic concerns of ill individuals experiencing safety and security needs. (p. 119)

TEACHING/LEARNING STRATEGIES

Lecture/Discussion

Ask students to identify the needs they feel are basic to life. Have them compare these to the basic human needs outlined by Maslow.

Lecture/Discussion

Help students understand the impact of unmet human needs on a person's ability to maintain health and prevent illness.

Encourage students to identify the unfulfilled needs that they experienced during their most recent encounter with illness.

Communication Activity

Have students interview an ill individual in their community. After all interviews have been completed, ask each student to share the problems they identified, and how these problems were affecting the person's homeostatic balance.

2.8 Discuss the impact illness can have on the fulfillment of love and belonging needs. (p. 120)

2.9 Identify basic concerns of ill individuals related to love and belonging needs. (p. 120)

2.10 Summarize the relationship of love and belonging needs to the satisfaction of esteem needs during illness. (p. 120)

2.11 Explore ways in which illness can interfere with the satisfaction of esteem needs. (p. 120)

2.12 Outline ways the nurse can promote the fulfillment of esteem needs during illness. (p. 121)

2.13 Identify the group of basic human needs that are the most difficult to fulfill during illness. (p. 121)

2.14 Describe behaviors associated with unmet self-actualization needs during illness. (p. 121)

3.0 Identify ways nursing care provides for the satisfaction of basic human needs during illness.

    3.1 Discuss the importance of assuming a supportive and protective nursing role when caring for ill individuals experiencing safety and security needs. (p. 119)

    3.2 Identify nursing measures useful in assisting ill individuals with the fulfillment of love and belonging needs. (p. 120)

    3.3 Describe nursing measures that can be utilized to assist individuals with self-actualization needs during illness. (p. 121)

## Class Activity

Ask students to analyze the nursing care given to a hypothetical hospitalized individual. Ask them to identify the actions that were taken by the nursing staff to help the person meet basic human needs.

## Clinical Laboratory Experience

Ask students to identify the unmet basic human needs experienced by an assigned person in the clinical area. Have them develop a plan of care to assist this individual in meeting their basic human needs.

---

| MULTIPLE CHOICE QUESTIONS | CORRECT ANSWER AND RATIONALE |
|---|---|
| 1. When illness occurs, a person's basic human needs:<br><br>  A. Are met in a sequential fashion<br>  B. For survival and security must be first<br>  C. Are totally unmet<br>  D. All of the above | B    Lower level human needs (e.g., physiologic and safety) must be minimally met before it is possible to satisfy higher level needs on the hierarchy. Needs may be totally unmet, partially met, or totally met. (p. 117) |
| 2. Mrs. Bell has been hospitalized for a critical illness. Nursing care for Mrs. Bell will primarily focus on the fulfillment of:<br><br>  A. Basic physiological needs<br>  B. Needs for safety and security<br>  C. Stimulation needs<br>  D. Aesthetic needs | A    A person's survival needs are the major concern during periods of critical illness. Other needs are less prominent during this time, but do not disappear entirely. (p. 119) |

3.  If a person shows an exaggerated concern over basic bodily functions, the nurse should:

    A.  Encourage further expression of the person's concerns.
    B.  Recognize that the behavior may indicate fear and anxiety.
    C.  Empathetically listen to the person's concerns.
    D.  All of the above

D.  When survival needs are threatened, people often display an exaggerated concern with basic body functions such as bowel elimination. A helpful nurse recognizes that such behavior is an expression of the person's fear and anxiety. The most helpful things to do are to listen empathetically to the person's concerns, to offer appropriate information, and to eliminate unnecessary concerns. (p. 118)

4.  When a person is ill, his stimulation needs:

    A.  May be more prominent
    B.  May be expressed in a sublimated fashion
    C.  Can be denied until he can express them normally
    D.  Are usually overtly expressed

B.  A person's needs for novelty, manipulation, exploration, and sexual expression may be less prominent during illness, but do not entirely disappear. Although illness and hospitalization may block the overt expression and satisfaction of some needs, evidence of the continued presence of such needs may appear in sublimated (disguised) form. (p. 119)

5.  A person whose safety and security needs are threatened by illness may feel:

    A.  Lonely and isolated
    B.  Helpless and not in control of the situation
    C.  Rejected by significant others
    D.  All of the above

D   When illness threatens a person's basic need for safety and security, they may experience all of the listed options. (p. 120)

6.  Which group of needs is most difficult to satisfy during illness?

    A.  Stimulation
    B.  Esteem
    C.  Self-actualization
    D.  Safety and security

C   The most difficult group of needs for a person to satisfy during illness are the self-actualization needs. These refer to: (a) expressing one's personality, and (b) developing one's ability. (p. 121)

7.  The nurse is aware that the ill individual often unconsciously looks to the health care professional for fulfillment of which basic human needs?

    A.  Stimulation; safety and security
    B.  Safety and security; esteem
    C.  Safety and security; love and belonging
    D.  Love and belonging; stimulation

C   Ill people may look for gratification of both love and belonging needs, and safety and security needs from health professionals who attend them. In doing so, they are attempting to fulfill the need for physical and psychosocial security. (p. 120)

# COPING WITH LOSS AND OTHER CHANGES

OBJECTIVES

TEACHING/LEARNING STRATEGIES

1.0 Identify losses commonly experienced by people throughout life.

1.1 Differentiate between the terms grief, mourning, and loss. (p. 123)

1.2 Compare definitions of loss described in this chapter by Engel and Carlson. (p. 123)

1.3 List and give examples of types of losses that may produce a grief reaction. (p. 123)

1.4 Explain ways in which the stage in the life cycle may influence responses to loss and subsequent grieving. (p. 124)

1.5 Utilizing the Holmes social readjustment scale, analyze the relationship between change and loss. (p. 124)

### Written Exercise

Ask students to outline the responses to loss and change at the various levels of the life cycle.

2.0 Explain that bereavement is just one kind of loss and may differ only in severity from other losses.

2.1 Compare and contrast the grief reactions provoked by bereavement to those produced through other losses. (p. 124)

2.2 Describe the terms: death, bereavement, preparatory grief, and anticipatory grief. (pp. 128-130)

2.3 Explain the significance of preparatory grief or anticipatory grief in individuals coping with loss. (p. 130)

### Communication Activity

Have students interview a person in the community who has experienced a loss, such as the loss of a job or significant other. Ask them to explore the individual's perceptions and feelings related to the loss.

3.0 List the signs and symptoms most often experienced by grieving people.

3.1 List and describe the three stages of the grieving as formulated by Engel. (p. 126)

3.2 Outline the somatic, psychological, and socials behavioral reactions, described by Lindemann, that are commonly associated with grieving. (p. 125)

### Lecture/Discussion

Ask students to describe the similarities and differences of various individual's responses to loss.

### Communication Activity

Request each student to select and conduct a 15 minute communication session with a family member or significant other of an individual receiving care in a critical care unit of a local hospital. Ask students to identify the personal feelings they encountered during the interview, as well as the behaviors and emotions displayed by significant other.

4.0 Describe the "coping mechanisms commonly used by grieving people.

    4.1 Identify coping mechanisms utilized by the individual experiencing a potential or actual loss of something significant. (p. 129)

    4.2 Compare and contrast the signs and symptoms of normal grief to abnormal grief reactions. (p. 132)

    4.3 Briefly discuss the grief reactions experienced from loss of: a terminally ill life partner, an infant from sudden infant death syndrome, a companion animal, and the sudden death of a significant other. (p. 130)

    4.4 Give examples of situations, and the coping mechanisms involved, in which individuals might experience "complicated" grief. (p. 132)

5.0 Apply the nursing process to the care of grieving people.

    5.1 Identify factors useful in assessing a person's needs related to loss. (p. 125)

    5.2 Provide examples of nursing diagnoses related to grief and loss. (p. 123)

    5.3 Identify common nursing goals related to care of grieving people. (p. 123)

    5.4 Discuss possible outcome criteria that can be utilized by the nurse to evaluate nursing care for grieving individuals and their significant others. (p. 123)

6.0 Identify your own reactions to loss and appreciate how these may influence the kind of missing care you offer.

    6.1 Explore past responses and reactions to a significant personal loss. (p. 124)

    6.2 Describe difficulties the nurse may encounter in coping with loss. (p. 124)

    6.3 Analyze personal responses, feelings, and reactions experienced while providing care for grieving individuals. (p. 124)

    6.4 Identify ways in which the reactions and feelings of the nurse to loss can influence nursing care. (p. 125)

    6.5 Discuss mechanisms the nurse can use to gain a sense of satisfaction in comforting and supporting individuals or groups through loss experiences. (p. 129)

## Guest Speaker

Invite a psychologist to discuss the coping mechanisms commonly displayed by grieving people.

## Panel Presentation

Invite nurses from the community to come to class for a panel discussion of nursing as it relates to the person coping with loss. Encourage participants to analyze effective methods of assisting the person at each stage of the grief process.

## Clinical Laboratory Experience

Develop a goal-directed plan of care for an actual person experiencing or anticipating a loss.

## Group Activity

Divide class into small groups and assign each group to develop a nursing plan of care for one of the following individuals experiencing loss of: a life partner, an infant from sudden infant death syndrome; a significant other, i.e., brother, sister, child, grandparent, close friend; and loss of a companion animal. Outline in class the similarities and differences in the care planned for each situation, and the special needs identified in each.

## Written Exercise

Ask students to write five words that describe their feelings related to loss. Display the responses to the entire group and discuss the impact of identifying personal feelings related to loss prior to administering nursing care to grieving individuals or groups.

## Values Clarification

Discuss personal feelings, beliefs, and attitudes related to loss and death. Ask students to analyze the impact these have had on the nursing care they administered to grieving individuals or groups.

7.0 Develop skills appropriate to helpful
relationships with grieving people.

    7.1 Describe actions the nurse might take to
help meet the needs of a terminally ill
person and their significant other as
they engage in each stage of the grief
process. (p. 128)

    7.2 Identify general principles the nurse
can utilize to guide nursing intervention for grieving people. (p. 128)

    7.3 Identify ways in which the nurse can
provide support for the significant
others of a dying person. (p. 129)

    7.4 Identify special needs and possible modes
of intervention for persons experiencing
problems related to the death of a: life
partner; child by sudden infant death
syndrome; and significant other by sudden
death. (p. 131)

    7.5 Outline special needs of children and
elderly individuals experiencing a loss.
(p. 131)

    7.6 Review techniques of therapeutic commun-
ication, emphasizing their importance in
caring for individuals coping with loss.
Chapter 5. (p. 82)

---

## MULTIPLE CHOICE QUESTIONS

1. All of the following statements about
grieving are true except:

    A. Is a typical reaction to the loss of a
valued object.
    B. Is a process reserved for those who have
lost a significant other.
    C. Is more severe when several loss factors
occur.
    D. Is a very personal experience that
follows certain predictable patterns.

2. Which of the following individuals will
suffer a more severe response to loss?

    A. Mr. Black whose wife has died after an
extended illness.
    B. Mrs. Smith whose lifelong friend died
suddenly from a "heart attack."
    C. Mrs. Jones whose son died yesterday in an
automobile accident.
    D. Miss Clayton who recently underwent
surgery for removal of a cancerous breast.

## CORRECT ANSWER AND RATIONALE

B    People grieve for other losses as well as
those associated with death. (p. 124)

C    The sudden loss of a family member will have
the greatest impact on significant others.
Two factors that are responsible for this
severe response pattern are: the closeness
of the relationship, and no anticipatory
grief possible. (p. 130)

SITUATION: Mrs. Smith has recently been diagnosed with a disease that is potentially fatal. Your nursing assessment of Mrs. Smith reveals the following information: loss of appetite for three days; inability to concentrate, and insomnia. Questions 3 through 5 relate to Mrs. Smith.

3.  The symptoms of grieving Mrs. Smith is experiencing are best termed:

    A.  Behavioral symptoms
    B.  Psychologic symptoms
    C.  Social symptoms
    D.  Somatic symptoms

D   Loss of appetite, lethargy, and inability to relax were categorized as somatic symptoms by Lindemann in his studies on responses to grieving. (p. 125)

4.  The most appropriate nursing diagnosis for Mrs. Smith at this time would be:

    A.  Grieving related to actual loss.
    B.  Grieving related to anticipated loss.
    C.  Inadequate emotional support while grieving.
    D.  Inability to control grief.

B   Grief responses are frequently initiated by the anticipated loss of life that occurs with a serious diagnosis. In this situation there has been no actual loss, nor is there any mention of the support systems available to the person. (p. 129)

5.  Nursing intervention for this person should include measures to help her:

    A.  Acquire appropriate support systems.
    B.  Express her feelings fully and appropriately.
    C.  Recognize her feelings as normal.
    D.  All of the above.

D   Possible goals of intervention related to grief include: understand the normal grieving processes; express feelings appropriately and fully; maintain control of their situation; experience hope; and obtain the kind of physical and emotional support they need. (p. 123)

6.  Dr. Holmes' life social readjustment scale suggests that:

    A.  A successful grieving process influences adjustment to loss.
    B.  All positive/negative life changes require the same amount of readjustment.
    C.  Any loss reaction equally predisposes the person to illness.

A   Holmes' social readjustment scale illustrates the following points: any change automatically involves a loss, either positive or negative; life readjustment is achieved through a successful grieving process; and the greater the readjustment required by the individual, the greater the person's susceptibility to illness. (p. 124)

7.  Select the statement that best exemplifies a person engaged in the restitution phase of Engel's grief process.

    A.  "John was such a good person, superior in every way."
    B.  "I always gave him my undivided attention."
    C.  "Without John, life has no purpose."
    D.  "The physician didn't really try to cure him."

A   Idealization of the lost object occurs during the restitution phase, with the individual suppressing all negative aspects of the lost object. Feelings of guilt are common. Feelings of emptiness, pointlessness in life, and anger are encountered in the stage of developing awareness. (p. 127)

8.  Mr. Ray's wife has recently expired. As you talk with him he states, "You nurses just didn't provide the care she needed." What would be the most therapeutic response you could make?

    A.  "I can understand how you must be feeling."
    B.  "Why do you say that, Mr. Ray?"
    C.  "We really did all that we could for her."
    D.  "What needs were unmet?"

A   Expressions of anger are often encountered in the stage of developing awareness. The most therapeutic way to handle such situations is with understanding, rather than defensiveness. (p. 127)

9.  A person tells you, "I can't be dying. I feel great!" This is best known as:

    A. Rationalization
    B. Denial
    C. Intellectualization
    D. Reflection.

B  The initial responses to a severe or anticipated loss are feelings of "shock" and "disbelief." This denial may include processes such as rationalization and intellectualization. (p. 126)

10. Choose the best initial response of the nurse in a suspected grief reaction:

    A. Identify circumstances that may have precipitated the feeling of loss.
    B. Acknowledge the loss.
    C. Emphasize grief as a normal process.
    D. Facilitate expression of feelings.

A  In suspected grief reactions the nurse should confirm the loss by listening carefully and empathetically in order to identify circumstances that may have provoked the loss. Other items (B,C,D) are important once the nurse is reasonably sure that a person is grieving. (p. 128)

11. Which of the following statements is false in regard to the dying person?

    A. The person anticipating death will experience preparatory grief.
    B. The person has more to grieve than their significant others.
    C. The person reaches the stage of acceptance prior to their significant others.
    D. The person may be a few steps ahead or behind their significant others in the grief process.

C  The dying person, experiencing preparatory grief, may be a few steps ahead or behind their significant others in the grief process. (p. 129)

12. The nurse can assist a dying person's significant others by:

    A. Providing all nursing care without assistance of family members.
    B. Informing a single family representative of impending death.
    C. Discouraging outbursts of emotions in the person's presence.
    D. Establishing a good family relationship prior to the actual death.

D  When possible, a helpful relationship should be established between the nurse and the significant others before the time of greatest stress, death, occurs. In response to items (A,B,C) the nurse should: permit significant others to assist in daily "caring" activities; give news of a death or impending death to a group of significant others if possible; and encourage expression of feelings. (p. 129)

13. Mr. Adams has just expired. The nurse can best assist his significant others by:

    A. Allowing them to spend time alone with their deceased loved one.
    B. Providing a private place for them to assemble.
    C. Permitting them to conduct significant cultural or religious practices.
    D. All of the above.

D  When death has occurred, the significant others need to be given time alone with their deceased loved one, to say their "goodbyes;" given a private place where they can express themselves; accepted and understood; and given the opportunity to carry out religious and cultural practices that are significant to them. (p. 130)

14. Identify the person who would be at greatest risk during the bereavement period:

    A. A person employed in an active law firm.
    B. A college student living away from home.
    C. A person of middle income status.
    D. All are equally at risk.

B  A college student away from home may feel isolated and lack a supportive network that actively encourages expression of grief. (p. 130)

15. Joe died instantly from massive injuries sustained in a motor vehicle accident. The nurse could assist his significant others by:

    A. Telling them what to expect prior to viewing the body, then leaving all injuries uncovered.
    B. Allowing them ten minutes alone with his body.
    C. Allowing them to touch the body.
    D. Making sure that all injuries are covered prior to their viewing the body.

C   Significant others should be given time to see and perhaps touch the body. This assists in making the death a reality. All mutilated areas of the body should be covered. If possible, they should be warned of any visible injuries. They should not be rushed in this important process. (p. 130)

16. All of the following data indicates a person experiencing "complicated grief" except:

    A. Avoids social engagements, preferring to be alone.
    B. Has feelings of guilt, self-blame, and worthlessness.
    C. Remembers both good and bad qualities of the deceased.
    D. Refuses to acknowledge that a loss has occurred.

C   The grieving person is able to remember both good and bad qualities of the deceased person in the last stage of the grief process, restitution. Symptoms of "complicated grief" include: prolonged social isolation; a persistent sense of worthlessness and self-blame; and prolonged denial of the loss. (p. 132)

17. Attendance and participation in the funeral ritual may benefit the grieving child if the child is over the age of:

    A. Four or five
    B. Five or six
    C. Six or seven
    D. Seven or eight

C   Children over the age of six or seven may be helped by attendance at the funeral. (p. 131)

18. In order to provide supportive care for grieving people, a nurse needs to understand that they:

    A. Should always attend to the person's needs, regardless of personal needs.
    B. Often experience the same despair and hopelessness as those in their care.
    C. Should immediately terminate the relationship with the family once death has occurred.
    D. Not overextend themselves in meeting family needs, limiting care to the person.

B   A nurse tends to equate "cure" with "success." It is not uncommon for them to experience the same feelings of despair and hopelessness felt by the person and their significant others. Nurses must avoid the tendency to overextend themselves, learning to say "no" sometimes, to allow time to attend to their own needs. It is important to remember that significant others need care too, often experiencing their greatest needs once death is imminent, or has occurred. (p. 130)

19. When providing care to the elderly, the nurse should be aware that:

    A. Age does not have an impact on grieving and ability to cope with loss.
    B. Grief sensations in the elderly are often displayed as physical symptoms/illnesses.
    C. Elderly people always express grief at a conscious level.
    D. All of the above.

B   The elderly person may not experience grief intensely at a conscious level, but may suppress feelings of grief, exhibiting them as somatic symptoms. (p. 131)

20. Factors to consider when assessing a person's needs related to grief and loss include:

    A. Available support systems
    B. Cultural beliefs and habits
    C. Personality characteristics
    D. All of the above

D   Many factors influence an individual's grief experience. These include: personality and cultural/social patterns. (p. 125)

# 9

# HISTORICAL INFLUENCES AND EXPANDING ROLES OF NURSES

## OBJECTIVES

1.0 Discuss major influences on a nurse's role throughout history.

    1.1 State the definition of role. (p. 140)

    1.2 Understand significant historical events that have influenced nursing and health care. (p. 140)

    1.3 Discuss the impact significant historical events have had on the present day professional role. (p. 140)

    1.4 Explore traditional historical images of the nurse that continue to influence the nursing profession today. (p. 140)

    1.5 Identify major influences on the development of the profession of nursing. (p. 141)

    1.6 Identify factors occurring within the last century that had a major influence on the development of the nursing profession. (p. 145)

2.0 Describe a variety of philosophies and definitions of nursing.

    2.1 Define the term philosophy. (p. 145)

    2.2 Explain the relationship of philosophy to nursing. (p. 145)

    2.3 Outline major components of Virginia Henderson's philosophy of nursing. (p. 145)

    2.4 State Virginia Henderson's definition of nursing. (p. 145)

    2.5 Identify major components of Dorothea Orem's philosophy of nursing. (p. 146)

    2.6 Briefly state Dorothea Orem's definition of nursing. (p. 146)

    2.7 State other significant definitions of nursing as formulated by: King, Peplau, Rogers, Vaillot, Kreuter, and the American Nurses' Association. (p. 146)

## TEACHING/LEARNING STRATEGIES

### Lecture/Discussion

Ask the students to identify factors they feel strongly influence the profession of nursing. Record responses on the board.

### Written Exercise

Encourage students to explore Florence Nightengale's influence on modern day nursing.

Ask students to write a brief paper summarizing significant events in the historical development of nursing.

### Lecture/Discussion

Ask the students to share their feelings on why they feel a definition of nursing is necessary.

### Written Exercise

Ask students to write their own personal definition of nursing. Instruct them to compare their own definition with those listed on page 145 to 147 in the text. What are the similarities and differences?

Have students write a three page paper on their philosophy of nursing at the beginning of the semester. Have them review the philosophy at the end of the semester to determine ways in which the philosophy has changed or evolved.

3.0 Analyze various nursing philosophies and
definitions according to their strengths and
weaknesses.

 3.1 Identify criteria useful in the
evaluation of models or philosophies of
nursing. (p. 147)

 3.2 Discuss common features of all
philosophies of nursing. (p. 147)

4.0 Identify factors that influence nurses' roles
in various health care settings.

 4.1 Identify the primary and secondary
functions of the nurse. (p. 147)

 4.2 Name and briefly describe five services
that are offered by a complete health
care system. (p. 147)

 4.3 Explore the relationship of the
cure-care concept of nursing to the
primary and secondary functions of the
nurse. (p. 147)

 4.4 Outline the nursing lines of authority
within the hospital system. (p. 148)

 4.5 Identify and discuss general inpatient
settings in which nurses work. (p. 148)

 4.6 List examples of community settings
where nurses practice. (p. 148)

 4.7 Briefly describe the concept of episodic
care. (p. 148)

 4.8 Describe basic methods used by the nurse
to organize care. (p. 148)

 4.9 Discuss the importance of developing
clear job descriptions for nurses
working in health care settings.
(p. 149)

 4.10 Identify essential attributes of an
effective health care service. (p. 149)

 4.11 Briefly explain the three categories of
working relationships. (p. 149)

 4.12 Explore the value of using a
collaborative approach in working
relationships. (p. 149)

 4.13 Identify prerequisites of an efficient
health care system. (p. 150)

 4.14 Enumerate various factors that affect
the nurse-physician relationship.
(p. 150)

## Group Activity

Divide students into small groups. Ask each group
to prepare an oral presentation on one major
philosophy of nursing.

After the presentation, ask students to identify
similarities and differences in the components of
the philosophies.

## Lecture/Discussion

Facilitate a discussion of the various roles of
the nurse: Manager, researcher, teacher, author,
and advocate. What are the perceptions of the
student in relation to each role. Which of these
roles can they participate in as a beginning
student in nursing?

5.0 Outline the variety of ways nurses prepare for their professional work.

    5.1 Define the term socialization and identify two ways in which it occurs. (p. 150)

    5.2 Name three levels of educational preparation in nursing. (p. 150)

    5.3 List and briefly describe three basic education programs in nursing. (p. 150)

    5.4 Describe the advantages of attaining higher nursing education at the master's and doctoral levels. (p. 151)

    5.5 Identify incidental learning situations that influence the process of socialization into the nursing profession. (p. 151)

6.0 Discuss the ways nurses' roles are expanding at the present time.

    6.1 Briefly discuss areas of expanded role functions in nursing. (p. 151)

    6.2 Describe specific expanded nursing roles: Nurse practitioner, nurse clinician, clinical nurse specialist, and certification. (p. 151)

    6.3 Discuss reasons the nurse should acquire continuing education upon graduation. (p. 151)

    6.4 Explore the future of the present-day nursing profession. (p. 155)

7.0 Describe the professional responsibilities of nurses.

    7.1 Discuss the role of the nurse manager. (p. 152)

    7.2 Identify requirements of the successful nurse manager. (p. 152)

    7.3 Describe the impact research can have on the advancement of the nursing profession. (p. 152)

    7.4 Discuss the teaching role of the nurse. (p. 152)

    7.5 Understand the nurse's responsibility to attempt to publish any new knowledge gained. (p. 152)

    7.6 Identify responsibilities of the nurse advocate. (p. 153)

    7.7 Identify three attributes characterizing a profession. (p. 153)

    7.8 Discuss the relationship of the attributes characterizing a profession to the profession of nursing. (p. 153)

### Lecture/Discussion

Encourage a discussion of the different types of nursing education programs. Ask students to identify the major differences in programs leading to the first degree in nursing: Associate, diploma, and baccalaureate.

### Lecture/Discussion

Discuss the expanded role of the nurse. Encourage students to compare this role with the role of the nurse in the early historical development of the nurse.

### Group Activity

After dividing students into work groups, assign each group one of the expanding roles of the nurse: Nurse practitioner, Nurse clinician, Nurse clinical specialist, and Certification. Ask each group to prepare a brief oral report on the responsibilities of the professional nurse within each role.

7.9 Give examples of professional organizations that have been developed for nurses. (p. 153)

7.10 Discuss basic functions of a professional organization. (p. 153)

7.11 Describe ways in which the nursing organization has achieved the functions of professional organizations. (p. 153)

7.12 Appreciate that the ultimate responsibility for professional nursing practice lies within the individual. (p. 154)

7.13 Explain what is meant by being accountable for the nursing care you give. (p. 154)

7.14 Explore ways in which the development of autonomous nursing practice has influenced nursing accountability. (p. 154)

8.0 Describe ways of evaluating standards of nursing care.

### Lecture/Discussion

Review the components of the Standards of Nursing Practice as listed on page 241 in the text.

8.1 Identify necessary requirements that must be fulfilled by standards of nursing practice. (p. 154)

8.2 State three purposes served by the systemic evaluation of nursing care. (p. 154)

### Clinical Laboratory Experience

Ask the student to review the standard of practice guiding the activities of nurses in their assigned clinical facility.

8.3 Describe three ways in which nursing care can be evaluated: Nursing audits, peer reviews, and "patient" audits. (p. 154)

9.0 Recognize the expectations the public has of the nursing profession.

### Lecture/Discussion

9.1 Discuss public expectations of nursing. (p. 154)

Have students identify their own personal expectations of nursing. How do these expectations compare with those of the general public.

9.2 Discuss legal requirements that govern or determine nursing responsibilities. (p. 155)

9.3 Understand the legal implications of increased nursing responsibility and accountability. (p. 155)

10. Discuss the relationship between nursing and traditional and changing sex roles.

### Lecture/Discussion

10.1 Explore the impact sexism has had on the nursing profession. (p. 155)

Ask students to share their feelings on the future of nursing. Have them identify ways in which they feel the nursing professional will change during their lifetimes.

Discuss sexism issues that have affected professional nursing: The women's movement and men in nursing.

1. Which of the following statements is <u>correct?</u>

   A. Historical images of the nurse emphasized the need for formal nursing education.
   B. Historical views of the nurse positively influenced the development of professional nursing.
   C. The religious image of nursing viewed the nurse as a saint.
   D. The nursing profession is no longer influenced by the traditional images of the nurse.

   **C**    The traditional historical images of the nurse were the folk image, religious image, and the servant image. Respectively, these images viewed the nurse as mother, saint, and servant. These images continue to present obstacles to the development of professional nurses as educated, well-paid respected, and independent practitioners. (p. 144)

2. A formal set of beliefs or attitudes upon which the nurse can base action is called:

   A. Philosophy of nursing
   B. Nursing theory
   C. Conceptual model of nursing
   D. All of the above

   **D**    Every nurse has a philosophy or set of beliefs that direct their nursing behavior. As the science of nursing has developed, a number of nursing theorists have composed formal philosophies of nursing (also called nursing theories or conceptual models). (p. 145)

3. Which theorist composed a philosophy of nursing based on the concept of self-care?

   A. Immogene King
   B. Dorothea Orem
   C. Hildegard Peplau
   D. Martha Rogers

   **B**    The basic premise of Orem's philosophy of nursing is self-care. "Self-care" refers to those activities that people (either individually or as groups) initiate and perform on their own behalf to maintain their life, health, and well-being. (p. 146)

4. A person in your care is unable to carry out any self-care activities. According to Orem, this person requires which type of nursing system:

   A. Complete Nursing System
   B. Fully Compensatory System
   C. Total Nursing System
   D. Wholly Compensatory System

   **D**    Orem defines three types of nursing systems: Wholly compensatory, partly compensatory, and supportive-education. The individual who is unable to perform any activities of daily living requires a wholly compensatory system, in which the nurse provides total health care needs. (p. 146)

5. The nurse is aware that factors influencing the development of community-based services include all of the following <u>except</u>:

   A. Increased focus on health prevention
   B. Decreased number of nurses working in hospital settings
   C. Spiraling costs of "inpatient" hospital care
   D. Growing awareness of the need for health maintenance

   **B**    Options A, C, and D all describe factors that have been significantly influential in the growth and development of health services outside the hospital setting. The majority of nurses continue to work in the acute care hospital setting, even though it has been documented that there are more individuals requiring assistance in community-type settings. (p. 148)

6. One nurse is completely responsible for the nursing care of an individual on a continuous 24-hour basis, in which type of nursing care delivery system.

   A. Functional nursing
   B. Holistic nursing
   C. Primary nursing
   D. Total care nursing

   **C**    A primary nurse is completely responsible for all the nursing care that a person requires until nursing care is no longer needed. (p. 149)

7. A health care team that exhibits a collaborative working relationship:

   A. Values each member's unique contribution to the group
   B. Demonstrates an understanding of each member's primary role in the group
   C. Is committed to people-centered care
   D. All of the above

   **D**    The collaborative working relationship is true partnership. An understanding and appreciation of each other's primary role, a commitment to people-centered care, and an ability to communicate clearly with each other are important factors to the success of the group. (p. 150)

8.  Which of the following statements about nursing education programs is <u>incorrect</u>?

    A.  Graduates from Diploma, Associate Degree, and Baccalaureate Programs take different licensing exams.
    B.  Students in baccalaureate programs receive a much broader background in basic and social sciences.
    C.  All three types of nursing education programs prepare a person to take a State Board examination to qualify for RN licensure.
    D.  None of the above

A   Students may study toward registered nurse (RN) qualification in three ways: Diploma programs, Associate Degree programs, and Baccalaureate Degree Programs. All three programs offer education based on physical and social sciences and clinical nursing instruction, but the baccalaureate program is longest and requires the greatest depth of general and nursing education. Graduation from each program allows a person to take the same licensing examination to qualify for RN status. (p. 150)

9.  The process of socialization into the nursing profession is:

    A.  Achieved through intentional interactions with other health care personnel
    B.  Achieved incidentally through the formal education process
    C.  Guided by formalized educational experiences and incidental interactions with other health care personnel
    D.  Usually an unconscious and unplanned process

C   Socialization into the nursing profession occurs in two ways: through intentional learning in formal nursing education program and through incidental learning interactions with other health care personnel. (p. 150)

C   Options A, B, and D are all factors that have contributed significantly to the professionalization of nursing practice. Traditional sexist roles have negatively influenced this professionalization by causing collaborative problems within the health care team. (pp. 144, 150)

10. All of the following have contributed positively to the advancement of the nursing profession <u>except</u>:

    A.  Advancement in medical education
    B.  Development of nursing philosophies
    C.  Traditional sexist attitudes
    D.  Changing societal values

11. Prior to his discharge from the hospital, Mr. Clark's primary nurse makes arrangements for follow-up home visits from a community health nurse. The primary nurse is demonstrating which nursing role?

    A.  Advocate
    B.  Adviser
    C.  Manager
    D.  Counselor

A   The nurse advocate is a person who speaks or acts for another person. (p. 153)

12. The professional nurse:

    A.  Demonstrates a commitment to people-centered care
    B.  Assumes accountability and responsibility for nursing actions
    C.  Maintains high academic standards
    D.  All of the above

D   The individual nurse must retain a commitment to people centered care, maintain a high academic standard, take responsibility, and be accountable for individual nursing practice. (p. 154)

13. A hospitalized individual is asked to evaluate the nursing care they are receiving. This is an example of a :

    A.  Nursing Audit
    B.  Nursing Review
    C.  Patient Audit
    D.  Patient Review

C   The "patient" audit allows the recipients of nursing care the opportunity to offer their evaluations of the nursing care they received or are receiving. (p. 154)

14. All of the following statements about the standards for nursing practice are true except:

    A. They outline criteria that can be used to evaluate nursing performance.
    B. They are standard indicators of quality care.
    C. They determine the education and examination requirements for nurses.
    D. Individual nursing agencies may formulate a set of standards to be used by their institution.

C    Options A, B, and C are correct statements about the standards for nursing practices. Option C is a function of the Nurse Practice Act. (p. 154)

# 10
# CHANGING CONCEPTS OF HEALTH, DISEASE, AND HEALTH CARE

## OBJECTIVES

1.0 Discuss why it is difficult to define the terms "health" and "disease" and describe those factors that influence how a person perceives these two entities.

   1.1 Identify reasons for the difficulty in defining health and disease. (p. 159)

   1.2 Discuss the impact an individual's values can have on definitions of health and disease. (p. 159)

   1.3 State the definition of health as described by the World Health Organization. (p. 159)

   1.4 Identify the biomedical, epidemiologic ecologic, sociologic, and consumer definitions of health and disease. (p. 161)

2.0 Describe several models of disease, identifying those that are holistic in scope.

   2.1 Briefly describe basic models of health and disease: Ancient Greek model, biomedical model, biopsychosocial model, stress model and nursing models. (p. 160)

3.0 List the social, historic, and economic trends that influence health care delivery.

   3.1 Explore the changing patterns of health care delivery. (p. 161)

   3.2 Identify trends affecting health care delivery. (p. 161)

   3.3 Define health and disease according to three differing view points. (p. 161)

   3.4 Identify significant events in the history of health care. (p. 162)

   3.5 Discuss major trends affecting the American health care industry. (p. 163)

   3.6 Cite examples of U.S. Federal health legislation. (p. 165)

   3.7 Appreciate the nursing professional's responsibility to acquire knowledge related to current economic, political, and cultural trends. (p. 169)

## TEACHING/LEARNING STRATEGIES

### Class Activity

Ask students to elicit definitions of health and disease from other health care professionals within their clinical facility: Respiratory therapist, physical therapist, laboratory specialists, occupational therapists, social worker, and other nurses. Share obtained definitions in class.

Have students interview a family member regarding their own personal definition of nursing. Report findings in class.

### Values Clarification

Ask students to write their own personal definitions of health and illness. Read the responses in class. Encourage a discussion of the similarities and differences in their personal definitions.

### Lecture/Discussion

Review various models of disease and health: Historical, medical, systems or biopsychosocial, stress and other holistic models, and nursing.

### Lecture/Discussion

Focus discussion on the impact of significant historical events that have influenced the Health Care Delivery System of today. (Outline of some of these events appears on page 162 in the text.)

Facilitate a discussion of the trends that are affecting the health care delivery system of today.

Discuss major trends that are presently affecting the American Health Care Delivery System. Have students identify the ways in which they feel these trends will affect the profession of nursing in the future.

### Class Activity

Ask several students to volunteer to visit the Bureau of Vital Statistics in their area. Ask them to obtain information on the leading causes of death in the state during the past five years. After presentation of this material in class, have students compare the findings with those listed on page 163 in the text.

4.0 List and describe the different levels in a comprehensive health care program.

    4.1 Give examples of nurse-managed health care centers. (p. 170)

    4.2 Briefly describe, using examples, the four levels of a comprehensive health care program: health promotion, primary prevention, secondary prevention and tertiary care. (p. 164)

    4.3 State the goal of comprehensive health care programs. (p. 164)

5.0 Discuss the different methods by which health care is financed.

    5.1 Explore changing patterns of health care financing. (p. 165)

    5.2 List four major types of health care financing. (p. 166)

    5.3 Describe the personal payment method of health care financing. (p. 166)

    5.4 Discuss the use of philanthropy as a means for financing health care. (p. 166)

    5.5 Discuss the use of private insurance for payment of health care services. (p. 166)

    5.6 Give examples of insurance organizations that provide payment for health care services. (p. 166)

    5.7 Discuss government involvement in the financing of health care services. (p. 167)

    5.8 Give examples and briefly describe health care financing programs sponsored by the U.S. government. (p. 167)

6.0 Describe some possible solutions to the financial crisis facing the health care industry today.

    6.1 Explore ways in which the crisis of rising costs and limited resources has affected the health care delivery system. (p. 167)

    6.2 Enumerate various reasons for the increase in health care spending. (p. 167)

    6.3 Describe ways in which health care costs may be cut without sacrificing the care given. (p. 168)

**Lecture/Discussion**

Encourage a discussion of the changing patterns in health care financing. Ask students to identify the ways in which these changing patterns will affect both nursing and the consumer.

**Guest Speaker**

Invite a person in the hospital who is responsible for obtaining financial payment for the services rendered by the hospital to a post-conference period. Have them discuss the various financial arrangements that are made by the hospital to assist the health care consumer with paying for hospital services. Also ask them to discuss other options that are available for individuals who cannot pay for health care services.

**Lecture/Discussion**

Ask students to identify their ideas on ways in which the financial crises facing the Health Care Delivery System could be managed.

7.0 Define diagnostic-related group (DRG) and discuss the impact of DRGs on nursing care.

    7.1 Explore the impact the Tax Equity and Fiscal Responsibility Act of 1982 may have on the Health Care Delivery System. (p. 168)

    7.2 Explain the DRG system for payment of health care services. (p. 168)

8.0 Discuss other crises influencing Health Care Delivery Systems.

    8.1 Discuss the impact that discrepancies between technology and health needs, ethical dilemmas arising from technological growth, and fragmentation of health care services is having on the Health Care Delivery System. (p. 168)

9.0 Describe the role of nursing in health care policy and planning.

    9.1 Identify measures that can be taken to assure adequate health care for minorities, the economically disadvantaged, and the elderly. (p. 169)

## Lecture/Discussion

Help students to understand the impact that the evolution of Diagnostic-related categories have had on the Health Care Delivery System. Facilitate a discussion of the ways in which DRGs are affecting the practice of nursing. What are the implications for the future? Ask students to identify current economic, cultural, and economic trends they feel are significantly influencing the practice of nursing.

---

## MULTIPLE CHOICE QUESTIONS

1. The nurse is aware that an individual's definition of health is greatly influenced by their:

    A. Personal attitudes and beliefs
    B. Social rank in society
    C. Cultural background
    D. All of the above

2. The World Health Organization defines health as:

    A. A state of high-level wellness in which one is free of illness
    B. A state of complete physical, mental, and social well-being and not merely the absence of disease or infirmity
    C. A state of high level biopsychosocial wellness
    D. A state of complete physical, mental, and social well-being

3. All of the following are holistic models of health and disease except:

    A. Biomedical model
    B. Biopsychosocial model
    C. Stress model
    D. Dunn model of high-level wellness

4. A nurse works in a community clinic that provides prenatal care to underprivileged women. The focus of this clinic's service is:

    A. Health promotion
    B. Primary care
    C. Secondary care
    D. Tertiary care

## CORRECT ANSWER AND RATIONALE

D    Individual definitions of health and disease vary according to personal values, peer group, cultural background, and social class. (p. 159)

B    Option B is a complete statement of the World Health Organization's definition of health. (p. 159)

A    The biomedical model deemphasizes the psychosocial component of disease. (p. 160)

B    The focus of primary prevention is to decrease an individual's chance of encountering disease. A prenatal clinic attempts to mitigate or prevent the complications of pregnancy. (p. 164)

5.  Which of the following statements about
    nursing models is _incorrect_?

    A.  They were developed to define nursing
        practice
    B.  Most models view health and illness
        holistically
    C.  They tend to emphasize disease rather
        than health
    D.  Most nursing models include or imply a
        definition of health

C   Nursing models place a greater emphasis on
    health than on disease. Nursing models are
    developed to define nursing practice, and
    have traditionally included a definition of
    health. In general, they are all based on a
    holistic theory. (p. 161)

6.  A number of factors have influenced changes
    in the health care delivery system. These
    include all of the following _except_:

    A.  Decrease in acute and infectious diseases
    B.  Better educated health care consumers
    C.  Decreased number of elderly people
        requiring extensive health care services
    D.  Increase in chronic and stress-induced
        illnesses

C   An increased life expectancy in developed
    countries has resulted in increased numbers
    of elderly people requiring extensive health
    care services. (p. 168)

7.  Which association is _incorrect_?

    A.  Private Insurance - Blue Cross/Blue Shield
    B.  Philanthrophy - Medicaid
    C.  HMO - Kaiser/Permanente
    D.  Personal payment - Consumer

B   Medicaid is a social insurance program
    funded by the government, not by charitable
    contributions. (p. 167)

8.  Health care designed to assist the disabled
    person with rehabilitation is called:

    A.  Primary Prevention
    B.  Tertiary Care
    C.  Health Restoration
    D.  Secondary Prevention

B   Rehabilitation is an integral part of
    tertiary care. Tertiary activities are
    designed to restore a disabled individual to
    the highest level of health possible. (164)

9.  Which statement about Medicare is _correct_?

    A.  Benefits are limited to people over the
        age of 65.
    B.  Originally designed to provide health
        services to the poor.
    C.  Consumer is restricted to providers and
        facilities that can be used.
    D.  Program is financed by Social Security
        taxes, general tax revenues, insurance
        premiums, and copayments made by
        beneficiaries.

D   Medicare provides benefits to people over
    the age of 65, some disabled people under
    65, and to people with end-stage renal
    disease. The consumer can still contact the
    practitioner of choice. Option D correctly
    describes the way in which the program is
    financed. (p. 167)

# EVOLVING LEGAL AND ETHICAL
# ASPECTS OF NURSING

**OBJECTIVES**

1.0 Describe sources of law.

    1.1 Briefly describe four major sources of the law: Statutes, administrative law, common law, and constitutional law. (p. 174)

**TEACHING/LEARNING STRATEGIES**

**Lecture/Discussion**

Review legal terminology listed on page 173 in the text.

Help students to understand major sources of the law: Statutes, administrative law, common law, and constitutional law.

Ask students to identify ways in which they feel statutes, administrative law, common law, and constitutional law affects the practice of nursing.

Describe the role of an expert nursing witness in the legal system.

**Guest Speaker**

Invite a legal representative to class who specializes in health care issues. Ask them to discuss the legal responsibilities of the various health care team members.

2.0 Identify at least two differences between a crime and a tort.

    2.1 Define the terms: Crime, tort, negligence, malpractice, and gross-negligence. (p. 174)

    2.2 Discuss the relationship of gross negligence to criminal liability. (p. 175)

    2.3 Discuss the nurse's legal and ethical responsibility for keeping all communication with an individual confidential. (p. 181)

**Lecture/Discussion**

Review examples of each of the following in class: Tort, crime, felony, malpractice, negligence, assault, battery, false imprisonment, invasion of privacy, and slander.

**Clinical Laboratory Experience**

Ask students to review the clinical record of a person in their care, identifying information they would consider to be confidential. Discuss findings in a clinical post-conference period.

3.0 Explain the use of the term "malpractice."

    3.1 Explore, using examples, areas of potential legal liability for the nurse: Crimes, torts, negligence, malpractice, and gross negligence. (p. 174)

**Lecture/Discussion**

Encourage students to explore ways in which the nurse can avoid litigation.

Ask students to compare and contrast the issues of gross negligence and malpractice.

**Written Exercise**

Ask students to prepare a brief report on legal accountability in nursing practice.

4.0 Identify reasons for carrying professional liability insurance: explain the concept of respondeat superior and to what extent, if at all, it protects the nurse against a malpractice suit.

4.1 Identify situations in which a nurse can incur liability for negligence. (p. 175)

4.2 Identify three common misconceptions related to the necessity of carrying professional liability insurance. Briefly discuss arguments used to discount each of these beliefs. (p. 176)

4.3 Describe the legal concept of respondeat superior. (p. 176)

4.4 Explain the importance of keeping accurate and complete nursing records. (p. 177)

4.5 Outline important guidelines for accurate record keeping. (p. 177)

4.6 Briefly explain components of the generic term, defamation: Libel and slander. (p. 178)

4.7 Briefly describe two defenses that may be used to an action for defamation. Truth and privilege. (p. 178)

4.8 Explore ways in which the nurse may violate the privacy of an individual. (p. 179)

4.9 Identify the nurse's role and responsibility in the administration of narcotics and other controlled substances. (p. 179)

4.10 Discuss the legal consequences of drug diversion by the nurse. (p. 179)

4.11 Identify four basic functions of the Nurse Practice Act. (p. 179)

4.12 Outline requirements for licensure as a registered nurse. (p. 180)

4.13 Identify two major offenses that may cause a nurse's license to be revoked or suspended by the board of nursing. (p. 180)

4.14 Compare and contrast the nursing student's legal responsibility for care rendered, to that of the licensed professional nurse. (p. 180)

4.15 Discuss the nurse's responsibility with regard to the witnessing of wills. (p. 180)

## Lecture/Discussion

Discuss the reasons why nursing students are held legally responsible for the care they render.

Impress upon students the importance of obtaining professional malpractice insurance. Review the concept of respondeat superior, helping students to understand how this might affect them in legal practice situations.

Emphasize the importance of adhering to the legal reporting requirements established for the state in which they reside.

Explore issues affecting legal accountability in nursing: Licensure and Nurse Practice Acts, self-regulation and professional associations, and the persons' rights and responsibilities.

## Group Activity

Assign a group of students to prepare an oral presentation on the various types of malpractice insurance that is available to the nurse.

## Values Clarification

Have students share their feelings on the ethical responsibilities related to various reporting requirements: Child abuse, communicable diseases, and gunshot wounds.

5.0 Explain what is meant by "Good Samaritan laws."

    5.1 Identify the purpose of the "Good Samaritan laws." (p. 176)

## Lecture/Discussion

Review the state Good Samaritan Law for your area.

Ask students to compare the legal protection offered a nurse who renders nursing care under the auspices of common law with those of the nurse rendering care under Good Samaritan laws.

## Values Clarification

Ask students to share what they would do if they encountered an emergency situation in which there were accident victims. Encourage them to explore the duties that they could perform as a beginning nursing student.

6.0 Define "assault" and "battery" and their implications for the nurse.

7.0 Define the responsibilities of a nurse asked to witness a will.

8.0 Explain what is meant by "passive euthanasia," and its legal implications.

    8.1 Describe the concepts of active and passive euthanasia. (p. 181)

    8.2 Cite examples of questions that may be used to evaluate the legal status of "passive euthanasia." (p. 182)

    8.3 Identify potential legal consequences of following a do not resuscitate or no-code order. (p. 182)

9.0 Identify the action that may be taken by a nurse who is asked to assist in an abortion and who does not wish to do so.

    9.1 Identify and briefly describe two sets of ethics that guide the actions of the nurse. (p. 182)

    9.2 Explore ways in which the nurse's personal ethical beliefs and values may conflict with legal obligations and duties. (p. 183)

    9.3 Briefly describe the three basic types of statutes designed to protect nurses from discrimination in employment based on their ethical obligations to assist with abortions. (p. 183)

    9.4 Explain the intent of the "Code for Nurses." (p. 183)

## Lecture/Discussion

Ask students to identify situations in which they feel "passive euthanasia" would be appropriate.

Discuss ways in which the nurse's personal values can conflict with their professional responsibilities.

1. A nurse discovers that she has administered the wrong dosage of a medication to Mr. Black. This act may be considered:

   A. A crime
   B. A tort
   C. Negligence
   D. None of the above

   C   The nurse's behavior is an act of negligence. This type of conduct may form the basis for a tort or a crime, if the actions cause damage to the individual. (p. 175)

2. If a nurse discovers that a physician has ordered five times the normal dosage of a medication for a person in their care, they should:

   A. Administer the medication as ordered
   B. Give the person a "normal" dosage of the medication
   C. Ask another nurse to give the medication
   D. Question the order and refuse to administer the drug

   D   If a physician orders a potentially harmful dosage of medication, it is the nurse's responsibility to question the order and refuse to administer the drug. A nurse cannot avoid responsibility for negligence in a situation simply because other members of the health care team have also been negligent. (p. 175)

3. According to law, if a nurse is employed by a health care facility and incurs liability for negligence while on the job, the facility is liable for the damages. This protection is provided by:

   A. Doctrine of Respondeat Superior
   B. Good Samaritan Law
   C. Malpractice Law
   D. Personal Liability Insurance.

   A   Under the legal doctrine of respondeat superior, an employer is liable for damages caused by the misconduct of an employee, within the scope of employment. The nurse can also be held personally liable for the action. (p. 176)

4. Accurate and complete nursing records should include all of the following except:

   A. Time, date, and signature on all entries
   B. Documentation in pencil only to allow easy correction of errors
   C. Documentation of all learning/teaching activities
   D. Routine documentation of nursing assessment and intervention

   B   Documentation should be made only in ink. When making corrections the nurse should draw one line through the error and add the corrected statement. The reason for the change should be noted and the entry dated and initialed. (p. 177)

5. Under the Good Samaritan law a nurse:

   A. Is legally obliged to provide aid to a person in distress
   B. Has complete immunity from damages that might occur as a result of voluntary emergency aid
   C. Can be held legally accountable for acts of gross negligence or more serious misconduct
   D. Can render emergency care only at motor vehicle accidents

   C   The Good Samaritan laws were established to provide immunity for damages as a result of voluntary emergency aid, with the exception of gross negligence and other more serious misconduct. The laws vary from one state to another. Some of the laws cover only roadside accidents or accidents outside the nurse's place of employment. No one can be made legally responsible to stop, but they can be made responsible to follow through with the emergency aid once they have begun to administer it. (p. 176)

6. A nurse administers an intramuscular injection against the will of a person who is oriented. The nurse's action constitutes:

   A. Assault
   B. Battery
   C. Invasion of privacy
   D. Negligence

   B   Battery is touching a person without their consent. Assault would occur prior to the act of battery, when the nurse approached the unconsenting individual with the hypodermic needle. (p. 177)

7. Mr. Winter wishes to leave the hospital, but is physically detained by a nurse because his physician has indicated that more hospitalization is needed. This nurse's behavior is an example of:

A. Defamation
B. False imprisonment
C. Invasion of privacy
D. Libel

**B**   False imprisonment is the unjustifiable restraint of an individual by force or threats of force. No one can be legally detained, but in many instances they may be asked to sign a statement saying that they are leaving the hospital "against medical advice." This releases the hospital from liability for damages that may occur as a result of the early departure. (p. 178)

8. During morning report, the night nurse tells oncoming staff that Mrs. Trail has been "stealing supplies again." The night nurse may be guilty of:

A. Libel
B. Slander
C. Perjury
D. Assault

**B**   A person may be charged with defamation of character if they make remarks (to another person) about another person that degrades or damages the reputation of the person who is the object of the remarks. If the remarks are made orally, they are slander. If they are stated in writing or on radio or television, they are called libel. (p. 178)

9. Nurses who take narcotics or other controlled substances from a hospital for personal use or sale may:

A. Lose their license to practice nursing
B. Be subject to criminal prosecution
C. Be required to attend a drug rehabilitation program
D. All of the above

**D**   Nurses who are guilty of drug diversion may lose their nursing license. The Board of Nursing may also choose to temporarily suspend the license if the nurse agrees to complete a drug treatment program and can prove that no further drug abuse has occurred. The nurse may also be subject to criminal prosecution. (p. 179)

10. In most states, the Nurse Practice Act allows the professional nurse to do all of the following except:

A. Supervise other health care personnel
B. Administer medications ordered by a physician or dentist
C. Make medical diagnoses and prescribe treatment
D. Perform treatment prescribed by the physician

**C**   Options A, B, and D include activities that are generally allowed by the Nurse Practice Act in most states. A nurse is never permitted to make a medical diagnosis or prescribe treatment, but is allowed to make a nursing diagnosis and carry out treatment prescribed by a physician or dentist. (p. 180)

11. In this country, a nurse's license is issued by:

A. American Nurses' Association
B. National League for Nursing
C. School of Graduation
D. State Boards of Nursing

**D**   In the United States, nurses are licensed by state boards of nursing. These boards determine which persons are legally qualified to practice as licensed nurses. (p. 180)

12. Nurses who witness a will have a responsibility to do all of the following except:

A. Be knowledgable of the contents of the will
B. Document the condition of the person at the time the will was signed
C. Observe the person making the will sign it
D. Sign their name in the designated place

**A**   When witnessing a will, the nurse has a responsibility to perform options B, C, and D. It is not necessary, however, for the witness (nurse) to read the will or be knowledgable of the contents. The witness is simply attesting that the person listed in the will signed it freely and was mentally competent at the time to do so. (p. 181)

13. When a person takes positive steps to terminate a person's life in order to end suffering, it is called:

A. Active euthanasia
B. Mercy killing
C. Murder
D. All of the above

**D**   Active euthanasia is also called "mercy killing." Legally it constitutes a first-degree murder in that it is a willful, deliberate, and premeditated murder. (p. 181)

# 12
# EMERGING RIGHTS OF HEALTH CARE CONSUMERS

## OBJECTIVES

1.0 Describe the rights of health care consumers, the rights of mentally retarded persons, and the rights of mentally ill persons.

   1.1 Briefly discuss the concept of consumer rights. (p. 187)

   1.2 Explore the impact of the consumer rights movement on the health care profession. (p. 187)

   1.3 Identify four general categories of health care consumer rights. (p. 187)

   1.4 List fifteen rights of the health care consumer as described by the National League for Nursing. (p. 188)

   1.5 Identify the specific purpose for the establishment of laws related to health care practices. (p. 188)

   1.6 Compare and contrast the rights of mentally ill or mentally retarded individuals with those of the normal, competent health care consumer. (p. 188)

   1.7 Identify sources of input that influence the development of legal standards of care. (p. 188)

2.0 Describe what is meant by a "reasonably prudent nurse."

   2.1 Explain the purpose of legal standards of care. (p. 188)

   2.2 Briefly describe the following concepts: Negligent; liable; and reasonably prudent nurse. (p. 189)

   2.3 Identify and briefly describe the two most common legal allegations made against nurses practicing in the health care setting. (p. 189)

3.0 State the five criteria of informed consent.

   3.1 Identify the role of the nurse in regard to the disclosure of information to the health care consumer. (p. 190)

   3.2 Summarize the nurse's responsibility with regard to the consumer's right to informed consent. (p. 191)

## TEACHING/LEARNING STRATEGIES

### Lecture/Discussion

Facilitate a discussion of the legal implications of standards of care.

Ask students to review the standards of care established by their clinical facility to guide the practice of nursing. Ask one student from each clinical facility to share information about these standards in class.

Review four general categories of consumer rights within the health care setting. The right for competent treatment; the right to information about their condition and treatment; the right to accept or refuse treatment; and the right to privacy.

Facilitate a discussion of nursing responsibilities with regard to the health care consumer's right to competent care.

Ask students to compare and contrast the rights of a mentally ill person with those of a well individual.

### Lecture/Discussion

Review the five criteria necessary for an informed consent.

Ask students to identify situations in which it would be necessary to obtain a written consent for care.

3.3 Outline five basic criteria of informed consent. (p. 191)

3.4 Give examples of individuals who might not be judged competent to give consent. (p. 191)

3.5 Articulate the nurse's responsibility with regard to obtaining consent for special procedures that will be performed by someone else. (p. 191)

3.6 Understand the health care consumer's right to withdraw consent. (p. 192)

3.7 Identify special situations in which an informed consent is not necessary. (p. 192)

Encourage discussion of nursing responsibilities in regard to the consumer's right to information.

Encourage students to review various consent forms used by their clinical facility.

4.0 Explain the right to privacy and the rule of confidentiality.

4.1 Explore the individual's right to privacy during the performance of special procedures. (p. 192)

4.2 Discuss the nurse's role in relation to the consumer's right to privacy. (p. 192)

4.3 Define the term, confidentiality. (p. 192)

4.4 Identify situations in which the health care professional has a legal duty to report confidential information about a person to state agencies. (p. 192)

### Lecture/Discussion

Review examples of ways in which the nurse could potentially violate a person's right to privacy.

### Written Exercise

Ask students to list the major advantages and disadvantages of consumer access to medical records. Facilitate discussion of this issue in class.

5.0 Define the role of the nurse advocate.

5.1 Briefly discuss the nurse's role as a consumer advocate. (p. 192)

### Lecture/Discussion

Have students discuss ways in which they can serve as a consumer advocate.

Ask students to share ways in which they would provide health care information to individuals in their care.

---

### MULTIPLE CHOICE QUESTIONS

1. All of the following statements about the American Hospital Association's "Patient's Bill of Rights" are true, except:

   A. It guarantees quality care to all individuals.
   B. It can be used as a standard against which to judge health care.
   C. It establishes the legal rights of health care consumers.
   D. It outlines the basic rights of health care consumers.

### CORRECT ANSWER AND RATIONALE

C    The "Patient's Bill of Rights," that was formulated by the American Hospital Association, outlined recommendations for the basic rights of health care consumers. The bill does not guarantee the kind of treatment a person will receive, but instead helps to set a standard against which to judge the acts of health care professionals. They are not law, however, so statement C is incorrect. (p. 187)

2.  Suzie, a new nursing graduate, fails to administer a medication to a person in her care because the physician's order was illegible. If this person suffers injury due to the medication omission, Suzie may be charged with:

    A. Liability
    B. Negligence
    C. Felony
    D. Misdemeanor

B   Negligence can result from an act or the failure to act. Options C and D are two specific types of crimes. An act is labeled a crime when it offends both the individual and society. (p. 189)

3.  In a court of law, Suzie's conduct would be judged according to the standard of care expected of:

    A. Nurses who work in the same setting
    B. Other new nursing graduates
    C. Any registered nurse
    D. All of the above

B   In the United States, a nurse is held to the standard of care as a reasonably prudent nurse. A nurse is, therefore, held to the same standard of care expected of other nurses with similar education and experience. (p. 189)

4.  If Suzie is charged with malpractice, who may be held responsible for the person's injuries?

    A. Suzie
    B. The hospital in which Suzie works
    C. The physician who wrote the illegible order
    D. All of the above

D   The physician, hospital, and nurse may be held liable for damages incurred by the individual. (p. 190)

5.  A nurse caring for a person is ultimately responsible to:

    A. Person
    B. Director of Nursing
    C. Hospital
    D. Physician

A   Ultimately, the nurse is responsible to the person for whom nursing care is being provided. (p. 189)

6.  Mr. Jones tells his nurse that he "can't decide which treatment to take for his newly diagnosed cancer." The nurse should:

    A. Tell Mr. Jones about the most successful treatments for his type of cancer
    B. Explain each recommended treatment to Mr. Jones
    C. Encourage Mr. Jones to take the lease invasive treatment
    D. Give Mr. Jones advice about the treatment he would select

B   The nurse should explain the prescribed health care measures, refraining from offering advice about which treatment the person should take. (p. 190)

7.  After administering a medication to sedate a person for surgery, the nurse realizes that the preoperative consent form has not been signed. The nurse's best response would be to:

    A. Notify the physician performing the surgery of the incident
    B. Immediately have the person sign the operative permit
    C. Ask the person's most immediate family member to sign the operative permit
    D. Send the person to surgery without the operative consent

A   The preoperative consent should be obtained before the person is sedated or given any medications that might affect mental ability. Upon failure to obtain a consent, the nurse should initially notify the physician performing the surgery, so that surgery can be rescheduled after the person has given written consent. (p. 191)

8. Which of the following individuals should the nurse consider the most legally competent to give consent for a surgical procedure?

   A. Mr. Clark, who has just been given a sedative medication
   B. John, a 16-year old male person
   C. Mrs. Johns, who has been hospitalized for a psychiatric disorder
   D. Stacey, a 23-year old mentally alert female

D  The 23-year old alert female would be most competent to give consent for a procedure for surgery. Consent should be obtained from individuals who are judged to be mentally competent to make a voluntary decision. It should never be obtained from an incompetent person. Most states rule that a person is incompetent to give consent until they have reached adulthood. (p. 191)

9. Sue Smith has agreed to undergo an intensive physical examination at a local hospital. The nurse caring for Mrs. Smith understands that this consent implies that:

   A. Nursing students assigned to Mrs. Smith may automatically observe the examination procedures
   B. Photographs may be taken during Mrs. Smith's examination for research purposes
   C. Information revealed during the examination can be shared with any other health personnel working in the hospital
   D. None of the above

D  All options listed could be considered an invasion of Mrs. Smith's right to privacy if carried out. (p. 192)

10. A nurse who serves as an intermediary between a health care consumer and the health care agency and its staff is functioning as a:

   A. Consumer advocate
   B. Health care counselor
   C. Resource advisor
   D. Consumer advisor

A  Many health care agencies now employ a person to serve as a consumer advocate. This person serves as an intermediary between the consumer and the health care agency. (p. 192)

# NURSING ASSESSMENT: GATHERING DATA AND MAKING NURSING DIAGNOSES

# NURSING MANAGEMENT: PLANNING, IMPLEMENTING, EVALUATING, AND MODIFYING NURSING CARE

# 15

# NURSING AND THE LEARNING/TEACHING PROCESS

## OBJECTIVES

1.0 Conduct a purposeful assessment interview.

1.1 State the major purpose of the nursing assessment interview. (p. 210)

1.2 Briefly list four reasons the nurse gathers data when planning nursing care. (p. 206)

1.3 Explore various factors that may have an influence on an individual's ability to give reliable data. (p. 207)

1.4 Explore the impact that human bias can have on data gathering. (p. 208)

1.5 Discuss reasons for the formulation of structured data base. (p. 208)

1.6 Discuss the importance of a review of the literature during assessment and throughout the nursing process. (p. 216)

2.0 Write a complete nursing history.

2.1 List Becknell and Smith's rules for complete, clear, objective, and accurate recording of the nursing history. (p. 212)

2.2 Identify and briefly discuss various nursing history formats. (p. 212)

2.3 Identify and briefly describe 11 components of a typical data base. (p. 206)

2.4 Explore eight attributes of the nursing history. (p. 212)

## TEACHING/LEARNING STRATEGIES

### Lecture/Discussion

Explore the specific assessment strategies that may be used by the nurse to gather each component of a typical data base: Demographic information, present symptoms and concerns, individual profile, social-cultural history, family medical history, interpersonal-communication patterns, activities of daily living, mental-emotional status, review of body systems, physical examination, and the review of laboratory-diagnostic tests.

Discuss ways in which an initial assessment interview may influence establishment of the nurse-individual relationship.

### Communication Activity

Ask students to role play a nurse conducting an assessment interview. Encourage students to critique each other as they take turns with the individual and nurse roles.

### Clinical Laboratory Experience

Have students accompany a nurse as she conducts an admission assessment interview.

### Lecture/Discussion

Analyze various assessment frameworks, such as those developed by Abdellah, Gordon, Henderson, and McCain.

Compare and contrast the nursing history to the medical history.

### Clinical Laboratory Experience

Instruct students to familiarize themselves with the nursing history form used by their clinical facility.

2.5 Compare components included in a medical history to those obtained in a nursing history. (p. 210)

2.6 Briefly describe assessment structures developed by: Abdellah, Gordon, Henderson, and McCain. (p. 208)

2.7 Explain the value of using secondary sources of information in the data base. (p. 208)

2.8 Describe the nurse's responsibility with regard to confidentiality and the data gathering process. (p. 208)

2.9 Explore the impact that the computer has had on the nursing history. (p. 212)

### Written Exercise

Ask students to outline essential information that should be obtained by the nurse when gathering a complete nursing history.

3.0 Assess the person's physical, mental, and psychosocial status (at a basic level).

3.1 List six methods of data collection. (p. 209)

3.2 Identify and briefly discuss the two steps of the assessment process. (p. 206)

3.3 Describe two approaches the nurse can utilize to ensure a systematic physical examination: Body system's approach and cephalocaudal approach. (p. 215)

3.4 Outline data to be included when conducting a nursing assessment of a person's psychosocial status. (p. 215)

3.5 Identify alterations in a typical adult data base that are required for pediatric assessment. (p. 206)

### Lecture/Discussion

Using hypothetical examples, review both a body system's approach and a cephalocaudal approach to systematic physical examination.

### Written Exercise

Ask students to identify data to be gathered during each phase of the physical examination process.

### Campus Laboratory Experience

Instruct students to conduct a physical examination on a classmate. Discuss findings in class.

4.0 Obtain subjective and objective data from primary and secondary sources of information.

4.1 Define subjective and objective data, and give an example of each. (p. 206)

4.2 Identify two major sources of data. (p. 207)

4.3 Give examples of primary and secondary sources of data. (p. 207)

4.4 Identify consultation sources available to the nurse during the assessment process. (p. 216)

### Lecture/Discussion

Discuss the process of consultation. Emphasize consultation as an important way to test the validity of an assessment and as a tool to increase the nurse's knowledge base.

### Clinical Laboratory Experience

Instruct students to review a completed admission assessment form for a person in their clinical facility. Require students to make separate lists of the subjective and objective data gathered. Include a review of appropriate sources of validation and proper methods of assessment for each piece of data listed.

5.0 Distinguish between a medical and a nursing diagnosis.

5.1 Explore the meaning of the concept nursing diagnosis. (p. 217)

5.2 Outline major differences between nursing and medical diagnoses. (p. 217)

### Lecture/Discussion

Compare and contrast the nursing diagnosis and medical diagnosis.

Review the admission assessment data for a hypothetical individual. Identify appropriate medical and nursing diagnoses.

6.0 Describe and explain the two components of a nursing diagnosis.

    6.1 Identify the relationship of the following terms: Problem, need, diagnosis, and data. (p. 219)

    6.2 Name and identify the three steps for identifying nursing diagnoses as formulated by Gordon. (p. 219)

    6.3 Describe Gordon's steps for identification of nursing diagnoses. (p. 219)

7.0 Write a nursing diagnosis.

    7.1 Identify tips for writing descriptive nursing diagnoses. (p. 221)

    7.2 Utilize approved nursing diagnostic statements when identifying a person's problems. (p. 218)

    7.3 Utilize appropriate abbreviations and symbols when writing nursing diagnostic statements. (p. 221)

    7.4 Identify criteria that can be used to evaluate the nursing diagnostic statement. (p. 221)

    7.5 Identify the relationship of accurate nursing diagnoses to the planning phase of the nursing process. (p. 224)

8.0 Differentiate between a nursing goal and a nursing objective.

    8.1 Define nursing objective and nursing goal. (p. 224)

    8.2 Explore reasons for the development of nursing goals and objectives. (p. 224)

    8.3 Briefly discuss the relationship of nursing goals to nursing objectives. (p. 224)

    8.4 State the general focus of nursing goals and objectives. (p. 231)

9.0 Designate priorities, develop goals and objectives for persons in your care, and set deadlines for the accomplishment of goals.

    9.1 Discuss the importance of setting priorities of care when planning nursing care. (p. 224)

    9.2 Identify factors that may influence the nurse when prioritizing person health care problems. (p. 224)

    9.3 Briefly describe the method used for the ranking of person health care problems and give examples of each. (p. 224)

## Lecture/Discussion

Briefly describe the two components of a well-developed nursing diagnostic statement: Statement of the problem and statement indicating the etiology of the problem.

Ask students to review the working list of approved nursing diagnoses on page 218 in the text.

## Clinical Laboratory Experience

Require students to gather a complete nursing history on a person in their clinical facility. From this history, identify the person's needs and formulate appropriate nursing diagnostic statements.

## Lecture/Discussion

Emphasize similarities and differences of nursing goals and objectives.

## Lecture/Discussion

Discuss essential facts related to the planning phase of the nursing process: Setting priorities, developing goals and objectives, setting deadlines, and formulating a plan of action.

## Campus Laboratory Experience

Provide students with a list of assorted person health care needs/problems. Ask them to rank the problems according to high, medium, and low levels of priority care.

9.4 Outline guidelines to be considered when formulating nursing objectives. (p. 231)

9.5 Differentiate between intermediate and long term nursing goals of care. (p. 231)

9.6 Explain the importance of setting deadlines for the accomplishment of nursing goals and objectives. (p. 225)

9.7 Explain the significance of unmet nursing objective deadlines. (p. 226)

10.0 Design a clear, precise, and realistic nursing plan of care based on principles of good management.

10.1 Identify common problem-solving methods and give an example of each. (p. 201)

10.2 Describe the seven major steps of the scientific method to problem solving. (p. 202)

10.3 Briefly discuss five reasons health care professionals must use a modified scientific approach for problem solving. (p. 202)

10.4 Compare and contrast the medical process approach to the nursing process approach for each step of the scientific problem solving process. (p. 203)

10.5 Describe the concept of a system within the context of problem solving. (p. 204)

10.6 Define and give the purposes for the following: Conceptual model of nursing and theory of nursing. (p. 205)

10.7 Identify models of nursing that have been used successfully by schools and hospitals to direct nursing care. (p. 205)

10.8 Outline four barriers to efficient problem solving that the nurse must overcome to deal effectively with nursing care and management. (p. 205)

10.9 State the definition of the nursing process. (p. 205)

10.10 Summarize five major purposes of the nursing process. (p. 209)

10.11 Briefly discuss attributes of the nursing process. (p. 209)

10.12 Identify the main steps of each phase of the nursing process. (p. 209)

10.13 Explore the relationship of a nursing process model to a philosophy of nursing. (p. 235)

## Clinical Laboratory Experience

Ask students to share examples of nursing diagnoses they have formulated for persons assigned to their care. Assist them in development of logical individual goals and objectives.

## Lecture/Discussion

Explore the relationship of basic management principles to the nursing planning and implementation processes.

Display a list of potential individual health care problems. Ask students to assist in development of appropriate nursing actions to solve the problems.

Discuss the impact of the written and oral plan of care on the coordination of person care.

## Clinical Laboratory Experience

Instruct students to develop a comprehensive written nursing care plan for a person in the clinical area.

10.14 State two attributes of a comprehensive nursing care plan. (p. 230)

10.15 Define nursing intervention. (p. 230)

10.16 List three steps the nurse-manager should utilize to assure effective problem resolution. (p. 227)

10.17 State four purposes of the planning phase of the nursing process. (p. 228)

10.18 List two steps for developing a nursing plan of action. (p. 230)

10.19 Discuss specific ways the nurse can develop alternatives for solving individual problems. (p. 231)

10.20 Identify five basic questions to be explored by the nurse when planning alternate problem solving methods. (p. 231)

10.21 Define nursing care plan. (p. 231)

10.22 Enumerate the disadvantages of an oral nursing plan of care. (p. 231)

10.23 Describe the advantages of using a written nursing plan of care. (p. 232)

10.24 Describe the responsibility of various nursing personnel in the development of the nursing care plan. (p. 232)

10.25 Identify and briefly describe three common nursing care plan formats. (p. 232)

10.26 Explore the concept of nursing implementation. (p. 238)

10.27 Identify major nursing responsibilities in the implementation phase of the nursing process. (p. 238)

10.28 Identify and give examples of specific methods for implementation of nursing intervention. (p. 239)

11.0 Differentiate between dependent, independent, and interdependent nursing actions.

   11.1 List three major classifications of nursing interventions. (p. 230)

   11.2 Give examples of dependent, independent, and interdependent nursing actions. (p. 230)

   11.3 List five components of a well-written nursing order. Summarize other requirements of a well-conceived nursing order (p. 238)

### Clinical Laboratory Experience

Instruct students to indicate on a written nursing care plan, whether designated nursing actions are dependent, independent, or interdependent in nature.

12.0 Evaluate the nursing care plan and modify as necessary.

    12.1 Define and state the purposes of the evaluation phase of the nursing process. (p. 243)

    12.2 Outline the five steps of the evaluation process. (p. 244)

    12.3 Identify eight essential guidelines for the evaluation process as established by Bailey and Claus. (p. 244)

    12.4 Explore implications of evaluation on both the individual and institutional levels. (p. 243)

    12.5 List criteria to be used by the nurse in evaluation of a person's discharge status. (p. 237)

    12.6 Outline guidelines for writing effective nursing discharge plans. (p. 238)

    12.7 Identify ways the nurse can assess achievement of discharge criteria. (p. 238)

13.0 Explain the precautions to take when writing on a legal document.

    13.1 Understand general principles guiding the legal requirements for medical documentation. (p. 247)

    13.2 Explain the significance of proper communication and documentation of person responses to care. (p. 240)

14.0 Maintain a concise, complete, and organized permanent record.

    14.1 Summarize the attributes of using abbreviations in the documentation of care. (p. 241)

    14.2 Utilize accepted abbreviations and symbols when documenting individual health care data. (p. 243)

    14.3 Summarize the benefits of using the problem-oriented medical record over traditional approaches to planning nursing care. (p. 240)

    14.4 Briefly describe the Problem-Oriented Medical Record. (p. 240)

    14.5 Identify and briefly explore the four major components of the Problem-Oriented Medical Record. (p. 240)

**Lecture/Discussion**

Provide students with a list of general person goals. Ask them to assist in the formulation of appropriate outcome criteria.

**Panel Presentation**

Invite a physician, a registered nurse, a dietician, and a social worker to class to provide a panel discussion of the various roles they play in the discharge process.

**Lecture/Discussion**

Discuss the legal guidelines for communication and documentation of care.

**Guest Lecturer**

Invite a nurse who has served as an expert legal witness to class to discuss their experiences related to the legal requirements of medical documentation.

**Lecture/Discussion**

Compare and contrast the traditional medical record with the problem-oriented medical record.

15.0 Define the nursing audit and explain its purpose.

    15.1 Describe the concept of the nursing audit. (p. 246)

    15.2 Identify five major goals of the nursing audit. (p. 246)

    15.3 Define the concept of accountability. (p. 246)

    15.4 Briefly describe the ANA's eight standards of nursing practice. (p. 245)

**Lecture/Discussion**

Review ANA's 8 standards of nursing practice.

**Clinical Laboratory Experience**

Encourage students to assess the functions of a hospital quality assurance program. Invite a representative from this department to speak in a clinical post-conference period to discuss the role they play in the health care delivery system.

16.0 Describe the three major domains of learning and give examples of each.

    16.1 Name and identify the three domains of learning and give an example of how each might be included in the learning/ teaching process. (p. 248)

    16.2 Identify and give examples of six distinct levels of learning within the cognitive domain of learning. (p. 249)

    16.3 Identify and give examples of four distinct levels of learning possible within the affective domain of learning. (p. 249)

    16.4 Explore challenges of the nurse in educating people within the affective domain. (p. 249)

    16.5 Identify and give examples of five distinct levels of learning available within the psychomotor domain of learning. (p. 250)

    16.6 Briefly outline general assumptions of adult learning theory. (p. 251)

    16.7 State four measures that the nurse can utilize to facilitate adult learning. (p. 251)

    16.8 Integrate all three domains of learning into a learning/teaching plan for a hypothetical person. (p. 248)

**Lecture/Discussion**

Emphasize to students the importance of incorporating/integrating the cognitive, affective, and psychomotor domains of learning into each teaching plan.

17.0 Identify the principles of learning.

    17.1 Identify 11 factors that facilitate learning in the adult, and give an example of each. (p. 251)

    17.2 Identify five major factors that hinder learning in the adult, and give an example of each. (p. 253)

**Lecture/Discussion**

Explore internal and external variables that influence/hinder the hospitalized individual's ability to learn.

18.0 Write and implement a learning/teaching plan based on thorough assessment of a person's learning needs and capabilities.

    18.1 List eight teaching strategies that may be used in individual health care education. (p. 256)

    18.2 State three characteristics of a well-written learning objective. (p. 256)

    18.3 Explain the intent of establishing learning goals and objectives. (p. 256)

    18.4 Explore the significance of using the proper teaching method for individual education. (p. 253)

    18.5 Plan and implement learning/teaching sessions at appropriate times during individual care. (p. 253)

    18.6 Give examples of inappropriate times for learning/teaching sessions. (p. 253)

    18.7 Identify five critical areas of assessment for the individual learner, as established by Cohen. (p. 254)

    18.8 Outline five steps in a systematic approach to applying nursing process to a learning/teaching situation. (p. 255)

    18.9 Discuss the significance of learning styles to learning/teaching theory. (p. 255)

    18.10 Explain the importance of mutual negotiation and planning in the learning/teaching process. (p. 255)

19.0 Evaluate the teaching plan and modify as necessary.

20.0 Describe strategies for evaluating both short-term and long-term learning.

    20.1 Explore the role of the nurse in evaluation of the teaching process. (p. 257)

    20.2 Describe ways in which evaluation relates to the desired type of learning outcome. (p. 258)

    20.3 Outline ways in which learning can be evaluated. (p. 258)

    20.4 Identify specific criteria used to evaluate the effectiveness of both short- and long-term learning/teaching processes. (p. 257)

## Group Activity

Divide the class into small groups of our or five students. Ask each group to prepare a learning/teaching plan to meet the educational needs of a hypothetical individual receiving nursing care.

## Clinical Laboratory Experience

Instruct students to develop a written teaching/learning plan for a hospitalized individual for whom they are providing care.

## Clinical Laboratory Experience

Require students to develop long- and short-term criteria to evaluate the effectiveness of each planned teaching session.

## Lecture/Discussion

Discuss ways in which long- and short-term outcomes of learning may be evaluated.

Review a teaching/learning plan for a hypothetical person. Discuss the specific criteria used to evaluate the effectiveness of the plan.

1. Problem solving is an essential component of the nursing process. The nurse can best assist people to meet their needs through the effective use of which of the following methods of problem solving?

   A. Intuitive problem solving
   B. Scientific method of problem solving
   C. Modified method of problem solving
   D. Trial and error problem solving

C  Nurses must use a modified scientific method of problem solving when working with people. The health care professional's work requires a problem solving approach that is systematic and scientific and, at the same time, flexible enough to deal with emergencies, unforeseen events, diverse personalities and life styles, and other problems. (p. 206)

2. Which of the following statements about nursing process are true?

   A. Use of the nursing process can improve the quality of individual care.
   B. The nursing process encourages individual participation in care.
   C. The nursing process helps provide continuity of individual care.
   D. All of the above.

D  All of the responses are true statements related to nursing process. (p. 209)

3. The assessment phase of the nursing process focuses on:

   A. Psychosocial needs of the individual
   B. Physiological needs of the individual
   C. Cultural needs of the individual
   D. Holistic needs of the individual

D  In the assessment phase of the nursing process, the nurse attempts to gather information about the individual's physical health, mental outlook, social circumstances, interpersonal relationships, and community life, as well as other factors. (p. 210)

4. The first step in the assessment phase is:

   A. Indentification of an existing problem
   B. Formulation of nursing diagnostic statements
   C. Collection of pertinent individual data
   D. Statement of a hypothesis

C  Assessment involves two steps. The first is data gathering and the second is problem identification or diagnosis. (p. 210)

5. Which of the following statements regarding the nursing diagnostic statement are true?

   A. Nursing diagnoses are always dependent on medical diagnoses.
   B. Nursing diagnoses indicate only the actual problems of the individual.
   C. Nursing diagnoses are alterations of medical diagnoses.
   D. Nursing diagnoses are summary statements based upon data gathered during the assessment process.

D  Response D is Sister Callista Roy's definition of the nursing process. Other responses are incorrect because: Nursing diagnoses include both actual and potential individual problems; nursing diagnoses are distinctly different from medical diagnoses, in that they focus on the individual's response to disease, not merely the disease process and its underlying pathologic processes; and nursing actions are both dependent and independent of the medical diagnosis. (p. 221)

6. In which stage of the nursing process does the nurse set priorities of care?

   A. Assessment
   B. Planning
   C. Intervention
   D. Evaluation

B  The first step in planning nursing care is to decide which problems require immediate attention and which ones are less threatening. (p. 228)

7. The written nursing care plan should be completed prior to which phase of the nursing process?

   A. Analysis
   B. Planning
   C. Implementation
   D. Evaluation

C  The implementation phase of the nursing process can begin once the written nursing care plan is completed. (p. 238)

8. Implementation of nursing intervention may
   include:

   A. Delegation of responsibilities to other
      health team members.
   B. Teaching the person and his significant
      others.
   C. Referring persons to other health care
      professionals.
   D. All of the above.

D  All of the responses are examples of specific
   methods of implementation of nursing
   interventions.  (p. 239)

9. Which step of the nursing process compares
   the person's behavioral outcomes to standard
   or expected outcomes?

   A. Assessment
   B. Nursing diagnosis
   C. Planning
   D. Evaluation

D  The evaluation process includes assessment of
   the individual's condition, and compares
   actual outcomes with standard or expected
   outcomes.  (p. 244)

10. Goals of care and expected outcomes of care
    are formulated in which phase of the nursing
    process?

    A. Assessment
    B. Planning
    C. Implementation
    D. Evaluation

B  Goals and objectives are developed in the
   planning phase of the nursing process.
   (p. 228)

11. The nursing plan of care is put into action
    in which phase of the nursing process?

    A. Intervention
    B. Implementation
    C. Planning
    D. Evaluation

B  Nursing interventions are put into action in
   the implementation phase of the nursing
   process.  (p. 238)

12. Priorities of care are established to:

    A. Ensure the provision of a high level of
       nursing care.
    B. Determine the order in which problems
       will be approached.
    C. Assure that higher level needs such as,
       self-actualization, are met first.
    D. Eliminate problems that are less
       life-threatening from the planning
       process.

B  The nurse determines priorities of care in
   order to determine which problems require
   immediate attention, and which ones are less
   life-threatening.  (p. 228)

13. When the nurse collects data related to the
    accomplishment of identified goals and
    objectives, the nurse is engaged in which
    phase of the nursing process?

    A. Assessment
    B. Data gathering
    C. Planning
    D. Evaluation

D  The evaluation phase of the nursing process
   enables the nurse to determine the progress of
   the person in relation to accomplishing
   identified goals and objectives.  (p. 243)

14. Which of the following best describes the
    purpose of documentation of nursing care?

    A. Provides the individual, health care
       system, and nurse with legal protection.
    B. Systematically describes the nursing
       process and an individual's response to
       care.
    C. Provides a record of an individual's
       health care status from shift to shift.
    D. Communicates and documents nursing care
       and person responses to that care.

D  Documentation of care is used to communicate
   and document the nursing care given, and the
   person's responses to that care.  (p. 240)

15. The ANA Standards of Practice were developed to:

   A. Provide outcome criteria for the evaluation of nursing practice.
   B. Provide a framework for standardized nursing care.
   C. Promote the development of a theory for nursing.
   D. Define the scope of nursing practice.

A   The ANA developed a set of broad standards to evaluate the extent to which the nursing process is being used in planning individualized nursing care. (p. 244)

SITUATION: Mr. James, a 55-year old banking executive has been admitted to the hospital for re-evaluation of his diabetes mellitus. Chief complaints upon admission include a 10 pound weight loss and loss of appetite. Questions 16 through 23 relate to this situation.

16. All of the following are primary sources of data the nurse can utilize to gather information about Mr. James except:

   A. The interview process
   B. The physical examination
   C. Mr. James's significant others
   D. Direct observations of Mr. James's behaviors

C   The person's significant others, such as family, friends, and the individual's business associates are examples of secondary sources of data. Responses A, B, D are primary sources of data. (pp. 211-213)

17. An important component of the nursing assessment is the medical history. An example of the medical history data you would gather is:

   A. Mr. James's previous hospitalizations, surgeries, and illnesses.
   B. Causes of death in Mr. James's close family members.
   C. Mr. James's present symptoms and concerns.
   D. Review of current laboratory tests performed on Mr. James.

A   The medical history includes: Discussion of previous hospitalization, surgeries, and illnesses; medications taken; chronic health problems; and allergies. (p. 210)

18. Results of diagnostic tests ordered for Mr. James are reviewed. This represents which stage of the nursing process?

   A. Assessment
   B. Planning
   C. Implementation
   D. Evaluation

A   A review of laboratory and diagnostic tests are components of a typical data base gathered by the nurse during the assessment phase of the nursing process. (p. 210)

19. Mr. James tells the nurse that he has recently experienced a loss of appetite. This represents which kind of data?

   A. Nutritional
   B. Secondary
   C. Subjective
   D. Objective

C   Subjective data are basically what individuals tell you they are experiencing: feeling, seeing, hearing, or thinking. (p. 210)

20. The nurse formulates several nursing diagnoses for Mr. James. Choose the problem that would assume the highest priority when planning his care.

   A. Activity tolerance.
   B. Nutrition, alteration in: less than body requirements.
   C. Communication, impaired: hearing.
   D. Home maintenance management, impaired.

B   According to Maslow's Hierarchy of needs, the lower physiological needs must be met to some degree before the higher level needs can be met. (p. 228)

21. When performing the physical examination, the nurse takes Mr. James's apical pulse. The data obtained represents which kind of data?

    A. Circulatory
    B. Objective
    C. Secondary
    D. Subjective

B   Data obtained through physical examination is objective in nature. It is derived from primary sources of information. (p. 211)

22. The nurse administers insulin to Mr. James each morning as ordered by the physician. This is an example of which type of nursing action?

    A. Dependent
    B. Independent
    C. Interdependent
    D. Intradependent

A   Dependent nursing actions are those functions that nurses perform in implementing the medical regime. (p. 230)

23. Which of the following information about Mr. James is considered to be subjective?

    A. Temperature of 99 degrees F
    B. Loss of appetite prior to admission
    C. Skin warm and dry to touch
    D. Apical pulse of 78

B   Responses A, C, and D are all examples of data gathered from a physical examination of Mr. James. Information related to Mr. James's loss of appetite would be obtained during the nursing interview process, therefore, making it subjective in nature. (p. 211)

24. The teaching/learning process allows the nurse to:

    A. Assist individuals to learn what they need to know in order to maintain or regain health
    B. Help individuals change unhealthy patterns of behavior
    C. Assist individuals to acquire new skills needed for effective self-care
    D. All of the above

D   All of the responses are purposes of the teaching/learning process. (p. 248)

25. Which of the following is an example of a level of learning within the affective domain?

    A. Characterization
    B. Comprehension
    C. Articulation
    D. Naturalization

A   Characterization is the highest level of affective learning. Option B is an example of cognitive learning. Options C and D are levels of learning within the psychomotor domain. (p. 249)

26. Prior to planning a teaching/learning program for the adult person, the nurse must understand that:

    A. The adult learner approaches new learning experiences with previous learning experiences.
    B. Mature individuals are often self-directed in meeting their learning needs.
    C. Adult learning is based on solving real-life problems.
    D. All of the above.

D   All responses are basic assumptions characterizing adult learning, as formulated by Malcolm Knowles, a leading authority on adult learning theory. (p. 251)

27. You have been assigned to provide health teaching to a person who speaks a different language from yours. This represents which type of barrier to learning?

    A. Cultural
    B. Emotional
    C. Environmental
    D. Psychological

A   Cultural barriers to learning/teaching occur when people speak a different language from the nurse. (p. 253)

28. Learning goals are developed to:

   A. Describe the intended results of learning
   B. Describe evaluation outcome criteria
   C. Describe competencies of learning
   D. Assist in the achievement of desired learning outcomes

D   The nurse formulates learning goals to help the person achieve the desired outcomes in the learning situation. Options A, B, and C are purposes of the learning objective. (p. 256)

# 16

# FROM CONCEPTION THROUGH CHILDHOOD YEARS

## OBJECTIVES

1.0 Describe the significance of genetic and environmental influences on human growth and development.

1.1 Briefly explore the influence of heredity and environment on the growth and development of an individual. (p. 261)

1.2 Identify human qualities that are genetically inherited. (p. 263)

1.3 Discuss the impact of altered nervous system functioning on the process of growth and development. (p. 263)

1.4 Describe the effect major endocrine glands have on the process of physiological growth and development: Pituitary, parathyroid, adrenals, pancreas, and gonads. (p. 263)

1.5 Discuss the impact of heredity and environment on the maturation process. (p. 263)

2.0 List and explain some basic principles common to all human growth and development patterns.

2.1 Identify and briefly describe common categories that are used to describe the growth and development process. (p. 261)

2.2 Outline and briefly discuss fundamental principles underlying the process of growth and development. (p. 261)

3.0 Discuss the relevance of homeostasis, motivation, learning, socialization, and the self to human growth and development.

3.1 Discuss major factors that influence the development of human function: Homeostasis, motivation, learning, socialization, and the self. (p. 262)

3.2 Summarize Freud's theory of human psychosexual development according to five major stages: Oral, anal, phallic, latency, and genital. (p. 263)

3.3 Differentiate between the three components of human personality as described by Freud: Id, ego, and superego. (p. 263)

## TEACHING/LEARNING STRATEGIES

### Lecture/Discussion

Emphasize the importance of genetic counseling.

### Guest Speaker

Invite a genetic specialist or counselor to class to discuss their role in the parenting process.

### Values Clarification

Have students individually list genetic and environmental factors they feel influence the process of human growth and development. Ask them to share their responses in class.

### Lecture/Discussion

Review basic principles common to all levels of human growth and development.

### Lecture/Discussion

Explore major factors that influence the development of human function: Homeostasis, motivation, learning, socialization, and the self.

4.0 Describe some major theories of psychosocial human development.

4.1 Summarize Erikson's theory of psychosocial development by stages: Infancy, early childhood, late childhood, school age, adolescence, young adulthood, adulthood, and old age. (p. 264)

4.2 Briefly discuss Piaget's theory of cognitive and intellectual development. (p. 264)

4.3 Identify human characteristics that are displayed at each stage of Piaget's theory of cognitive and intellectual development: Sensorimotor, preoperational, concrete operational thought, and formal operational thought. (p. 264)

4.4 Summarize Kohlberg's theory of moral development according to levels: Preconventional, conventional, and postconventional. (p. 269)

4.5 Briefly summarize Havinghurst's theory of developmental tasks according to levels: Infancy and early childhood, Middle childhood, adolescence, early adulthood, middle age and later maturity. (p. 268)

4.6 Identify major concepts in other theories of psychosocial development: Adler, Bijou and Baer, Dreihers, Cumming and Henry, Gesell, Heider, Lewin, Neugarten, and Sears. (p. 269)

4.7 Identify six major commonalities shared by all theories of psychosocial development. (p. 269)

5.0 Identify implications for nursing practice from the theoretical approach to human growth and development.

5.1 Briefly discuss, using examples, ways in which a nurse can use Piaget's theory of cognitive and intellectual development to facilitate and enhance interactions with children. (p. 264)

6.0 Discuss general patterns of physical growth and development through the neonatal infancy, early childhood, play-age, and school-age life stages.

6.1 State the length of the prenatal period. (p. 270)

6.2 Define the following concepts: Conception, fertilization, embryo, fetus, and neonate. (p. 270)

## Lecture/Discussion

Facilitate a discussion of the similarities and differences that exist between the major psychosocial theories of development.

## Written Exercise

Ask students to outline basic principles of growth and development for individuals from conception through the childhood years.

## Written Exercise

Ask students to identify the major developmental tasks for a person in their care. Encourage them to outline a plan for assisting the individual with any identified developmental needs.

## Lecture/Discussion

Have students interview the parent of a small child within the community regarding the child's physiological and psychological growth and development. Ask them to compare the parent's conception of normal growth and development with those identified by Erikson. Share findings in class.

6.3 Discuss the role of the umbilical cord, placenta, fetal membranes, and amniotic fluid in the development of a human being. (p. 270)

6.4 Briefly discuss physiological development that occurs during the embryonic period. (p. 270)

6.5 Define the term teratogen. (p. 270)

6.6 Identify teratogens that can adversely affect embryo and fetal development. (p. 270)

6.7 Describe the major physiological characteristics of a neonate at birth. (p. 272)

6.8 Briefly describe normal reflexes demonstrated during the neonatal period: Sucking; rooting; swallowing; gag, cough, and sneeze; moro; tonic neck; stepping; placing; grasp reflexes; and babinski. (p. 272)

6.9 Briefly discuss two common conditions of a newborn's skull; Caput succedaneum and cephalhematoma. (p. 272)

6.10 Identify neonatal reflexes that normally disappear, and discuss the significance of reflexes that do not disappear within the expected time. (p. 273)

6.11 Summarize the growth and development of the neonate in the physical domain. (p. 272)

6.12 Summarize the normal physical development of a person during the period of infancy. (pp. 276-277)

6.13 Summarize the normal physical development of a preschool child. (p. 280)

6.14 Summarize the normal physical development of a person in the early childhood years. (p. 280)

7.0 Discuss general patterns of psychosocial development through the neonatal, infancy, early childhood, play-age, and school-age life stages.

7.1 Describe three major psychosocial tasks of development during the neonatal period: Bonding, building trust, and communication. (p. 273)

7.2 Summarize the normal development of the neonate within the psychosocial domain. (p. 272)

7.3 Describe the four major psychosocial tasks of development during infancy: Building trust, communication, cognitive development, and emotional development. (p. 275)

## Clinical Laboratory Experience

As a part of a clinical experience, arrange for students to conduct a basic psychosocial assessment on a child in a local day-care center.

7.4 Summarize the growth and development of the infant in the psychosocial domain. (p. 275)

7.5 Identify key criteria used to evaluate the development of trust in an infant. (p. 279)

7.6 Briefly discuss the psychosocial tasks of development during the period of early childhood: Developing autonomy, developing toilet independence, and developing other social controls. (p. 280)

7.7 Summarize the growth and development of a preschool child in the psychosocial domain. (p. 282)

7.8 Summarize the psychosocial development that occurs during early childhood. (p. 280)

7.9 State outcome criteria that can be used to evaluate the development of autonomy in early childhood. (p. 280)

7.10 Discuss the major psychosocial tasks of development for the play-age child: Developing initiative, communication, play, and moral development. (p. 282)

7.11 Briefly describe the major psychosocial developmental tasks of a school-age child: Cognitive development, developing industry, relationships, communication, and moral development. (p. 285)

7.12 Identify criteria that can be used to evaluate the achievement of a sense of initiative in the play-age child. (p. 284)

8.0 Identify and apply implications for nursing practice from physical and psychosocial growth and development patterns.

8.1 Identify two alternative methods of human sexual fertilization. (p. 270)

8.2 Explain Nagele's method for calculating the expected date of birth. (p. 270)

8.3 Identify crucial adjustments that must be made by the neonate during the first 24 hours of extrauterine life. (p. 271)

8.4 Discuss the purpose of obtaining an apgar score at birth. (p. 271)

8.5 Outline normal measurement and vital sign ranges for the neonatal period. (p. 274)

8.6 Identify criteria that can be used by the nurse to evaluate a neonate's adjustment to extrauterine life. (p. 275)

## Lecture/Discussion

Discuss common reactions to illness for each period of development from conception through the childhood years.

Help students identify ways in which the nursing process can be used to help individuals to cope with normal growth and developmental changes.

## Written Exercise

Instruct students to formulate appropriate guidelines that can be used to teach a child about an upcoming diagnostic procedure or surgery.

8.7 Describe nursing management of an individual during the neonatal period of life. (p. 275)

8.8 Outline normal measurement and vital sign ranges during the period of infancy. (p. 275)

8.9 Describe basic nursing management measures during the period of infancy. (p. 279)

8.10 Plan appropriate nursing intervention for individuals in stage of early childhood. (p. 280)

8.11 Identify four major causes of accidents in childhood, and outline measures for the prevention of each. (p. 282)

8.12 Describe nursing activities that are useful in the management of play-age children. (p. 285)

8.13 Summarize nursing management activities for a school-age child. (p. 288)

8.14 Discuss nursing measures useful in decreasing the trauma of hospitalization for children and their significant others. (p. 289)

8.15 Summarize important immunizations that should be obtained during childhood. (p. 288)

9.0 Identify the factors involved in child abuse.

9.1 Outline signs of child neglect. (p. 289)

9.2 Identify family situations that may trigger or promote child abuse. (p. 290)

9.3 Identify common indicators of child abuse. (p. 290)

9.4 Discuss the responsibilities of the nurse if child abuse or neglect is suspected. (p. 290)

**Lecture/Discussion**

Review common indicators of child abuse.

**Class Activity**

Instruct students to obtain information on the procedure for reporting child abuse in their clinical facility.

**Values Clarification**

Ask students to explore their feelings related to the person who is a child abuser. Ask them how they would handle an incident of child abuse.

---

MULTIPLE CHOICE QUESTIONS

1. Mrs. Todd tells the nurse that she can't believe how much 7-year-old Johnny has grown in the past year. She also comments that he used to be so shy, but now talks to everyone. The nurse understands that Johnny's physical and psychosocial changes are appropriately called:

   A. Maturation
   B. Growth
   C. Development
   D. Learning

CORRECT ANSWER AND RATIONALE

C   Development refers to the orderly and predictable changes (physical and psychosocial) that occur over time as a result of maturation and learning. (p. 260)

2.  Which of the following associations related to categories of growth and development is incorrect?

    A.  Cognitive - intellectual knowledge and understanding
    B.  Emotional - feelings and subjective experiences
    C.  Social - interactions with other people
    D.  Spiritual - beliefs and values of right and wrong

D   Spiritual growth and development refers to a person's beliefs about the creation and purpose of existence. A person's beliefs and values about right and wrong are moral issues. (p. 261)

3.  An individual's attitudes, traits, life style, behavior, and growth patterns develop during:

    A.  Adolescence
    B.  Early childhood and adolescence
    C.  Early childhood
    D.  Infancy and early childhood

D   Basic personality factors (attitudes, traits, life style, behavior, and growth patterns) develop during the periods of infancy and early childhood. (p. 262)

4.  The central theme of Freud's life cycle theory is:

    A.  Intellectual growth and development
    B.  Moral development
    C.  Psychosexual development
    D.  Psychosocial development

C   Using the medium of psychoanalysis to observe human behavior, Freud developed what is now known as the Freudian theory of psychosexual development. (p. 263)

5.  According to Freud, a 5-year-old male child may develop an attraction for his mother in which stage of development?

    A.  Anal
    B.  Genital
    C.  Odedipus
    D.  Phallic

D   The odedipus complex is experienced during Freud's phallic stage of psychosexual development. According to Freud, the child's energy is concentrated on genitalia with primary sexual feelings that are directed toward the parent of the opposite sex. (p. 264)

6.  A small child imitates his father while playing. At which period of Paiget's theory of cognitive development is this most likely to occur?

    A.  Concrete operations
    B.  Formal operations
    C.  Preoperational
    D.  Sensorimotor

C   According to Jean Piaget, a child uses fantasy or imitation of others in behavior and play during the preoperational period of cognitive growth and development. (p. 266)

7.  In what stage of Erikson's theory of psychosocial development does an individual attempt to develop a "coherent sense of self?"

    A.  Adolescence
    B.  Adulthood
    C.  School age
    D.  Young adulthood

A   During adolescence a child attempts to develop a coherent sense of self and plans to actualize personal abilities. Alternately, the child is confronted with feelings of confusion, indecisiveness, and possibly antisocial behavior. The conflict is also known as the stage of identity vs. role diffusion. (p. 265)

8.  As a nurse, you are aware that the process of growth and development:

    A.  Occurs in steps of increasing complexity
    B.  Progresses in an orderly sequence
    C.  Is influenced by both heredity and environment
    D.  All of the above

D   All of the listed options are correct. (p. 269)

9.  A nurse should plan to teach a pregnant person to avoid:

    A.  Excessive intake of coffee
    B.  Exposure to individuals with rubella
    C.  Use of products containing alcohol
    D.  All of the above

    D   Certain teratogens can adversely affect embryo and fetal development. Among the most common are: Infectious organisms, drugs, caffeine, maternal smoking, poor maternal nutrition, radiation, and lead. (p. 270)

10. Which of the following reflexes can the nurse expect to disappear by 6 weeks of age?

    A.  Grasp
    B.  Moro
    C.  Rooting
    D.  Stepping

    D   The stepping reflex normally disappears by the age of six weeks. Neonatal reflexes listed in options A, B, and C disappear as follows: Grasp (6 weeks to 3 months), Moro (1-4 months), and Rooting (3-4 months in awake neonate, 7-8 months in sleeping neonate). (p. 272)

11. In Erikson's theory of psychosocial development, trust is to mistrust as industry is to:

    A.  Generativity
    B.  Inferiority
    C.  Isolation
    D.  Stagnation

    B   During the school age years (from 6-12 years) a child undergoes the period of industry vs. inferiority. Basic conflicts during this period resolve around the resolution of one's realization of competence and perseverance versus feelings that one will never be "any good." (p. 265)

12. According to Erikson, a sense of identity begins to develop at which stage in the life cycle?

    A.  Adolescence
    B.  Late childhood
    C.  School age
    D.  Young adulthood

    A   During the adolescent stage of development, the individual struggles for resolution of the crisis of identify vs. role diffusion. (p. 265)

13. Nursing care for a neonate might include measures to:

    A.  Decrease the neonate's risk of eye infection
    B.  Facilitate bonding between the neonate and parents
    C.  Maintain the neonate's temperature while adjusting to extrauterine environment
    D.  All of the above

    D   Nursing management during the neonatal period of development is directed toward all of the listed options. (p. 275)

14. If posture and locomotion develop as expected, an infant should be able to sit with support at what age?

    A.  2-3 months
    B.  4-5 months
    C.  5-6 months
    D.  6-1/2 to 7-1/2 months

    C   An infant normally sits with support, holds the head erect and is alert at 5-6 months of age. (p. 278)

15. Major needs manifested by a child during early childhood include all of the following except:

    A.  Developing socially acceptable patterns of behavior
    B.  Developing a sense of initiative
    C.  Learning to eat independently
    D.  Accomplishing toilet training

    B   Psychosocial tasks of early childhood include: Development of autonomy; toilet independence and other social controls, such as: interacting with others, eating independently, developing routine sleeping patterns, and participating in self-care. Development of a sense of initiative is a task of the play-age child. (p. 280-282)

16. At what age does a child normally develop a sense of right and wrong, good or bad?

    A.  2-3 years
    B.  2-1/2 to 3-1/2 years
    C.  3-5 years
    D.  4-5 years

    C   The play-age years (from 3-5 years) are important times for the moral and spiritual development of the child. (p. 284)

17. The theorist who describes the school-age years as a time for industry-absorption in physical and mental activities is:

    A. Erikson
    B. Havinghurst
    C. Kohlberg
    D. Piaget

A   According to Erikson, the fourth stage of psychosocial development (school age) resolves around the crisis of industry vs. inferiority. (p. 285)

18. When planning recreational activities for a seven-year-old girl who is hospitalized, the nurse should remember that the six- to seven-year old child:

    A. Dislikes playing with members of the opposite sex
    B. Enjoys projects and working with the hands
    C. Plays well alone, but enjoys small groups of the same sex
    D. Prefers imaginary, dramatic play

D   A child between the ages of six and seven plays well alone but enjoys small groups of both sexes; begins to prefer the same sex peer during the seventh year. This age child prefers imaginary, dramatic play with real costumes. It is not until the 11-12th years that a child is particularly interested in projects and hand work. (p. 286-287)

19. Six-year-old Molly has just been admitted to the hospital to correct a heart abnormality. All of the following nursing actions would be useful in decreasing the trauma of hospitalization for Molly except:

    A. Allow Molly's parents to visit as often as possible
    B. Avoid telling Molly about procedures that may be uncomfortable
    C. Explain upcoming events in terms Molly can understand
    D. Take Molly on a tour of the operating room

B   Children should be given explanations that are appropriate to their age and developmental status. Always tell the truth. The child should be told when he can expect discomfort. This facilitates a therapeutic, trusting relationship between the child and care giver. (p. 289-290)

20. Which of the following statements is incorrect?

    A. Parents who abuse their children were often abused themselves
    B. Child abuse occurs primarily in families of socioeconomic status
    C. Child abusers often have unrealistic expectations of their children
    D. Adults who abuse children have totally varied backgrounds

B   Child abuse occurs in families of all socioeconomic groups. For a complete list of factors that potentiate the occurrence of child abuse see page 290 in text. (p. 290)

# 17

# FROM ADOLESCENCE THROUGH ADULT YEARS

OBJECTIVES

1.0 Describe the physical and psychosocial changes that occur at puberty and through the adolescence period.

    1.1 Summarize physical growth and development changes that occur for the male and female during the period of adolescence. (p. 292)

    1.2 Identify secondary male and female characteristics that develop during prepubescence and continue to develop through the first half of adolescence. (p. 293)

    1.3 Briefly discuss the major psychosocial developmental tasks of adolescence: Cognitive development, relationships, vocational choices, and moral development. (p. 293)

    1.4 Identify six criteria used to evaluate the achievement of self-identity in an adolescent. (p. 294)

    1.5 Briefly explore major health concerns during the adolescent period of life: Accidents, eating disorders, sexual concerns, substance abuse, and depression. (p. 294)

2.0 Discuss the adjustments necessary as a person leaves childhood behavior and takes on adult behavior.

    2.1 Identify three major periods of life in which nutritional needs are the greatest. (p. 293)

    2.2 Identify physical growth and development changes that occur during early adulthood and middle age. (p. 295)

    2.3 Briefly discuss major psychosocial tasks of adulthood: intimacy and generativity. (p. 295)

    2.4 Describe three ways in which the young adult can achieve intimacy. (p. 295)

    2.5 Briefly explore major issues/concerns that are significant during adulthood: Shared life, pregnancy/childbearing, and mid-life changes. (p. 295)

    2.6 Identify factors that are involved in one's selection of a life partner. (p. 296)

TEACHING/LEARNING STRATEGIES

Lecture/Discussion

Discuss the health concerns that are particularly significant during the adolescent years. Accidents, eating disorders, sexual concerns, substance abuse, and depression.

Lecture/Discussion

Review the common indicators of spouse abuse. Encourage a discussion of the nurse's role in expected spouse abuse situations.

Encourage students to explore the centers for spouse abuse that are available within their community.

Identify common reactions to illness for each period of development from adolescence through the adult years.

Values Clarification

Ask students to list the desirable traits they feel are necessary for their "perfect" mate. Encourage them to explore the factors that influence their decisions regarding a suitable life partner.

Clinical Laboratory Experience

Ask students to assess the developmental needs for an adult person in their care. Instruct them to incorporate any developmental needs into their nursing plan of care for the individual.

3.0 Describe the process of physical aging as it occurs through adulthood and into the senior years.

    3.1 Explore the influence of the aging process on "mid-life crises." (p. 298)

    3.2 Summarize major physiologic changes that occur with aging during the senior years. (p. 299)

    3.3 Outline appropriate nursing measures to assist a person who is experiencing the physiologic changes due to aging. (p. 299)

4.0 Discuss the responsibilities and life decisions required of people through the adult years.

## Lecture/Discussion

Assist students in identifying appropriate ways in which they can assist an individual to meet the growth and developmental needs encountered during adolescence, adulthood, and the senior years.

## Values Clarification

Ask students to identify their long and short term lifetime goals. Have them discuss their progress toward meeting these identified goals.

## Group Activity

Divide students into groups. Ask each group to plan appropriate intervention that can be used to address the specific health concerns during pregnancy. Assign each group to one of the following: accidents, eating disorders, sexual concerns, substance abuse, and depression.

## Communication Activity

Have students interview a pregnant individual within the community regarding her expectations of pregnancy. Ask them to compare these expectations with those of the spouse.

5.0 Discuss the process of pregnancy from both the pregnant woman's point of view and the point of view of her significant others.

    5.1 Outline major physiologic changes that occur during pregnancy. (p. 297)

    5.2 Describe the major psychosocial changes that occur as a result of pregnancy. (p. 297)

6.0 Identify factors involved in spouse abuse.

    6.1 Describe the concept of spouse abuse. (p. 298)

    6.2 List possible signs of spouse abuse that the nurse should be aware of when caring for adult persons. (p. 298)

    6.3 Briefly discuss the nurse's role in providing assistance to an abused individual. (p. 299)

7.0 Discuss changes required at the time of retirement from full-time employment.

    7.1 Summarize common psychosocial changes occurring during the senior years. (p. 299)

## Lecture/Discussion

Help students to identify the local, regional, and national organizations whose primary purpose is the support of aging individuals.

7.2 Briefly discuss significant factors/ issues that have an impact on the individual during the senior years: Retirement, accommodation, and loss. (p. 299)

7.3 Identify criteria that can be used to evaluate the achievement of a sense of integrity during the senior years. (p. 303)

**Group Activity**

Divide students into groups. Ask each group to prepare an oral report on one of the organizations designed to assist the elderly.

**Values Clarification**

Ask students to imagine that they are retiring in five years. Have them identify the requirements they feel are necessary for a satisfactory retirement.

**Clinical Laboratory Experience**

As a part of a clinical experience, have students observe activities at a local senior citizen facility.

8.0 Discuss the effect of loss on the psychosocial adjustment of an elderly person.

**Lecture/Discussion**

Ask students to identify common types of losses encountered by the elderly individual. Have them develop criteria for dealing with each type of identified loss.

9.0 Identify factors involved in the abuse of elderly people.

9.1 Recognize the main characteristics or indicators of elderly abuse. (p. 303)

**Lecture/Discussion**

Ask students to identify data useful in assessing the occurrence of elderly abuse. Have them explore the nurse's role in suspected cases of elderly abuse.

---

MULTIPLE CHOICE QUESTIONS

1. All of the following are secondary sexual characteristics the nurse would expect to find in an adolescent female, except:

   A. Growth of axillary, perineal, and facial hair
   B. Deepened voice
   C. Onset of menstruation
   D. Continued enlargement of breasts

2. The period in life in which nutritional requirements are greatest is:

   A. Adolescence
   B. Infancy
   C. Pregnancy and Lactation
   D. Same for all three periods

3. All of the following are expected to occur during the adolescent period except:

   A. Increased concern with self-image
   B. Beginning independence from parents
   C. Choice of eventual life occupation
   D. Development of masculinity or femininity

4. Health problems frequently encountered during the adolescent period of development include:

   A. Alcohol abuse
   B. Malnutrition
   C. Venereal diseases
   D. All of the above

CORRECT ANSWERS AND RATIONALE

A   The adolescent female is expected to experience the growth of axillary and pubic hair. Growth of facial hair would be an abnormal finding. (p. 293)

C   Nutritional needs are increased during the two great growth periods in life, infancy and adolescence, but are greatest during pregnancy and lactation. (p. 293)

C   Decisions about future occupations are often made during adolescence, but do not necessarily determine an individual's life occupation. (p. 294)

D   A number of health concerns arise during the adolescent period of development. These include: Accidents, eating disorders (often leading to malnutrition), sexual concerns (sexually transmitted diseases), substance abuse (alcohol), and depression. (p. 295)

5.  The major cause of death during the adolescent years is:

    A.  Automobile accidents
    B.  Suicide
    C.  Homicide
    D.  Drug overdose

    A    Accidents (particularly automobile and motorcycle accidents) are the major cause of death during the adolescent period. (p. 294)

6.  The maximum potential for physiological intellectual growth and development is most likely to have been achieved by which of the following individuals?

    A.  A 19-year-old male with paralysis due to polio
    B.  An 18-year-old intellectually gifted female
    C.  A 40-year-old female experiencing menopause
    D.  A 29-year-old professional football player

    D    Early adulthood (from approximately 20-45 years) is usually a time of peak physical and mental functioning. For the healthy adult, all body systems are fully developed and functioning efficiently. Relatively little physical change occurs during this period. (p. 295)

7.  Generativity is most easily accomplished by middle-age persons who have:

    A.  Produced and raised offspring
    B.  Been successful in their chosen occupation
    C.  Developed a strong sense of intimacy
    D.  Successfully fulfilled major psychosocial developmental tasks

    D    Generativity is the creative production or contribution to life. It generally refers to having and raising children, but can refer to creativity in occupation, social relationships, and other social contributions. Option D encompasses all of these factors, as generativity is really the consequence of success in a person's psychosocial life tasks. (p. 295)

8.  The nurse should plan to teach every adolescent individual about all of the following except:

    A.  Menstrual cycle
    B.  Common sexual misconceptions
    C.  Normal physiologic changes occurring during adolescence
    D.  All of the above

    A    The nurse should provide the adolescent with health information related to: Nutrition, normal growth and development, common sexual misconceptions, and the physiological/psychosocial changes they can expect to occur during this period. Information related to birth control could be provided to adolescents of both sexes, but it would generally be necessary to provide information about the menstrual cycle to female individuals. (pp. 292-295)

9.  Physiological changes caused by pregnancy include all of the following except:

    A.  Increased appetite
    B.  Absence of menstruation
    C.  Nausea during first two months
    D.  Alterations in body image

    D    The changes in body image that frequently occur during pregnancy are emotional, not physiological, in origin. (p. 296)

10. Psychosocial issues that may require the nurse's special attention during adulthood include:

    A.  Pregnancy and childbearing
    B.  Mid-life changes
    C.  Spouse abuse
    D.  All of the above

    D    Issues of great psychosocial importance during adulthood include: Making a commitment to others, sexuality, shared life, pregnancy and childbearing, mid-life changes/crises, and spouse abuse. (pp. 295-296)

11. Mrs. Wood, a 78-year-old female, recently lost her husband. Since his death, Mrs. Wood has found it increasingly difficult to communicate with her "adult" children. She tells the nurse that "they just can't wait to put me in a nursing home." When providing care for Mrs. Wood, the nurse's primary goal of care would focus on:

A. Facilitating communication between Mrs. Wood and her children
B. Assisting Mrs. Wood in coping with her husband's death
C. Encouraging Mrs. Wood to make the "move" to the nursing home
D. Assisting Mrs. Wood to maintain as much independence as possible

A  According to the information provided, Mrs. Wood's greatest concern is related to communication problems with her children. It is, therefore, appropriate for the nurse to focus actions on the alleviation of this problem. (p. 302)

# 18
# THE EXPERIENCE OF DYING

## OBJECTIVES

1.0 Discuss current attitudes toward death.

   1.1 Identify major factors that influence a person's attitudes toward death. (p. 308)

   1.2 Briefly describe three broad cultural attitudes toward death: Death-accepting, death-defying, and death-denying. (p. 308)

   1.3 Explore common views and beliefs about the existence of life after death. (p. 309)

2.0 Identify various ways people cope with anxieties about death.

   2.1 Explore the meaning of the following statement: "Death is a reality which most cannot believe." (p. 310)

   2.2 Identify and discuss three major psychologic adaptive mechanisms people use to protect themselves from the reality of death. (p. 310)

   2.3 Briefly describe, using examples, defense mechanisms often used by the nurse to cope with personal reactions to the death of individuals in their care. (p. 311)

   2.4 Briefly discuss major psychologic coping mechanisms used by the dying individual, as described by Kubler-Ross: Denial, anger, bargaining, depression, and acceptance. (p. 312)

3.0 Identify your personal reactions toward death.

   3.1 Explore your own personal feelings related to controversial death-related issues. (p. 307)

   3.2 Identify specific death situations that may be particularly stressful for the nurse. (p. 311)

## TEACHING/LEARNING STRATEGIES

### Group Activity

Divide students into groups. Ask each group to research the practices of a different religious group at the time of death. Encourage them to explore ways in which the nurse can assist each group in meeting these needs. Allow each group to briefly discuss the way in which their assigned religion influences the care of an individual after death.

### Lecture/Discussion

Review the stages of death as described by Kubler-Ross. Help students to understand the characteristic behaviors elicited during each stage.

### Values Clarification

Ask students to explore the way in which they would like to be informed of a potentially unfavorable diagnosis.

### Lecture/Discussion

Ask students to share their feelings they encountered in personal experiences with death.

### Values Clarification

Ask students to explore their own personal feelings about death and dying.

Ask students to examine their feelings about working with a dying person and their family.

4.0 Identify ways your personal reactions toward death influence the nursing care you offer.

**Lecture/Discussion**

Ask students to identify common defense mechanisms frequently used by the nurse dealing with a person in a dying situation.

Encourage a discussion of the ways in which the nurses own personal feelings about death and dying can influence the care given to dying individuals.

5.0 Identify various reactions a terminally ill person may have about dying.

    5.1 Briefly discuss the influence of age on a person's view of death. (p. 309)

    5.2 Explore the advantages and disadvantages of disclosing a terminal diagnosis to a dying individual. (p. 314)

    5.3 Define the concepts of grieving and grief work. (p. 314)

    5.4 Briefly discuss common fears experienced by dying individuals: Fear of isolation, abandonment, loneliness, loss of control, loss of privacy, invasion into one's body, and concern over the welfare of significant others. (p. 318)

**Lecture/Discussion**

Focus discussion on the ways in which various age groups approach death.

Explore ways in which the nurse can approach the issue of death at each stage in the life cycle.

6.0 Apply the nursing process in planning care appropriate to the reactions a terminally ill person is experiencing.

    6.1 Discuss nursing measures that can be used to facilitate communication about death. (p. 315)

    6.2 Outline appropriate guidelines that can be used in interactions with dying individuals and their significant others. (p. 318)

    6.3 Discuss nursing intervention that can be utilized to reduce or alleviate a dying person's fears and concerns. (p. 318)

    6.4 Identify six major characteristics of hospice care. (p. 315)

    6.5 Briefly describe the standards and principles of hospice care programs. (p. 316)

**Lecture/Discussion**

Focus discussion on the ways in which the nurse can offer support to terminally ill individuals and their significant others during the various stages of grief.

**Guest Speaker**

Arrange for a nurse from a local hospice to speak in class about the role of a hospice facility in the care of the dying.

7.0 Provide appropriate physical and psychosocial support for terminally ill people and their significant others.

    7.1 Utilize commonly identified nursing diagnoses when planning nursing care for the terminally ill individual. (p. 321)

**Written Exercise**

Instruct students to outline a physical care program for a terminally ill person.

7.2 Identify ways in which the nurse can assist a person through each stage of the dying process: Denial, anger, bargaining, depression, and acceptance. (p. 312)

7.3 Identify ways in which the nurse can provide psychologic support to the dying person and their significant others. (p. 314)

7.4 Briefly explore the care of a dying person's significant others. (p. 319)

7.5 Outline appropriate nursing intervention for identified terminally ill individuals. (p. 321)

7.6 Identify measures that can be used to reduce the stress and anxiety of a dying person and their significant others. (p. 320)

7.7 Discuss the role of the physician and nurse in maintaining an appropriate medication regime for the dying individual experiencing pain. (p. 320)

7.8 Briefly describe four major groups of medications that are frequently used to relieve the symptoms associated with terminal illness: Antianxiety drugs, antiemetics, antidepressants, and corticosteroids. (p. 327)

7.9 List major side effects encountered with use of antianxiety agents, antiemetics, antidepressants, and corticosteroids. (p. 327)

7.10 Discuss five major methods of pain control: Modification of the environment, mind-body techniques, physical methods, collaborative methods, and pharmacologic agents. (p. 328)

8.0 Apply the nursing process for someone experiencing the last few days of life.

8.1 Describe the ultimate role of the nurse when working with an individual who is dying. (p. 306)

8.2 Discuss factors that might be considered when deciding the place of death for an individual (home or hospital). (p. 314)

8.3 Outline the dying person's "Bill of Rights." (p. 313)

8.4 Identify factors that may influence a person's reaction to the knowledge of impending death. (p. 313)

8.5 Describe the anticipatory guidance or pro-active approach to nursing care of the terminally ill. (p. 320)

8.6 Summarize physical changes indicative of imminent death. (p. 328)

## Lecture/Discussion

Discuss signs that indicate approaching death.

Discuss commonly used diagnostic aids used to pronounce death.

Ask students to identify the role of the nurse in care of a person after death.

Have students discuss the advantages and disadvantages of hospice care programs for the terminally ill.

## Written Exercise

Instruct students to outline a plan of care for meeting the needs of a person during the final hours of life.

8.7 Outline appropriate nursing intervention that should be carried out for an individual in the final hours of life. (p. 328)

8.8 List criteria that can be used to establish a diagnosis of death, when heart beat and respiration are being artificially stimulated. (p. 331)

8.9 Identify situations in which it is more difficult to determine death. (p. 328)

8.10 Describe the nurse's primary responsibility at the moment of death. (p. 328)

8.11 Outline major responsibilities of the nurse in care of an individual after death. (p. 331)

## Class Activity

Ask a group of students to visit a local funeral home. Instruct them to observe the physical facilities, obtain information on the supportive services available to the significant others of a deceased person, and the general costs of funeral services. Have them share their findings in class.

---

## MULTIPLE CHOICE QUESTIONS

1. The nurse should be aware that an individual's feeling about death, may have been influenced by which of the following factors?

   A. Early childhood experiences with death
   B. Exposure to "symbolic representations" of death
   C. Cultural affiliation
   D. All of the above

2. In order to provide effective nursing care for a dying individual, the nurse should possess which of the following attitudes toward death?

   A. Death is an inevitable process in the life cycle
   B. Death should be defined, or "gotten the better of"
   C. Death is an intrusion; man should exist eternally
   D. None of the above

3. A nurse has been assigned to provide care for a terminally ill, five-year-old child. The nurse knows that a child of this age:

   A. Tends to view death as something that happens to other people
   B. Understands that death is the final process of life
   C. Does not view death as permanent
   D. Is unable to understand that they are dying

## CORRECT ANSWER AND RATIONALE

D    Many factors influence a person's attitudes toward death. For complete discussion of these factors, see page 308 in text. (p. 308)

A    Professional responsibilities of the nurse require a death-accepting attitude. The nurse who attempts to deal with death by running from it, denying it, or trying to conceal it, will ultimately reject the dying person in the hour of greatest need. (p. 308)

C    Children perceive death according to their developmental stage in life. A five-year-old child does not view death as permanent. Children are, however, able to understand that they are dying, as early as three years of age. (p. 309)

4. In response to the overwhelming reality of death, all of the following individuals display psychologic coping mechanisms. The nurse will probably find it most difficult to deal with the person who:

A. Refuses to recognize that they are dying
B. Transfers their angry feelings related to death onto other people
C. Takes a casual, intellectual approach to their death
D. Openly discusses their feelings and anxieties related to death

**B** The person who displaces, or transfers, their feelings may be more difficult to cope with than the one who uses denial or intellectualization, because these feelings are directed outward at other people. (p. 310)

5. Mr. Author tells his nurse that he knows he doesn't have long to live. Which of the following statements would best facilitate communication with this person?

A. "How long do you think you have?"
B. "I'm sure that everything is going to be all right."
C. "Why do you feel that way?"
D. "You feel as though you don't have long to live. . ."

**D** By restating the person's comment, the nurse encourages the person to continue. It gives the person permission to share their feelings. Other options may be used by the nurse to discourage the person from talking about death. (pp. 87, 311)

6. A terminally ill person frequently summons nursing personnel to their room. Each time a nurse enters the room, the person complains bitterly about the care he is receiving. This person is using which of the following psychologic defense mechanisms to cope with death?

A. Denial
B. Anger
C. Objection
D. Depression

**B** According to Kubler-Ross, this person is in the second stage of the dying process called anger. Anger is not actually directed at the nurse, but rather arises out of the person's feelings of helplessness and fear. (p. 312)

7. Which statement best reflects a person who is in the bargaining stage of the dying process?

A. "I have so many things to do before I die."
B. "I'll finish college next year."
C. If I take this medicine, will you give me more later?"
D. "If only I were a better person. . . maybe I'd live longer."

**D** In the bargaining stage of the death and dying process, the person attempts to barter for more time. This bargaining is often covert, and may go completely unnoticed by health team members. (p. 312)

8. Impending death becomes a reality that cannot be ignored, in which stage of the dying process?

A. Anger
B. Bargaining
C. Depression
D. Acceptance

**C** A person acknowledges a terminal illness in the depression stage of the dying process. During the stage, the person may cry and express other indications of grief. (p. 312)

9. Which of the following associations is incorrect?

A. Acceptance - Detachment
B. Anger - Emotionalism
C. Denial - Belief
D. Depression - Awareness

**C** Denial is the stage of disbelief. All other options are correct. (p. 312)

10. When a terminally ill person uses anger as a coping mechanism, the best nursing approach is to:

A. Avoid the person until they are no longer angry
B. Tell the person that they should not act so angry
C. Retaliate with expressions of anger
D. Maintain contact with the person, rather than avoiding them

D    The nurse should remain with the person when appropriate so that they will not feel that the anger has driven them away. (p. 312)

11. Which of the following is a true statement related to the stages of dying as outlined by Kubler-Ross?

A. The terminally ill person and their significant others experience the stages simultaneously
B. All persons progress sequentially through the various stages
C. It is uncommon for a person to regress back to earlier stages in the process
D. The stages do not always follow one another, and may overlap in many instances

D    Options A, B, and C are all incorrect. The stages of the dying process should never be viewed as "fixed stages" through which the person passes in a sequential order. The person, their significant others, and health care providers will pass through the various stages, but at different times and rates. (p. 313)

12. According to Kubler-Ross, a dying person reaches the stage of acceptance when they have:

A. Acknowledged the reality of their death
B. Completed all unfinished business
C. Resigned themselves to their fate
D. Exhausted all alternative outcomes

B    The person who experiences acceptance, feels that they have taken care of all unfinished business. They are ready to accept their death, with all fear, anxiety, and pain gone. (p. 312)

13. Common concerns and fears that are frequently expressed by those who are dying include:

A. Abandonment
B. Isolation
C. Loss of control
D. All of the above

D    Common fears and concerns frequently experienced by dying individual's include: Fear of abandonment, isolation, loneliness, pain, loss of control, loss of privacy, and concern over the welfare of significant others. (p. 318)

14. Which of the following nursing measures is least likely to reduce the fear and anxiety frequently experienced by a dying individual?

A. Attentively listening as the person verbalizes feelings and identifiable fears
B. Encouraging the person to ventilate concerns
C. Identifying fears and concerns for the person
D. Teaching meditation and relaxation techniques

C    The nurse should help the person to identify their personal concerns and fears. The person must be allowed to identify their concerns for themselves, otherwise the nurse may suggest anxieties that the person has not even thought about. (p. 318)

15. A terminally ill individual has recently expired. Appropriate nursing intervention for this person's significant others would include all of the following except:

A. Allowing time for the performance of personal rituals
B. Providing an opportunity for the body to be viewed
C. Allowing time alone with the body for 10 minutes
D. Allowing final good-byes in any way they wish

C    The significant others should be allowed the opportunity to complete options A, B, and C. They should not, however, be hurried at this time. They need to be given time to complete the essential tasks of this period. (p. 328)

# 19
# BASIC PSYCHOSOCIAL ASSESSMENT

OBJECTIVES

1.0 Discuss purposes and value of psychosocial assessment for people receiving nonpsychiatric care.

   1.1 Define the process of psychosocial assessment. (p. 336)

   1.2 Identify the principal purpose for conducting a nursing assessment. (p. 337)

   1.3 Identify the nurse's primary purpose for gathering psychosocial data from medical-surgical individuals. (p. 339)

   1.4 Briefly describe the value of conducting a psychologic assessment. (p. 342)

   1.5 Discuss the primary reasons for gathering a social nursing assessment. (p. 345)

2.0 Identify components of your personal value system that may influence the psychosocial assessment you make.

   2.1 Explore the importance of displaying a nonjudgmental attitude when caring for a person and their significant others. (p. 338)

   2.2 Explore factors that may influence a nurse's initial reaction to a person. (p. 339)

   2.3 Discuss factors that may hinder the creation of a therapeutic environment, and narrow the nurse's perception of psychosocial information. (p. 341)

3.0 Discuss psychologic and social areas important in psychosocial assessment.

   3.1 Outline psychosocial data that can be gathered during an initial individual interview. (p. 339)

   3.2 Discuss the basic components of a psychologic assessment. (p. 342)

   3.3 Identify additional psychosocial information the nurse should gather in order to individualize person care. (p. 344)

TEACHING/LEARNING STRATEGIES

Lecture/Discussion

Differentiate between a person's psychologic patterns and social experiences.

Lecture/Discussion

Focus discussion on the concepts of bias, discrimination, and stereotyping. Ask students how they feel each might influence the delivery of nursing care.

Values Clarification

Ask students to complete the "Identification of Personal Values" tool on page 342 in the text. Encourage them to explore the ways in which their own personal values can influence their perception of psychosocial information.

Written Exercise

Instruct students to outline the basic components of a psychosocial assessment.

3.4 Identify the principal areas assessed when conducting a mental status examination. (p. 343)

3.5 Differentiate between two types of behavior: Verbal and nonverbal. (p. 343)

3.6 Discuss the components of a sociologic assessment. (p. 345)

3.7 Discuss ways in which the nurse can gather useful information about an individual's social network. (p. 345)

3.8 Identify information the nurse should gather in order to assess a person's socioeconomic status. (p. 346)

3.9 Describe information that should be gathered by the nurse to assess a person's life style. (p. 346)

3.10 Identify information included in a sociologic assessment of an individual's sexuality. (p. 346)

3.11 Identify information the nurse should gather to assess a person's psychosocial development. (p. 347)

3.12 Discuss the benefits of obtaining spiritual data in a basic psychosocial assessment. (p. 347)

3.13 Identify questions that can be asked in an assessment of a person's spiritual beliefs. (p. 347)

4.0 Make psychosocial assessments with supervision.

## Campus Laboratory Experience

Using the material listed on Page 340 in the text, instruct students to perform a psychosocial assessment on a classmate. Ask them to share any difficulties they encountered during the process.

## Clinical Laboratory Experience

With guidance, instruct students to perform a psychosocial assessment of a person in their care. Ask them to identify ways in which any psychosocial problems might be affecting the person's present illness.

5.0 List formal psychosocial assessment tools.

5.1 List common uses of formalized psychologic tests. (p. 344)

5.2 Describe two general classifications of psychologic tests: Objective and projective. (p. 344)

## Lecture/Discussion

Review Barry's Psychosocial Assessment Interview Guide in class. Focus discussion on the areas of the assessment that you feel will be most difficult for the student to obtain.

6.0 Describe factors that influence the validity of psychosocial assessment.

   6.1 Briefly discuss factors that influence a person's self-disclosure of personal psychosocial information. (p. 337)

   6.2 Identify criteria that can aid the nurse in gathering appropriate psychosocial information. (p. 338)

   6.3 Summarize factors that can minimize the accuracy and usefulness of psychosocial assessment data gathered by the nurse. (p. 341)

**Lecture/Discussion**

Ask students to identify factors that they feel influence a person's disclosure of psychosocial information.

**Clinical Laboratory Experience**

Have students identify factors in their clinical facility that could hinder the development of a therapeutic environment. Ask them to explore ways in which these factors influence the nurse's psychosocial assessment of an individual. What could be done to eliminate these problems.

7.0 Use information gathered through psychosocial assessment appropriately.

   7.1 List and briefly describe factors that influence the uniqueness of a person's responses to illness and hospitalization. (p. 341)

   7.2 Discuss important functions of a person's social network: intimacy, social integration, nurturing behavior, reassurance, and assistance. (p. 345)

   7.3 Identify information gained from a basic psychosocial assessment that would indicate the need for psychiatric assistance. (p. 349)

**Lecture/Discussion**

Discuss ways in which psychosocial assessment data can be used to plan effective nursing care.

8.0 Practice using a psychosocial assessment guide and applying the data in planning nursing care.

   8.1 Analyze the importance of performing a holistic nursing assessment. (p. 337)

   8.2 Compare and contrast the focus of a physical assessment, with that of a psychosocial assessment. (p. 337)

   8.3 Identify and briefly describe factors that the nurse must consider when attempting to reduce environmental stress. (p. 341)

**Lecture/Discussion**

Ask students to identify ways in which they can effectively meet the psychosocial needs of a person in their care.

---

**MULTIPLE CHOICE QUESTIONS**

1. Which of the following best describes the process of psychosocial assessment?

   A. An objective assessment of a person's intellectual, social, and emotional needs.
   B. The assessment of a person's social and psychological well-being
   C. A data-gathering process that focuses on the intellectual, social and emotional needs of an individual.
   D. The assessment of psychological and sociological factors affecting a person's health status.

**CORRECT ANSWERS AND RATIONALE**

C   Statement C is the most complete statement. Psychosocial assessment focuses on subjective and objective information related to a person's intellectual, social, and emotional needs. (p. 373)

2. A person will be less willing to share personal, psychosocial information with the nurse who:

A. Sympathizes with the person's problems and needs
B. Has shown professional expertise in meeting their physical needs
C. Occasionally leaves the room during the interview to assist other persons
D. Approaches the assessment in a calm, unhurried manner

C    The sharing of personal, psychosocial information depends upon many factors. These include: The amount of trust that the person has in the nurse; how genuine the nurse is in communication; the nurse's mastery and use of effective listening skills; and the ability of the nurse to make accurate observations and have them validated by the nurse. (p. 337)

3. Which of the following would be the most appropriate way for a nurse to address a new person?

A. "Hello, Mrs. James. I'm Sally Smith, an R.N., and I'll be in charge of your nursing care while you're in the hospital."
B. "Jan, I'll be your nurse while you're in the hospital."
C. "My name is Sally Smith. I'll be providing your nursing care for the next few weeks."
D. "I'm Sally Smith, an R.N., and I'll be helping you with your nursing needs during your hospital stay."

D    In option D the statement includes the name, title, and role of the nurse. Unlike option A, the person is not addressed using a title that designates marital status. (p. 339)

4. The nurse knows that a person will be less reluctant to share person information in an environment that:

A. Promotes privacy and confidentiality
B. Is free of unpredictable and unexplained noises
C. Produces a minimal amount of stress and anxiety
D. Familiar and non-threatening

C    Nurses can make more accurate psychosocial assessments if they reduce the amount of environmental stress experienced by the people and their significant others. These stress-provoking factors include: inadequate orientation, lack of privacy, feeling that they don't belong, and noise. (p. 341)

5. Questions used to assess a person's psychosocial status:
A. Are the same for every individual and situation
B. Are largely determined by the person's reason for seeking health care
C. Are directed entirely at those parts of a person's life that are affected by other people
D. Always contain sexual information

B    The nurse should be aware of the common types of psychosocial information that are available, but should thoughtfully gather information specific to the pertsonbeing interviewed. (p. 341)

6. Which of the following statements about behavior is false?

A. Behavior is the way in which a person responds to a stimulus
B. Behavior is all the activities of an organism that can be observed by others
C. Behavior can be displayed both verbally and nonverbally
D. Behavior is usually meaningless and related to childhood experience

D    All behavior has meaning. It is, however, sometimes difficult to determine what that meaning is exactly. (p. 342)

7. All of the following are common components of a psychosocial history except:

A. Person's position in home relationships
B. Family history of psychiatric illness
C. Patterns in which a person copes with stress
D. Activities of daily living

B    The psychosocial history would contain information about the person's history of physical illness, but not that of the family. (p. 348)

8.  The statement, "A bird in the hand is worth two in the bush" could be used during a psychosocial assessment to determine a person's:

    A.  General knowledge level
    B.  Orientation to person, place, and time
    C.  Ability to do abstract reasoning
    D.  Ability to make judgments

C   Common proverbs are used during a mental status examination to judge a person's ability to do abstract reasoning. (p. 343)

9.  When a person displays inappropriate behavior during a psychosocial assessment, the nurse should:

    A.  Omit the information from the assessment summary, as anxious behavior is often displayed during interviews
    B.  Document the behavior in the assessment summary, labeling it as abnormal
    C.  Describe the person's behavior and the situation in which it was produced
    D.  Summarize an interpretation of the meaning of the behavior

C   When abnormal behavior is observed, the nurse should attempt to accurately describe the behavior. This reduces the likelihood of making invalid and inaccurate assumptions about the person. The behavior should never be labeled as abnormal. (p. 343)

# 20
# BASIC HEALTH ASSESSMENT

## OBJECTIVES

1.0 Define various terms used in basic health assessment.

    1.1 Utilize terminology related to basic health assessment. (p. 353)

    1.2 Correctly utilize common abbreviations used during the assessment process. (p. 353)

2.0 Discuss the similarities and differences between the way nurses use assessment and the way physicians use assessment.

    2.1 Identify the major purpose for conducting a physical assessment. (p. 364))

3.0 Discuss the diagnostic process.

    3.1 Identify two basic functions of the diagnostic process. (p. 354)

    3.2 Discuss factors that influence the occurrence of diagnostic errors. (p. 354))

    3.3 Distinguish between an organic and a functional disorder. (p. 354)

    3.4 Compare the diagnostic process with the "crime-solving" process. (p. 354)

    3.5 Identify the main objective of the diagnostic process. (p. 354)

4.0 Practice taking medical and psychiatric histories.

    4.1 Identify information included in a typical history and health assessment data-base. (p. 381)

## TEACHING/LEARNING STRATEGIES

### Lecture/Discussion

Ask students to review the terminology and abbreviations listed on page 353 in the text.

Ask students to review the list of commonly accepted abbreviations used in their clinical facility.

### Lecture/Discussion

Help students to differentiate between a medical diagnosis and a nursing diagnosis.

### Written Exercise

Ask students to write a paper comparing and contrasting the components of the medical history with those of the nursing history.

### Class Activity

Review a hypothetical individual situation in class. Identify the medical diagnoses that were established for the person, and the nursing diagnoses that were formulated.

### Lecture/Discussion

Explore factors that influence the occurrence of diagnostic errors.

### Lecture/Discussion

Briefly describe the components that should be included in the assessment of a person with a psychiatric disorder: History interview, mental status examination, assessment of pertinent social environmental factors, and complete physical assessment. (p. 354)

4.2  Identify factors that influence an
individual's personal account of
symptoms related to their illness.
(p. 356)

4.3  Summarize the major components of a
medical history. (p. 356)

4.4  List and briefly describe the major
components of a complete psychiatric
history. (p. 358)

5.0  Identify common diagnostic tools.

5.1  Describe the purpose and uses of various
diagnostic tools for physical
assessment: Stethoscope, scopes,
mirrors, speculums, and instruments of
measurement. (p. 360)

6.0  Practice, with supervision, the four basic
assessment maneuvers.

6.1  Briefly describe, using examples,
assessment maneuvers used during a
physical examination: Inspection,
palpation, percussion, and
auscultation. (p. 360)

7.0  Assist another health professional in
physical assessment.

7.1  Identify the nurse's responsibility when
assisting with a complete physical
assessment. (p. 364)

7.2  Identify nursing activities used to
prepare an individual for physical
assessment. (p. 365)

7.3  Summarize activities of the nurse during
a physical assessment. (p. 365)

7.4  Summarize the positions assumed by the
examiner and individual during a
physical examination. (p. 365)

7.5  List supplies the nurse should gather in
preparation for a physical examination.
(p. 380)

7.6  List actions the nurse might take upon
completion of a physical examination.
(p. 380)

8.0  Practice making physical assessments yourself.

8.1  Identify individual symptoms that
warrant immediate investigation.
(p. 355)

8.2  Identify symptoms displayed by the
individual that can be investigated at a
later date. (p. 355)

## Clinical Laboratory Experience

Have students review the physician's history and
physical write-up for a person in their care.

## Lecture/Discussion

Bring commonly used assessment tools to class.
Discuss the purposes and use of each.

## Campus Laboratory Experience

Allow students to practice the use of common
diagnostic tools listed on page 359 in the text.

## Campus Laboratory Experience

Provide a demonstration of the various assessment
maneuvers: inspection, palpation, percussion, and
auscultation.

Allow students to practice the assessment
maneuvers: inspection, palpation, percussion, and
auscultation.

## Lecture/Discussion

Compare and contrast the roles of the nurse and
physician in the physical examination process.

## Lecture/Discussion

Ask students to outline the major characteristics
they should observe in each anatomical area when
performing a physical assessment.

8.3 Discuss normal ranges for weight in adult men and women. (p. 357)

8.4 Describe the procedure for determining an individual's body frame size. (p. 357)

8.5 List the usual sequence of assessment activities. (p. 360)

8.6 Identify organs that are anatomically placed in each abdominal quadrant. (p. 361)

8.7 Identify characteristic odors detectable during a physical assessment and their possible causes. (p. 363)

8.8 Outline the major components of a complete physical examination. Describe methods used to assess each area. (p. 366)

8.9 Briefly describe the purpose of including ancillary or adjunctive assessments in the examination of a person's health status. (p. 380)

9.0 List and describe various ancillary assessment procedures.

9.1 Identify examples of ancillary or objective tests that are commonly utilized to evaluate a person's health status. (p. 380)

9.2 Identify the components of an ancillary psychiatric assessment. (p. 380)

9.3 Discuss two major uses of ancillary physical assessment examinations. (p. 382)

9.4 Discuss the role of roentgenography, fluoroscopy, and computerized transaxial tomography in a complete physical examination. (p. 382)

9.5 Briefly discuss the role of radioactive-tracer materials in identifying the location of some malignancies. (p. 383)

9.6 Describe two types of radioactive scanners used in evaluation of malignancy location. (p. 384)

9.7 Identify body substances that may be sent for examination to the clinical laboratory. (p. 384)

9.8 Discuss the importance of properly handling any specimen that is to be sent to the clinical laboratory for diagnostic purposes. (p. 384)

9.9 Discuss major uses of ultrasonography. (p. 386)

Explore techniques that can be used to facilitate the physical examination process for individuals throughout the lifespan.

Have students outline guidelines to be used when assessing a person's presenting symptoms.

## Campus Laboratory Experience

Ask each student to conduct a physical assessment on another class member.

## Lecture/Discussion

Focus discussion on the various ancillary procedures that are commonly used in health assessment.

Give examples of diagnostic procedures used to assess the various body systems: Cardiovascular/hematopoietic systems, kidney/urinary tract, respiratory system, reproductive system, digestive system, musculoskeletal system, nervous system, and the endocrine system.

## Clinical Laboratory Experience

Arrange for students to visit various ancillary departments within their clinical facility.

9.10 Describe the function of biopsies in the diagnostic examination of an individual. (p. 386)

10.0 Plan nursing care for a person experiencing common ancillary assessment procedures.

10.1 Discuss the importance of becoming familiar with normal value ranges for laboratory tests at each different clinical facility. (p. 385)

10.2 Discuss responsibilities of the nurse in conjunction with common ancillary diagnostic tests. (p. 386)

10.3 Describe various ancillary tests and the nursing responsibilities associated with each: Abdominal paracentesis, angiography, blood analysis, bone marrow biopsy, bronchography, cholecystography, cisternal puncture, colonoscopy, cystoscopy, electrocardiography, electroencephalography, electromyelography, esophagoscopy, gastric analysis, gastroscopy, intravenous cholangiography, intravenous pyelogram, laryngoscopy, liver biopsy, lower gastrointestinal x-rays, lumbar puncture, mammography, myelography, proctoscopy, pulmonary function tests, scans, secretion analysis, sigmoidoscopy, small bowel x-ray series, thermography, thoracentesis, ultrasonography, uppergastrointestinal x-rays, and urinalysis. (p. 387)

## Lecture/Discussion

Discuss the role of the nurse in assisting with ancillary diagnostic processes.

## Clinical Laboratory Experience

Ask students to incorporate information obtained from the ancillary diagnostic studies performed on their assigned clinical person into their assessment.

---

## MULTIPLE CHOICE QUESTIONS

1. A diagnosis that focuses on a person's response to disease and the resulting pathologic changes is called a:

   A. Differential diagnosis
   B. Medical diagnosis
   C. Nursing diagnosis
   D. Psychiatric diagnosis

2. Which of the following associations is incorrect?

   A. LLQ - Left lower quadrant
   B. OS - Left eye
   C. Post - Posterior
   D. Tx - Treatment

3. When conducting a basic physical assessment, the nurse should immediately investigate symptoms that:

   A. Are unrelated to the current reason for hospitalization
   B. Occur frequently in other disorders
   C. The person appears concerned about
   D. All of the above

## CORRECT ANSWERS AND RATIONALE

C  A nursing diagnosis focuses on a person's physical and emotional responses to disease and the resulting pathologic changes. (p. 353)

D  The correct abbreviation for treatment is Rx. (p. 353)

C  The nurse should investigate symptoms that: Have objective proof; are localized to a specific body part or organ; have obvious clinical relationships; and that the person identifies as giving concern. Symptoms that can be temporarily "put aside" include: Those that are known to occur in many disorders; those that are vaguely defined; those arising from causes unrelated to the main problem or reason for hospitalization. (p. 355)

4. When assessing a person's respiratory status, the nurse should perform basic assessment maneuvers in which of the following sequences?

   A. Auscultation, percussion, inspection, and palpation
   B. Auscultation and percussion
   C. Inspection, auscultation, percussion, and inspection
   D. Inspection, palpation, percussion, and auscultation

D   The usual sequence of assessment activities is to: Inspect, palpate, percuss, and auscultate. (p. 360)

5. A person complains of left upper abdominal pain. The nurse knows that the organs found within this quadrant include all of the following <u>except</u>:

   A. Descending colon
   B. Liver
   C. Gallbladder
   D. Stomach

C   The gallbladder is situated in the right upper abdominal quadrant. Organs found in the LUQ include: Adrenal gland, colon (splenic flexure, transverse, and descending), kidney, liver, pancreas, spleen, and the stomach. (p. 361)

6. A person complains of decreased sensation in the right lower extremity. The nurse can check this area for temperature changes that would denote decreased sensation by using which of the following?

   A. Auscultation
   B. Inspection
   C. Palpation
   D. Percussion

C   Temperature changes can be detected by running the backs of the fingers or the dorsum of the hand over the skin. This is called palpation. (p. 360)

7. A stethoscope is required to perform which basis assessment maneuver?

   A. Direct auscultation
   B. Indirect percussion
   C. Direct percussion
   D. None of the above

D   The indirect method of auscultation requires the use of a stethoscope. (p. 362)

8. A complete physical assessment is performed for which of the following reasons?

   A. To assess healthy individuals at regular intervals for early signs of disease
   B. To identify deviations in a person's health care status
   C. To assess the type and extent of a disease process
   D. All of the above

D   The physical assessment is used for all of the listed reasons. Its major purpose is to identify deviations from normal in healthy individuals and in individuals experiencing symptoms of disease. (p. 364)

9. When assisting with a physical examination, the nurse's <u>primary</u> responsibility is to:

   A. Assemble equipment and prepare the examination area
   B. Supply the examiner with necessary tools and supplies
   C. Observe and meet the holistic needs of the person being examined
   D. All of the above

C   When assisting with a physical examination, the nurse may perform all of the listed options. The nurse's primary responsibility is, however, to assist the person receiving care. (p. 365)

10. The nurse instructs a person to lie on their back, with knees bent and feet flat on the bed. This position is called:

   A. Dorsal recumbent
   B. Lithotomy
   C. Knee-chest
   D. Sims

A   The position described is the dorsal recumbent. A special table is required to place the person in a lithotomy position. (p. 364)

11. To facilitate a complete examination of the heart, the nurse will need to assist a person into which of the following positions?

  A. Sitting only
  B. Sitting and lying flat on the bed
  C. Sitting, lying on the back, and on the right side
  D. Sitting, lying on the back, and on the left side

D  Three positions must be assumed by the person during an examination of the heart. These are: Sitting, lying on the back, and on the left side. (p. 365)

12. An examiner uses the six cardinal positions of gaze to determine abnormalities in:

  A. Intraocular pressure
  B. Ocular movement
  C. Visual acuity
  D. Visual field

B  The six cardinal positions of gaze are used to determine abnormalities in ocular movement. (p. 369)

13. Intraocular pressure should be assessed regularly in which population?

  A. Newborns and infants
  B. Adolescence through young adulthood
  C. Middle age through elderly
  D. Elderly

C  Adults over the age of 40 require tonometry regularly to ascertain the development of glaucoma. (p. 369)

14. When assessing the lymph nodes draining the breast, the nurse knows that:

  A. Any complaint of tenderness should be considered abnormal
  B. Some of the lymph nodes are normally palpable
  C. Male breasts do not normally have to be examined
  D. Female breasts should be examined just after the menstrual period

D  Statements A, B, and C are all incorrect. Statement D is correct. Due to physiological changes in the female breast just prior to the menstrual cycle, it is deemed best to examine the breasts just after the menstrual period. (p. 375)

15. When examining the lungs, the nurse should be especially alert for abnormal findings which may include:

  A. Areas over the lung dull when percussed
  B. Adult respiratory rate ranging from 8-18 times per minute
  C. Vesicular sounds when auscultating area over lungs
  D. Equal bilateral movement of the diaphragm

A  The lungs should normally sound resonant when percussed. (p. 373)

16. What is the nurse's responsibility upon discovering abnormal data during a physical examination?

  A. Document the significant findings in the person's clinical record
  B. Formulate appropriate nursing diagnoses for the identified individual needs
  C. Notify other appropriate health personnel of the significant findings
  D. All of the above

D  The nurse should document all significant findings from physical assessment. These findings should be used to identify nursing diagnoses and to plan appropriate intervention. In addition, the nurse should make appropriate referrals for abnormal findings. (p. 379)

17. Which of the following diagnostic tests is not used to assess the functioning of the kidneys and urinary tract?

  A. Cholangiography
  B. Cystometry
  C. Nephrotomography
  D. Renogram

A  A cholangiography is an x-ray examination of the bile ducts. (p. 387)

18. When examining a person, the nurse notes the presence of rhythmic oscillations in both eyes. This is called:

   A. Diplopia
   B. Nystagmus
   C. Stabismus
   D. Pitosis

B   Nystagmus is the rhythmic oscillations of the eyes. (p. 369)

# CARING FOR PEOPLE UNDERGOING NONSURGICAL THERAPIES

| OBJECTIVES | TEACHING/LEARNING STRATEGIES |
|---|---|
| 1.0 Define various types of treatments. | **Lecture/Discussion** |
| | Ask students to review the terminology used to describe the various types of treatment that are listed on page 397 in text. |
| 1.1 Briefly describe the following types of treatment: causal, empiric, conservative, curative, palliative, preventive, rational, specific, supportive, and symptomatic. (p. 397) | Provide examples of the various types of treatment: Causal, empiric, conservative, curative, palliative, preventive, rational, specific, supportive, and symptomatic. |
| | Ask students to identify the various types of treatment being received by a person in their care. |
| 2.0 Describe the meaning of the term "treatment." | **Lecture/Discussion** |
| | Discuss the meaning of the term "therapeutic activity." |
| 3.0 Identify factors that influence the type of treatment a person seeks. | **Values Clarification** |
| | Ask students to share factors that have influenced their past health care decisions in regard to treatment. |
| 3.1 Briefly discuss variables that have a significant influence on an individual's choices related to health maintenance and treatment, activities: past experience, social network patterns, personal concepts of health and illness, belief about what treatment is appropriate for which problems, and beliefs about which activities are important, for health maintenance and which are not. (p. 397) | **Clinical Laboratory Experience** |
| | Have students identify factors influencing the choice of treatment by a person in their care. |
| 4.0 Discuss the responsibilities of health care professionals as administrators of treatment modalities. | **Lecture/Discussion** |
| | Discuss factors that influence the health care practitioner's choice of treatment. |
| 4.1 Identify knowledge needed by a health professional prior to engagement in the treatment process. (p. 397) | Focus discussion on the professional responsibilities of the nurse in the treatment process. |
| 4.2 List major factors the health care professional should take into consideration when selecting an individual's method of treatment. (p. 397) | |

5.0 Describe what is meant by the therapeutic use of self.

**Lecture/Discussion**

Explore ways in which the nurse can act as therapeutic agent to enhance the effectiveness of the various types of traditional treatment: therapeutic radiation, pharmaceutical treatments, physical medicine, nutritional therapy, and psychiatric therapies.

6.0 Discuss the issue of compliance with treatment regimens.

    6.1 Outline information needed by an individual in preparation for scheduled treatment activities. (p. 398)

    6.2 Discuss the importance of individual compliance with any proposed plan of care or treatment. (p. 398)

**Lecture/Discussion**

Explore the various factors that influence a person's compliance with various treatment modalities.

7.0 List and briefly describe various nonsurgical treatment modalities commonly used in traditional health care systems.

    7.1 Discuss the benefits of various nonsurgical therapeutic approaches: Therapeutic radiation, pharmaceutical treatments, physical medicine, nutritional therapy, and psychiatric therapies. (p. 399)

**Lecture/Discussion**

Review various traditional treatment modalities: therapeutic radiation, pharmaceutical treatments, physical medicine, nutritional therapy, and psychiatric therapies. Provide a clinical example of each.

**Written Exercise**

Ask students to outline the responsibilities of the nurse in relation to the various traditional treatment modalities: Therapeutic radiation, pharmaceutical treatment, physical medicine, nutritional therapy, and psychiatric therapies.

8.0 List and briefly describe various therapeutic approaches not usually part of traditional health care systems.

    8.1 Briefly describe various nontraditional therapeutic modalities: Acupressure, acupuncture, ayurveda medicine, chiropody, chiropractic, chromotherapy, electrolyte regeneration program, herbalism, homeopathy, iridology, kinesiology, macrobiotics, mechanotherapy, naprapathy, naturopathy, osteopathy, reflexology, shiatsu, therapeutic touch, and yoga. (p. 401)

**Lecture/Discussion**

Have students explore the advantages and disadvantages of using nontraditional therapeutic modalities.

9.0 Discuss iatrogenic disorders.

    9.1 Discuss, using an example, the etiology of iatrogenic disorders. (p. 400)

**Lecture/Discussion**

Give clinical examples of iatrogenic disorders.

10.0 Discuss the meaning and scope of preventive medicine.

    10.1 Describe the role of preventive medicine in the conservation of health and prevention of disease. (p. 400)

    10.2 Identify factors that influence the usefulness of a program designed for the prevention of disease. (p. 400)

**Lecture/Discussion**

Emphasize the importance of preventive health care techniques. Ask students to incorporate appropriate techniques into the care of individual's in the hospital and the community.

Ask students to identify measures useful in prevention of illness at each stage in the life cycle.

10.3 Identify areas of current focus in preventive medicine. (p. 400)

11.0 Discuss the growing health care consumer trend toward self-care.

    11.1 Briefly describe Breslow and Somers' system for monitoring health over the life span. (p. 400)

    11.2 Summarize recommendations for preventive health care during the period of middle age. (p. 401)

    11.3 Explore the role of self-care in the prevention of illness and disease. (p. 402)

## Communication Activity

Have students interview a person in the community regarding their preventive health care practices.

## Clinical Laboratory Experience

Have students identify ways in which they can promote self-care in a person they are presently caring for in the clinical environment. Ask them to use the nursing process as their guide.

---

## MULTIPLE CHOICE QUESTIONS

1. As a nurse, you are aware that treatment is best described as:

    A. An activity that promotes a person's well-being, not merely the curing of disease
    B. Any procedure used to cure a disease or pathological condition
    C. A therapeutic activity for disease prevention and health maintenance
    D. Holistic management techniques used to cure disease processes

SITUATION: Mrs. Fernandez, a person in your care, is receiving radiation therapy for an abdominal tumor. The physician tells you that this will not cure the person, but will merely lessen her pain and discomfort by reducing the size of the tumor. Questions 2 through 4 apply to this situation.

2. Mrs. Fernandez is receiving which type of treatment?

    A. Casual
    B. Conservative
    C. Palliative
    D. Rational

3. One day while talking with Mrs. Fernandez, she tells you that another physician recommended surgery for her "tumor" two years ago, but she had thought that method of treatment was a "little too drastic." You understand that her choice of treatment may have been influenced by:

    A. The similar health experiences of her significant others
    B. Her beliefs about the type of treatment that was appropriate for her condition
    C. Her personal concepts of health and illness
    D. All of the above

## CORRECT ANSWER AND RATIONALE

A   In its broadest sense, treatment is considered to be an activity that promotes a person's well-being, not merely the curing of disease. (p. 396)

C   Palliative treatment is directed at relieving pain and distress, but does not attempt a cure. (p. 396)

D   All of the factors listed could have influenced Mrs. Fernandez's treatment decisions. Other factors that have a potential influence on a person's treatment decisions are their past experience and beliefs about what is necessary for health maintenance and what is not. (p. 397)

4. The physician who selected Mrs. Fernandez's treatment modality, should have made a decision based upon all the following factors except:

   A. The known advantages and disadvantages of treating a person with radiation therapy
   B. The person's willingness to comply and understanding of the goals of radiation therapy
   C. The person's previous refusal to undergo surgical intervention methods
   D. Current therapies available for the person's specific type of abdominal tumor

C  If surgery continued to be a viable treatment option for Mrs. Fernandez, then it was the professional responsibility of the physician to discuss it with her before assuming she would again refuse.  (p. 397)

5. Which of the following statements is correct?

   A. An individual is more likely to comply with nontraditional forms of treatment if informed.
   B. The health care practitioner should independently select appropriate methods of treatment.
   C. Very rarely are several methods of treatment combined to treat an individual.
   D. Treatment should never be initiated before a definitive diagnosis has been established.

A  The individual should be included in treatment decisions. An informed individual is more likely to cooperate with treatment plans. (p. 398)

6. Choose the one that doesn't belong:

   A. Acupuncture
   B. Convulsive therapy
   C. Hydrotherapy
   D. Dietary therapy

A  Options B, C, and D are all traditional forms of treatment.  Option A is a nontraditional form of treatment.  (p. 399)

7. According to the Lifetime Health Monitoring Plan, a middle-age adult should be screened for visual impairment:

   A. Once a year
   B. Every two years
   C. Every 3-4 years
   D. Every 4-5 years

D  The LHMP recommends a visual examination every 4-5 years for the middle-age adult.  (p. 401)

# 22

## CARING FOR PEOPLE UNDERGOING SURGERY

OBJECTIVES

1.0 Describe the three phases of the perioperative experience.

2.0 Discuss the roles and responsibilities of the
surgical team.

2.1 Summarize the role of the nurse during
each phase of surgery: Preoperative,
intraoperative, and postoperative.
(p. 406)

2.2 Identify and discuss the role of various
surgical team members throughout the
phases of surgery: Preoperative,
intraoperative, and postoperative.
(p. 406)

3.0 List the purposes and types of surgery.

3.1 Identify six purposes of surgery.
(p. 405)

3.2 Briefly describe the following types of
surgical intervention: Exploratory,
curative, ablative, reconstructive,
constructive, palliative, emergency,
urgent, required, imperative, elective,
and optional. (p. 406)

3.3 Briefly describe the system used to
classify or measure the degree of hazard
associated with a surgical procedure:
Major surgery and minor surgery.
(p. 406)

4.0 Describe alterations in psychophysiologic
function that result from surgery.

4.1 Identify and briefly discuss potential
psychophysiologic alterations resulting
from surgery. (p. 408)

4.2 Discuss methods of assessing factors
that may influence a person's degree of
surgical risk: Age, general health,
medications, mobility, nutritional
status, fluid and electrolyte balance,
and psychosocial condition. (p. 411)

4.3 Identify other factors that influence
the degree of surgical risk (p. 412)

TEACHING/LEARNING STRATEGIES

Clinical Laboratory Experience

Arrange for students to observe a surgical
procedure in their clinical facility. Ask them to
prepare a report on the various roles of members
of the surgical team.

Lecture/Discussion

Review the purposes for performing surgical
procedures: Diagnostic, curative, ablative,
constructive, reconstructive, and palliative.

Provide clinical examples of the different types
of surgery: Major, minor, emergency, urgent,
required, and elective.

Lecture/Discussion

Facilitate a discussion of the psychophysiologic
alterations that result from surgery. Ask them to
identify the presence of any of the alterations in
a surgical individual they have cared for in the
past.

Have students explore ways in which the purpose of
a surgical procedure can influence the reactions
displayed by an individual.

Clinical Laboratory Experience

Ask students to identify individuals in their
clinical facility who would be high risk surgical
candidates.

5.0 Discuss the developmental needs of children, adolescents, and adults undergoing surgery. Describe nursing intervention appropriate for each developmental stage.

    5.1 Identify factors that influence a person's response to surgery. (p. 407)

    5.2 Explore the impact of surgery on the holistic needs of an individual. (p. 407)

    5.3 Explore the influence of a person's developmental stage on the response to surgery. (p. 409)

6.0 Describe stress and life style alterations that can result from surgery.

    6.1 Outline appropriate nursing intervention for individuals during the extended postoperative stage. (p. 425)

7.0 Discuss the preoperative, intraoperative, and postoperative needs of the person undergoing surgery and nursing intervention and expected outcomes.

    7.1 Describe the affect surgery can have on an individual's homeostatic stress response. (p. 407)

    7.2 List factors that are of legal significance to the nurse caring for an individual during surgery. (p. 410)

    7.3 Briefly explain the purpose of obtaining an informed consent for surgery. (p. 410)

    7.4 Discuss the responsibilities of the nurse when witnessing a consent to surgery. (p. 410)

    7.5 Describe basic nursing intervention useful in assisting a person with admission to the health care facility. (p. 410)

    7.6 Identify essential sources of data to obtain when conducting a preoperative nursing assessment. (p. 410)

    7.7 List information that should be included in the health history of a person who is to undergo a surgical procedure. (p. 411)

    7.8 List and briefly describe the function of common preoperative diagnostic procedures. (p. 412)

    7.9 Discuss reasons the nurse should perform preoperative teaching to an individual before surgery. (p. 412)

    7.10 Identify specific concepts and principles related to preoperative teaching and assessment. (p. 412)

## Lecture/Discussion

Ask students to identify factors that should be taken into consideration when participating in the perioperative care of children, adolescents, and adults.

Briefly discuss the impact of personal factors on a person's response to surgery.

## Clinical Laboratory Experience

Assist students in developing a plan to prevent long-term postoperative complications for an individual in their care. Use the table listed on pages 423-424 in the text as a guide.

## Lecture/Discussion

Ask students to differentiate between the various phases of surgery: Preoperative, intraoperative, and postoperative.

Ask students to review anesthetic agents and their nursing implications listed on page 420-421 in the text.

## Campus Laboratory Experience

Have students practice the technique for preoperative removal of hair.

## Clinical Laboratory Experience

If possible, arrange for students to follow an individual throughout the entire perioperative period. Ask them to identify the individual's needs at each phase of the process.

Instruct students to identify the preoperative teaching needs of a surgical individual in their care. Ask them to develop a plan for meeting these identified needs.

Encourage students to observe the preoperative teaching performed by the nurse for an individual in their assigned clinical facility.

Have students review the forms used to document and evaluate the postanesthesia recovery of an individual in their assigned clinical facility.

## Clinical Laboratory Experience

Allow students to participate in the physical preparation of an individual going to surgery: Preoperative skin assessment, preparing the gastrointestinal tract, preparation for anesthesia, and the promotion of rest and sleep.

7.11 Discuss nursing intervention to facilitate the preparation of the gastrointestinal tract prior to surgery. (p. 416)

7.12 Identify measures that are instituted to prepare a person for anesthesia before surgery. (p. 416)

7.13 Outline nursing measures to promote rest and sleep prior to surgery. (p. 416)

7.14 Identify important intervention the nurse should carry out the day of surgery. (p. 416)

7.15 Describe the morning care of an individual the day of surgery. (p. 416)

7.16 Describe the pharmacologic action of various agents used as premedication for surgery: Sedatives, tranquilizers, narcotic analgesics, vagolytic agents, and antinausea agents. (p. 418)

7.17 Discuss the responsibilities of the individual who transports a person to surgery. (p. 418)

7.18 Describe the nurse's responsibility for care of an individual during the intraoperative phase of surgery. (p. 418)

7.19 Explain the importance of proper positioning of an individual who is to receive anesthesia. (p. 418)

7.20 Briefly discuss the pharmacologic action of the three different categories of anesthetic agents: Local, regional, and general. (p. 419)

7.21 Explain the importance of maintaining a sterile environment during surgery. (p. 419)

7.22 Summarize anesthetic agents commonly used during surgery and the nursing implications related to each. (p. 420)

7.23 Describe basic nursing care of an individual during the postoperative phase of surgery. (p. 421)

7.24 Identify precautions necessary when transporting a person from the operating room to the recovery room. (p. 421)

7.25 List assessment data that should be gathered about an individual immediately upon arrival to the recovery room. (p. 421)

7.26 Describe the basic components of a preoperative teaching plan: Deep breathing exercises, coughing exercises, extremity exercises, and movement/ambulation. (p. 413)

7.27 List nursing actions that should be carried out in preparation of a person for surgery. (p. 414)

7.28 Discuss the purpose of proper preoperative skin preparation. (p. 414)

7.29 Outline guidelines for preoperative hair removal. (p. 414)

7.30 List reasons for cleansing or emptying the gastrointestinal tract prior to surgery (p. 416)

7.31 Discuss nursing intervention measures to prevent complications during the intermediate postoperative stage. (p. 423)

7.32 Explain the purpose of immediate postoperative physician orders. (p. 422)

7.33 Discuss nursing care of an individual who has had "ambulatory surgery." (p. 422)

7.34 Describe nursing assessment and intervention activities during the intermediate postoperative phase. (p. 422)

7.35 Discuss the importance of discharge planning and teaching for an individual who has had surgery. (p. 425)

---

## MULTIPLE CHOICE QUESTIONS

## CORRECT ANSWER AND RATIONALE

1. If a person has surgery to remove a diseased gallbladder, it is called:

   A. Ablative surgery
   B. Curative surgery
   C. Diagnostic surgery
   D. Palliative surgery

   A   The purpose of ablative surgery is to remove diseased organs. (p. 406)

2. All of the following are characteristics of minor surgery except:

   A. Display a low risk for complications after the procedure
   B. Have a potential for moderate blood loss
   C. Involve uncomplicated alterations in major body organs
   D. Length of the procedure is of short duration

   C   Typically, minor surgery includes procedures that are uncomplicated, of short duration, have the potential for minimal blood loss, and involve a low degree of risk. Statement C is incorrect because it involves surgery to a major body organ, which is considered major surgery. (p. 406)

3. The phase of surgery that begins with the administration of anesthesia and terminates when surgery is complete is called the:

   A. Constructive phase
   B. Intraoperative phase
   C. Perioperative phase
   D. Surgical phase

   B   The intraoperative phase of surgery begins when anesthesia is administered and ends when the surgery is completed. (p. 406)

4. When preparing to teach an adolescent individual about an impending surgery, the nurse should understand that:

    A. Body image is very important to this age group.
    B. Separation from parents is usually the child's main concern.
    C. Fears of pain and mutilation are typical in this age group.
    D. The child should be given minimal information about any physical changes occurring as a result of surgery.

A   Adolescents are acutely aware of their physical appearance and may fear changes in body image as a result of surgery. They should be given clear explanations of any body changes that can be expected to occur as a result of surgery. (p. 409)

5. Which of the following is a true statement regarding informed surgical consents?

    A. Consent can be obtained at any point in time prior to the administration of anesthesia.
    B. Verbal consent may be given for minor surgical procedures.
    C. It is always the physician's responsibility to see that a surgical consent form has been signed prior to surgery.
    D. Surgery can be refused, even after an informed consent has been signed.

D   An individual has the right to refuse surgery, even after giving an informed consent. All other statements are incorrect because: Consent cannot be obtained if a person has received preoperative medications prior to anesthesia; consent must be in written form for both major and minor surgery; and the nurse sometimes obtains the written consent. (p. 410)

6. Which of the following individuals would be considered the greatest surgical risk?

    A. An individual taking a antihypertensive medication
    B. An obese middle-aged individual
    C. An elderly person
    D. A neonate with a respiratory dysfunction

D   Surgical risks are greatest among the very young and elderly. The neonate would display the highest risk because of its decreased capacity to endure surgical trauma and the additional respiratory problems. (p. 411)

7. Which of the following definitions is incorrect?

    A. Blood urea nitrogen - assesses urinary excretion
    B. Complete blood count - establishes blood type in the event a blood transfusion is needed
    C. Fasting blood sugar - determines metabolic disorders such as diabetes mellitus
    D. Serum electrolytes - determines electrolyte balance

B   A complete blood count determines hemoglobin, red blood cell count, and white blood cell count. A blood grouping and crossmatching determines the blood type. (p. 412)

8. The nurse should plan to teach a postoperative individual:

    A. Coughing and deep breathing exercises
    B. Leg exercises
    C. To turn in bed and ambulate early
    D. All of the above

D   Preoperative teaching should include all of the above. Coughing and deep breathing exercises will help prevent postoperative pulmonary complications. Leg exercises will help to prevent thrombophlebitis caused by postoperative venous stasis. Turning in bed and early ambulation will stimulate respiratory functioning, improve blood circulation, and reduce gastric distention. (p. 412)

9. When shaving an operative area in preparation for surgery, all of the following would be appropriate except:

    A. Lather skin well with a soap solution
    B. Shave against the direction of hair growth
    C. Stretch the skin and hold it taut
    D. Wipe excess hair and soap off with sponges

B   The nurse should shave in the direction of hair growth to prevent nicks and cuts. (p. 414)

10. A preoperative analgesic has been ordered for a person in your care. This medication is given to:

    A. Produce sedation and amnesia
    B. Provide mild relaxation and sedation
    C. Reduce the amount of anesthesia required during surgery
    D. Relax the individual and reduce anxiety

D   Narcotic analgesics are administered preoperatively to relax the individual and to reduce anxiety. A discussion of other pharmacologic medications used preoperatively appears on page 418 in the text. (p. 418)

11. Laryngeal spasm, nausea, vomiting, and hypotension are adverse effects associated with the use of which anesthetic agent?

    A. Entrance
    B. Ether
    C. Fluothane
    D. Nitrous Oxide

B   A number of adverse effects have been associated with the use of ether. These include: Laryngeal spasm, hypersecretion, postoperative nausea and vomiting, urinary retention, paralytic ileus, and hypotension. (p. 420)

12. The nurse knows that food and fluids are restricted prior to surgery to reduce the risk of:

    A. Aspiration during anesthesia
    B. Postoperative gastric distention
    C. Postoperative nausea and vomiting
    D. All of the above

D   Food and fluids are restricted eight to ten hours prior to surgery for all of the listed reasons. (p. 416)

13. All of the following nursing actions should be performed the day of surgery except:

    A. Administering morning hygienic care
    B. Asking the person to void before the preoperative medication
    C. Performing preoperative teaching
    D. Removing all jewelry and placing it in the hospital safe

C   Preoperative teaching should be performed several days prior to surgery, to allow time for individual participation and discussion. (pp. 412, 416)

14. When receiving a person in the recovery room, the nurse's initial responsibility is to:

    A. Appraise the person's respiratory status
    B. Assess the person's level of consciousness
    C. Review the postoperative orders
    D. Verify the person's identity

A   The recovery room nurse's first responsibility is to assess the individual's respiratory status. This includes; Ensuring a patent airway, preventing respiratory distress, and promoting adequate oxygen exchange. (p. 422)

15. Measures to prevent thrombophlebitis in the postoperative person would include all of the following except:

    A. Carefully massaging the lower extremities
    B. Discouraging dependent leg positions
    C. Encouraging early ambulation
    D. Increasing oral intake of fluids

A   The nurse should avoid massaging the lower extremities because it might encourage the migration of a clot to the pulmonary system. (p. 424)

16. A person experiences wound evisceration several days after abdominal surgery. The nurse's initial reaction should be to:

    A. Cover the area with sterile wet dressings
    B. Notify the physician
    C. Replace any abdominal organs that are protruding
    D. Prevent further increases in abdominal pressure

A   The eviscerated area should be covered with wet sterile dressings moistened in saline before other actions are taken. (p. 424)

17. You notice small openings in a person's suture line several days after surgery. This is correctly reported as:

    A. Dehiscence
    B. Eviceration
    C. Separation
    D. None of the above

A  Separation of the wound margins is called dehiscence. (p. 424)

# CARING FOR PEOPLE THROUGH REHABILITATION

OBJECTIVES

1.0 Discuss the basic philosophy of rehabilitation.

   1.1 Identify and briefly discuss factors that influence a person's ability to complete a rehabilitation program. (p. 432)

2.0 Discuss the role of nurses in the rehabilitation process.

   2.1 Discuss the role of the nurse in the rehabilitation process. (p. 428)

   2.2 List the potential members of the rehabilitation team and their principal functions. (p. 429)

   2.3 Briefly describe activities of the nurse in the rehabilitation setting. (p. 432)

3.0 Make useful nursing assessment of people requiring rehabilitation.

   3.1 Identify information that should be obtained during the nursing assessment of an individual receiving rehabilitation care. (p. 430)

4.0 Develop nursing care plans (with supervision) for people requiring rehabilitation.

   4.1 Outline appropriate nursing intervention to maintain normal body functioning in a person requiring rehabilitative care. (p. 434)

   4.2 Formulate appropriate nursing diagnoses for the health problems of people with disabilities. (p. 430)

   4.3 Identify factors that influence the plan of care for an individual requiring rehabilitative care. (p. 430)

   4.4 Outline long- and short-term goals of nursing care that can be utilized for individuals with rehabilitation needs. (p. 430)

TEACHING/LEARNING STRATEGIES

### Lecture/Discussion

Ask students to identify agencies in their community whose primary purpose is assisting the disabled person.

### Lecture/Discussion

Facilitate a discussion of the potential members of the rehabilitation team and their principal functions.

Discuss the various roles of the nurse in the rehabilitation process: Advocate, coordinator, and care-giver.

### Guest Speaker

Invite a professional nurse working in rehabilitation nursing to class to discuss their role in the rehabilitation process.

### Clinical Laboratory Experience

Assist students in interviewing disabled individuals within the community. What major lifestyle changes has their disability caused?

### Written Exercise

Given hypothetical situations, ask students to create a nursing plan of care for a person requiring rehabilitation.

4.5 Discuss the impact a person's developmental life stage can have on the rehabilitation process. (p. 431)

4.6 Explore nursing intervention effective in dealing with a person's response or reaction to a disability. (p. 432)

4.7 Describe criteria used to evaluate the effectiveness of a rehabilitation program. (p. 439)

5.0 Initiate appropriate environmental and equipment adaptation for people with disabilities.

5.1 Outline guidelines that can be used to prevent complications in an individual receiving rehabilitative care. (p. 431)

5.2 Identify essential teaching/learning needs of individuals receiving rehabilitative care. (p. 431)

5.3 Discuss the role of discharge planning and vocational rehabilitation for a person who is completing a rehabilitation program. (p. 435)

## Class Activity

Solicit volunteers to visit local community agencies for the disabled. Ask them to identify the populations served and the types of services rendered. Have them report their findings in class.

## Clinical Laboratory Experience

Arrange for students to observe a discharge planning session for a rehabilitation person returning to the community.

---

## MULTIPLE CHOICE QUESTIONS

1. Rehabilitation is best described as a process that:

   A. Assists the handicapped person to achieve total independence
   B. Assists a person to use their abilities
   C. Maximizes a person's capabilities and minimizes their limitations
   D. Restores a person to their previous level of health

   C   Rehabilitation focuses on the use of a person's capabilities, thereby minimizing their limitations. (p. 427)

2. The occupational therapist's primary role of the rehabilitation team is to:

   A. Assist the person in the development of skills necessary for daily living
   B. Assist with job placement of handicapped individuals
   C. Evaluate the self-care capabilities of the rehabilitated individual
   D. Test individuals for vocational aptitudes, skills, and interests

   A   The occupational therapist's role in the rehabilitation process is to develop functional living skills, e.g. activities of daily living, household maintenance, and child care. (p. 429)

3. If the nurse plans and supervises the daily activities of a rehabilitation person, they are functioning in which of the following roles?

   A. Advocate
   B. Coordinator
   C. Liaison
   D. Supervisor

   B   The role of the nurse coordinator is to plan and cooperate the overall schedule of activities for the rehabilitation person on a daily basis. (p. 429)

SITUATION: Mr. Hopkins, who is engaged in a cardiac rehabilitation program, expresses great concern about his ability to resume sexual concerns after discharge from the hospital. He states, "I sure don't want to have another attack!" Questions 4 through 6 relate to this situation.

4.  Based on this information, the nurse might make which of the following nursing diagnoses?

    A.  Ineffective coping related to lack of knowledge and fear of health problem recurrence.
    B.  Knowledge deficit regarding sexual capabilities after myocardial infarction
    C.  Physiologic changes in sexual response cycle due to change in body image
    D.  Sexual dysfunction: Change in belief about sexual capabilities related to fear of health problem recurrence

C  Mr. Hopkins is obviously concerned that sexual activity may provoke another MI. He is associating activity with the disease process, therefore, option C is the best response. (p. 438)

5.  The nurse's best response to this person would be:

    A.  "Do you feel that your recent heart attack was brought on by sexual activity?"
    B.  "I'm sure that your physician would be happy to discuss this issue with you."
    C.  "You shouldn't worry about that right now."
    D.  "You're afraid that sexual activity might cause another heart attack."

D  Option D encourages the person to continue the conversation. (p. 438)

6.  All of the following assessment data could be used to evaluate Mr. Hopkins's success in a progressive exercise program except:

    A.  Diastolic BP no greater than 85
    B.  Free from symptoms
    C.  Pulse no greater than 100 or less than 60
    D.  Systolic BP no greater than 140 or less than 90

C  The pulse rate after exercise can vary from 100 to 50 beats per minute. (p. 438)

7.  The most effective way to teach a paralyzed person self-catheterization would be:

    A.  Demonstration
    B.  Diagrams
    C.  Programmed media instruction
    D.  Return demonstration

D  Skills are most effectively learned by demonstration and practice. In this instance, the person would probably benefit from return demonstration. (p. 434)

8.  The nurse should plan to begin discharge planning for a rehabilitation person:

    A.  Several weeks before the scheduled discharge
    B.  The day that they enter the rehabilitation facility
    C.  When all short-term rehabilitation goals have been accomplished
    D.  When the physician writes a preliminary discharge order

B  Discharge planning begins upon admission for the rehabilitation person. All activities are geared toward their usefulness at home. (p. 435)

# ASSESSING AND PROMOTING A POSITIVE HEALTH CARE ENVIRONMENT

## OBJECTIVES

1.0 Describe factors composing a therapeutic environment for people requiring nursing care.

    1.1 List factors that should be considered when assessing the environment of a Health Care Facility. (p. 444)

    1.2 Outline the use of the nursing process in the admission of a person to a Health Care Facility. (p. 445)

    1.3 Identify factors that influence an individual's adaptation to the hospital environment. (p. 455)

    1.4 Describe nursing intervention designed to promote a person's adaptation to the hospital environment. (p. 456)

2.0 Apply the nursing process to promoting physical safety and comfort for people requiring nursing care.

    2.1 Identify important personal assessment data that should be gathered about a person when planning to ensure proper planning for a safe and therapeutic environment. (p. 444)

    2.2 Identify health care recipients who may have an increased risk of injuries due to falls. (p. 446)

    2.3 Briefly discuss nursing interventions that can be utilized to prevent falls in home environments adapted for care and in health care facilities. (p. 447)

    2.4 Identify factors contributing to development of thermal injuries within the health care environment. (p. 448)

    2.5 Discuss the important precautions the nurse should take with administering heat for therapeutic purposes. (p. 448)

    2.6 Identify factors that influence the hospitalized person's feelings of psychosocial safety and comfort. (p. 451)

    2.7 Identify nursing interventions that promote psychosocial safety and comfort in the hospitalized person. (p. 451)

## TEACHING/LEARNING STRATEGIES

### Lecture/Discussion

Discuss factors that influence the degree of anxiety experienced by a person entering a hospital facility.

If students in the class have experienced hospitalization, ask them to voluntarily share their feelings upon admission and during the hospital period. Encourage them to explore measures that would have been useful in increasing their comfort level.

### Lecture/Discussion

Discuss factors that influence the comfort level felt by hospitalized individuals: Room temperature, room humidity, room light, noise, and contamination. Describe important nursing implications for each factor.

### Clinical Laboratory Experience

Ask students to identify hospitalized persons who they feel are more susceptible to accidents. Have them devise measures to prevent the occurrence of accidents in each identified situation.

3.0 Apply the nursing process to promoting psychosocial safety and comfort for people requiring nursing care.

## Lecture/Discussion

Focus discussion on the factors influencing a hospitalized person's psychosocial safety and comfort: Personal control, personal loss, emotional support, external factors, and sensory disturbances. Ask students to identify the important nursing implications for each factor.

4.0 Plan environmental modifications appropriate to an individual's age, sensory status, mobility status, belief system preference, sociocultural background, health care needs, and personal preference.

    4.1 Discuss environmental adaptations that can be made to provide optimal physical safety and comfort for a person. (p. 446)

## Lecture/Discussion

Ask students to identify ways in which they could adapt the hospital environment to meet the individual needs of persons in their care.

## Group Activity

Divide students into small groups. Ask each group to explore the impact of one of the following on the promotion of a positive health care environment: Age, sensory status, mobility status, belief system preference, health care needs, and personal preferences. Have them identify special nursing implications for each. Allow each group to make a brief oral presentation.

5.0 Recognize and list environmental comfort hazards and plan practical means to reduce or alleviate them.

    5.1 Discuss the safety needs of the nurse working in a health care environment. (p. 446)

    5.2 Identify environmental factors that influence a person's comfort level in the Health Care Facility. (p. 449)

    5.3 Briefly discuss the impact environmental room temperature can have on a person's comfort level. (p. 449)

    5.4 Identify ways in which the nurse can modify the environmental temperature to promote individual comfort. (p. 450)

    5.5 Briefly describe the influence room humidity can have on a health care recipient's level of comfort. (p. 450)

    5.6 Discuss nursing intervention useful in maintaining an appropriate room humidity level. (p. 450)

    5.7 Discuss the importance of monitoring room light and noise levels to ensure the comfort of hospitalized individuals. (p. 450)

    5.8 Discuss measures that would be effective in the maintenance of appropriate light and noise levels in a hospital environment. (p. 450)

## Clinical Laboratory Experience

Ask each student to assess the health care environment of a person in their care. Instruct them to include in this assessment: External environmental factors, safety factors, psychosocial factors, and microbial factors. If problems are identified, ask to describe ways in which the safety of the environment could be enhanced.

6.0 Recognize and list environmental safety
    hazards and plan practical means to reduce or
    alleviate them.

    6.1 Identify a variety of safety hazards
        that may be present in health care
        environments. (p. 446)

    6.2 Identify areas within the Health Care
        Facility that display a higher risk for
        the development of fires. (p. 448)

    6.3 Outline measures that should be used in
        health care environments to reduce the
        possibility of fire. (p. 448)

    6.4 Outline the responsibilities of the
        nurse in the event of a fire in a Health
        Care Facility. (p. 448)

    6.5 Identify sources of chemical injury
        commonly present in health care
        environments. (p. 448)

    6.6 List common guidelines that should be
        used to care for medications stored
        within the Health Care Facility.
        (p. 449)

    6.7 Identify major causes and effects of
        electric shock in a health care
        environment. (p. 449)

    6.8 Discuss ways of reducing the potential
        for electric shock injuries in the
        health care environment. (p. 449)

    6.9 Identify the impact functioning
        microwave equipment can have on a person
        with a pacemaker. Describe nursing
        measures to alleviate the occurrence of
        these problems. (p. 449)

    6.10 Describe nursing measures to prevent
        injuries associated with the therapeutic
        use of x-rays and radioactive
        substances. (p. 449)

7.0 Describe basic principles for assessing and
    promoting microbial safety for people
    requiring nursing care.

    7.1 Identify potential sources of
        contamination in a Health Care
        Facility. (p. 451)

    7.2 Identify measures to reduce the
        possibility of contamination in the
        Health Care Facility. (p. 451)

    7.3 Identify essential information to obtain
        when assessing the microbial safety of
        the hospital environment. (p. 453)

    7.4 Discuss the importance of using proper
        handwashing techniques when working in a
        health care environment. (p. 453)

## Lecture/Discussion

Have students list the major causes of hospital
fires. Facilitate a discussion on how these
hazards can be prevented.

## Guest Speaker

Invite a local hospital safety control officer to
class to discuss their role in promoting a
positive health care environment.

## Clinical Laboratory Experience

Instruct students to identify the safety needs of
a person in their care. Incorporate this need
into the nursing plan of care for the individual.

## Lecture/Discussion

Discuss measures that could be used within the
hospital to prevent the occurrence of nosocomial
infections.

## Campus Laboratory Experience

Have students demonstrate proper handwashing
technique.

7.5 Briefly discuss interventions that promote the microbial safety of a health care environment. (p. 453)

    7.6 Outlines the steps in the chain of infection. (p. 453)

    7.7 Identify the basic characteristics of each link in the infection chain: infectious agent, reservoir, portal of exit, mode of transmission, portal of entry, and susceptible host. (p. 454)

    7.8 Describe ways of weakening links in the infection chain. (p. 454)

    7.9 List nursing situations that demand effective handwashing. (p. 455)

    7.10 Outline guidelines for effective handwashing. (p. 455)

---

## MULTIPLE CHOICE QUESTIONS

1. A recently hospitalized person appears restless and uncomfortable. Which of the following factors would contribute most to the person's apparent anxiety?

   A. Has recently been told that the hospital stay will be indefinite
   B. Third hospitalization in the past year
   C. Scheduled for major surgery in one week
   D. Significant others able to visit only twice a week because they live 75 miles away

A All of the listed factors could contribute to the person's anxiety, but the fact that they are told that the hospital stay will be longer than expected is most significant. (p. 445)

2. Measures that would be useful in the creation of therapeutic hospital environment include all of the following except:

   A. Altering the intensity of room lighting according to planned activities
   B. Maintaining the room temperature between 20 to 22 C
   C. Positioning persons away from windows to avoid outside light
   D. Offering quiet, piped in music to promote rest and relaxation

C Whenever possible, the person should have a window facing outside, so they can see natural day to night cycles. This facilitates the person's level of orientation. (p. 449)

3. On several occasions, Mrs. First has attempted to get out of bed to a portable bedside commode, barely escaping injury each time. Which of the following nursing actions would be the most useful in this situation?

   A. Give Mrs. First a call light to summon for assistance and remove the commode from the room
   B. Position the commode close to the bed, so Mrs. First doesn't have to walk so far
   C. Place the commode across the room to discourage further unassisted attempts
   D. Tell Mrs. First that she must not use the commode without assistance

A Since Mrs. First has made several attempts to get out of the bed to the portable commode without assistance, it is probably best to remove the commode from the room and give her a viable means of obtaining assistance. (p. 446)

4. Which of the following individuals is least likely to experience an injury due to falls? The person who:

A. Is normally hypotensive
B. Is receiving continuous intravenous infusions
C. Has been confined to bed for one week
D. Wears corrective eyeglasses

D   The individual wearing eyeglasses would display the least potential for injury, as their vision problem has been corrected. Other individuals are still at risk for falls because the factors that have increased their risk have not been eliminated. (p. 446)

5. The nurse's first responsibility in the event of a fire is to:

A. Call for assistance from other health personnel
B. Notify the local fire department
C. Remove individuals in immediate danger
D. Use a fire extinguisher on the fire

C   The nurse's primary responsibility when a fire is noticed is to remove all individuals that are in immediate danger. Assistance then should be obtained and a fire extinguisher used on the fire. (p. 448)

6. The pharmacy at your hospital labels all medications by their generic names. If a physician orders a medication by a trade name you are unfamiliar with, how should you select the correct medication?

A. Call the physician and ask for the generic name
B. Consult another more knowledgeable nurse
C. Contact the pharmacy and request the alternate name
D. Obtain the generic name from available drug text resources

D   The nurse should attempt to utilize available resources. If unable to obtain the information in this way, the pharmacy should then be contacted. (p. 449)

7. When performing any treatment or procedure, the nurse should always:

A. Explain all necessary information in understandable terms
B. Proceed in a calm, professional manner
C. Protect the person's dignity by using curtains, screens, and drapes when appropriate
D. All of the above

D   All listed actions should be used by the nurse to assure an individual's comfort during special procedures and treatments. (p. 452)

8. A person in your care has an autoimmune disorder that makes him more susceptible to infection. To reduce the spread of microorganisms to this person, the nurse should:

A. Clean exposed room surfaces frequently with antiseptic agents
B. Practice good handwashing technique before administering care
C. Provide care for this person before caring for others
D. All of the above

B   The single, most effective way the nurse could prevent the spread of microorganisms to this person would be to use careful handwashing technique. A disinfectant could be used to clean exposed surfaces in the room; antiseptics are used on living tissue. (p. 453)

9. Which of the following is the best definition of medical asepsis?

A. Measures used to eliminate all microorganisms
B. Measures used to reduce the number of microorganisms and prevent their spread
C. Practices used to render a person free of all microorganisms
D. Techniques used to prevent infection

B   Medical asepsis refers to those practices aimed at controlling and reducing the number of microorganisms. (p. 453)

10. If a person acquires an infection while hospitalized, it is most appropriately referred to as a:

    A. Clinical infection
    B. Community-acquired infection
    C. Hospital-acquired infection
    D. Nosocomial infection

D   Infections acquired while staying in the hospital are called nosocomial infections. (p. 455)

11. After changing the dressing on an infected wound, you carefully dispose of contaminated articles in an appropriate manner. Your actions are aimed at weakening which link in the "infection chain?"

    A. Infectious agent
    B. Mode of transmission
    C. Portal of exit
    D. Reservoir

C   The proper disposal of dressings and wound coverings intercepts the "chain of infection" at the portal of exit. (p. 454)

# 25

# INFECTION CONTROL: MEDICAL ASEPSIS

## OBJECTIVES

1.0 Describe the historical development of the prevention and control of infections.

 1.1 Briefly discuss the historical development of measures to promote control of infection. (p. 460)

 1.2 Describe the role of Ignaz Semmelweis in the development of infection control and prevention measures. (p. 460)

2.0 Describe the "chain of Infection."

 2.1 Outline typical body responses to the exposure to infectious agents. (p. 461)

 2.2 Identify and briefly describe sources of infection. (p. 461)

 2.3 Define the terms: Pathogen, infectious agent, and normal flora. (p. 461)

 2.4 Discuss variables that influence the virulence of a microorganism. (p. 461)

 2.5 Identify factors that influence a person's risk or probability for the development of an infection. (p. 462)

 2.6 Identify areas of the body that contain normal bacterial flora. (p. 463)

 2.7 Identify normal bacterial flora commonly found within various human body sites. (p. 463)

 2.8 List common infectious agents (pathogens) that may be found in various human body sites. (p. 463)

 2.9 Explain the etiology of nosocomial infections. (p. 646)

 2.10 Describe the links in the chain of infection (p. 464)

 2.11 Identify microorganisms that display a great potential for producing infection. (p. 464)

 2.12 Identify sources or reservoirs that promote the reproduction of microorganisms. (p. 464)

## TEACHING/LEARNING STRATEGIES

### Lecture/Discussion

Facilitate a discussion of the historical factors that have influenced the present infection control practices of today.

### Guest Speaker

Invite the hospital quality assurance nurse in each clinical facility to a postconference period to discuss their role in the preventing and controlling infection within the hospital environment.

### Lecture/Discussion

Ask students to identify the most common organisms causing disease. Assist them in exploring the factors that influence a microorganism's ability to produce disease.

Discuss factors that increase a person's susceptibility to infection. Ask students to identify ways to strengthen the body's barriers to infection.

### Written Exercise

Ask students to outline the stages in the infectious disease process. Have them outline nursing measures used to break the chain of infection at each stage.

Instruct students to identify environmental factors that contribute to the growth of microorganisms. Ask them to formulate a plan for reducing these environmental hazards.

### Class Activity

Ask two students to volunteer to visit a local community health department. Ask them to review the statistics for the incidence of communicable disease in their area. Have them present their findings in class. Afterwards, facilitate a class discussion on the measures that could be used to reduce the occurrence of communicable diseases.

2.13 Identify common portals of exit by which
      microorganisms may exit the body.
      (p. 465)

2.14 Briefly discuss four major ways in which
      infectious agents are transmitted from
      reservoirs. (p. 465)

2.15 Identify portals used by infectious
      agents to enter the body of susceptible
      hosts. (p. 465)

2.13 Identify common portals of exit by which
      microorganisms may exit the body.
      (p. 465)

2.14 Briefly discuss four major ways in which
      infectious agents are transmitted from
      reservoirs. (p. 465)

2.15 Identify portals used by infectious
      agents to enter the body of susceptible
      hosts. (p. 465)

3.0  Behave in ways that reduce risks of
     transmitting infectious agents.

     3.1  Describe risk factors that increase a
          person's risk of contracting a
          nosocomial infection while hospitalized
          (p. 464)

     3.2  Discuss the nurse's role in interrupting
          the transmission of potentially
          infectious agents from one person to
          another. (p. 467)

4.0  Plan, implement, and evaluate nursing care
     using sound principles of infection
     prevention and control.

     4.1  Discuss intervention used to control and
          eliminate infectious agents. (p. 464)

     4.2  Describe the impact drug-resistant
          microorganisms can have on intervention
          designed to control infection. (p. 462)

     4.3  Describe strategies that are commonly
          employed to eliminate reservoir sites
          that encourage the reproduction of
          microorganisms. (p. 464)

     4.4  Discuss measures used to eliminate
          environmental reservoirs that harbor
          microorganisms. (p. 465)

     4.5  Identify mechanical barriers that
          protect a potential host from the
          development of an infection. (p. 466)

     4.6  Discuss nursing intervention to reduce
          the susceptibility of a host to
          infection. (p. 466)

     4.7  Identify major body defenses used to
          protect a person from the development of
          an infection, should mechanical barriers
          fail. (p. 466)

## Lecture/Discussion

Discuss factors that should be considered by the
nurse when choosing a roommate for a person
requiring isolation.

## Communication Activity

Ask a student to volunteer to interview a local
health inspector regarding the health inspection
of local restaurants. Ask them to obtain
information on the assessment criteria used during
the inspection. Allow them to share their
findings in class.

## Lecture/Discussion

Ask students to give examples of people with
infectious diseases that should not be transported
from their rooms. Have them identify appropriate
measures for transferring other individuals with
infections within the health care environment.

## Clinical Laboratory Experience

Have students obtain information of the procedure
used to handle the postmortem bodies of individuals
with infection in their clinical facility. Ask
them to share their findings in class.

4.8 Outline nursing activities to prevent and control the transmission of infectious agents. (p. 466)

4.9 Identify essential data to be gathered by the nurse when planning intervention to prevent and control the transmission of infectious agents. (p. 466)

4.10 Summarize the proper care and handling of soiled equipment and supplies: Needles, dishes, trash, thermometers, linen, and laboratory specimens. (p. 470)

4.11 Outline guidelines for transporting an individual with an infection outside of the isolation environment. (p. 471)

4.12 Describe daily cleaning procedures that should be used to care for isolation environments. (p. 471)

4.13 Discuss the postmortem care of an infected body upon death. (p. 471)

5.0 Implement specific isolation precautions.

5.1 Explain the role of various isolation systems in the prevention and control of the transmission of infectious agents. (p. 467)

5.2 Briefly discuss two types of isolation systems that are used to combat infection: Category specific and disease-specific. (p. 467)

5.3 Identify common features of the various isolation precaution procedures. (p. 467)

5.4 Summarize category-specific isolation precautions as formulated by the Centers for Disease Control: Strict, contact, respiratory, AFB, enteric, drainage/secretion, and blood/body fluid precautions. (p. 469)

5.5 Discuss the role of gowns, masks, and isolation carts in various isolation procedures. (p. 469)

5.6 Identify factors that are taken into consideration when selecting a roommate for a person requiring isolation. (p. 470)

6.0 Use gloves, gowns, and masks effectively and appropriately while providing nursing care.

7.0 Describe the psychosocial reactions that often accompany infections.

7.1 Describe nursing assessment and intervention techniques useful in assisting a person with psychosocial aspects of infection control. (p. 471)

## Campus Laboratory Experience

Demonstrate nursing procedures for donning gloves, gowns, and masks. Afterwards allow each student to practice the techniques.

## Clinical Laboratory Experience

Have students review the isolation cart used in their clinical facility.

Allow students to participate in the care of person on isolation precautions. In the clinical postconference period ask them to share the precautions taken in the care of each person.

## Lecture/Discussion

Focus discussion on the psychosocial implications of care for the individual requiring isolation.

7.2 Identify educational needs of persons
    requiring isolation for infectious
    processes.  (p. 472)

8.0 Teach others about infection prevention and
    control.

Written Exercise

Instruct students to outline guidelines for
teaching other individuals about the infectious
process.

---

## MULTIPLE CHOICE QUESTIONS

1. Which of the following does not belong in the
   group?

   A. Cross-contamination
   B. Cross-transmission
   C. Colonization
   D. Transmission of infectious agents

2. A pathogen is:

   A. A microorganism that causes disease
   B. An infectious agent
   C. A substance capable of producing disease
   D. All of the above

3. Which of the following statements is false?

   A. A person's normal bacterial flora can
      cause an infection
   B. A person's normal bacterial flora cause
      infection only if body immune defenses
      are compromised
   C. Certain areas of the body have abundant
      microorganisms or normal flora
   D. Normal bacterial flora are part of the
      body's natural defense mechanism

4. Which of the following individuals displays
   the greatest risk for the development of an
   infection?

   A. A person receiving care in the
      physician's office
   B. A health college student
   C. AN acutely ill person who has been
      hospitalized
   D. A terminally ill person being cared for
      at home

5. "Normal flora" commonly found in the bladder
   and upper urinary tract, include all of the
   following except:

   A. Enterobacter species
   B. Escherichia coli
   C. Staphylococcus aureus
   D. Streptococcus faecalis

6. Nosocomial infections occur more often in
   hospitalized individuals who:

   A. Are experiencing severe illness
   B. Are taking antimicrobials or other drugs
   C. Have treatment devices inserted into
      normally sterile body areas
   D. All of the above

## CORRECT ANSWER AND RATIONALE

C  Items A, B, and D are all terms used to
   describe the process of transmitting
   infectious disease from one person to
   another.  (p. 459)

D  Options A, B, and C represent both the
   historical and current day definitions of a
   pathogen.  (p. 461)

B  The body's normal bacterial flora can produce
   an infection if the body's immune defenses are
   compromised, or if they migrate to a body area
   where they are not normally found.  (p. 461)

C  The microorganism present in hospitals are
   often more virulent, or more drug-resistant
   than those generally found in other types of
   care facilities or the community.  (p. 462)

C  Staphylococcus aureus are normally found only
   in the following areas:  Skin, hair, and
   perineal skin areas.  (p. 463)

D  All of the listed factors contribute to the
   development of nosocomial infections in the
   hospital environment.  (p. 464)

7. Which of the following statements about antimicrobial agents is false?

   A. Antimicrobial agents reduce infection by destroying "sensitive" microorganisms
   B. Antimicrobials can become ineffective against certain pathogens
   C. Drug resistant microorganisms are easily treated with other available antimicrobial agents
   D. Antimicrobial agents can reduce the body's normal bacterial flora

C  Drug-resistant microorganisms are a serious treatment problem since some microorganisms become resistant to all available drugs and the resultant infection cannot be treated or controlled. (p. 464)

8. Nursing measures used to disrupt the chain of infection at the infectious agent link, include:

   A. Administering antimicrobial agents as ordered for individuals experiencing infection
   B. Removing visible dust, soils, and foreign material from an individual's health care environment
   C. Using disinfectants to clean inanimate objects in the person's health care environment
   D. Wearing gloves when handling any substance excreted by the body

D  The nurse creates a barrier to the transmission of disease at the infectious link by: Using disinfectants, antiseptics, antimicrobial drugs, and by using proper handwashing techniques. Gloves are used to disrupt the mode of transmission link. (p. 465)

9. Isolation techniques are initiated by the nurse to disrupt the infection chain at which link?

   A. Infectious agent
   B. Portal of exit
   C. Reservoir
   D. Transmission

D  Isolation techniques (handwashing, use of gloves and gowns) can be initiated to prevent the transmission of disease. (p. 465)

10. The nurse plays an important role in the prevention of infection at the portal of entry by:

   A. Exercising measures to prevent any breaks in the skin or integument
   B. Properly handling all body substances
   C. Using clean technique when the skin is not intact
   D. All of the above

A  In order to prevent the introduction of pathogens to the body through a portal of entry, the nurse should institute measures to protect the body's defenses and utilize good handwashing techniques. (p. 465)

11. As you examine Mrs. Peters, you notice redness, swelling, and warmth at her peripheral IV site. This is correctly reported as:

   A. Congestion
   B. Edema
   C. Infection
   D. Inflammation

D  Redness, swelling, warmth, and pain are classic examples of inflammation. (p. 467)

12. If an individual is admitted to the hospital with acquired immunodeficiency syndrome, which type of isolation precautions should be initiated?

   A. AFB precautions
   B. Blood and body fluid precautions
   C. Drainages and secretion precautions
   D. Enteric precautions

B  AIDS necessitates the use of blood and body fluid precautions since this is the primary mode of transmission for the disease. (p. 469)

13. The nurse should always wear a gown when caring for an individual with:

A. Chickenpox
B. Measles
C. Meningitis
D. Rubella

A   Gowns should be worn by all persons entering the room of a person who has been placed on strict isolation. Strict isolation is used specifically for pharyngeal diphtheria, chickenpox, and zoster. The nurse should wear a gown when caring for a person with rubella, only if soiling is likely. (p. 468)

14. Nurses have failed to use appropriate isolation technique when they:

A. Changes gloves after handling potentially contaminated drainage
B. Covers the nose and mouth with a mask before entering the isolation room
C. Practices appropriate aseptic measures when removing all articles from the isolation room
D. Removes an isolation gown immediately after leaving an isolation room

D   Articles worn in an isolation room should be discarded prior to exit from the room. (p. 468)

15. Before transferring a person with respiratory isolation precautions to another area in the hospital, the "receiving" staff should be asked to wear:

A. Gloves
B. Gowns
C. Masks
D. None of the above

C   Masks are necessary for those who come close to an individual with a respiratory disorder requiring isolation precautions. (p. 468)

16. You begin to notice signs of sensory deprivation in a four-year-old child who has been placed on isolation precautions. Which of the following activities would not be beneficial in reducing sensory deprivation in a child of this age?

A. Being read to
B. Craft projects and number games
C. Creative drawing and painting activities
D. Listening to records and rhythmic play

B   Craft projects and number/letter games are usually enjoyed by the older, school-age child. (p. 283, 471)

# 26

# INFECTION CONTROL: SURGICAL ASEPSIS

## OBJECTIVES

1.0 Explain the differences between medical asepsis and surgical asepsis.

    1.1 Describe the major differences in medical and surgical asepsis. (p. 475)

2.0 List procedures during which surgical asepsis is necessary.

    2.1 Identify situations that demand the use of sterile techniques. (p. 475)

    2.2 Briefly describe the rationale for using sterile technique with immunosuppressed individuals. (p. 476)

    2.3 Identify special procedures that do not require the use of sterile technique. (p. 476)

3.0 Explain the difference between disinfection and sterilization. Describe different methods of sterilization and list indications for each method.

    3.1 Discriminate between the various methods used to prepare sterile equipment: Sterilization, disinfectants, and antiseptics. (p. 476)

    3.2 Identify disinfectant agents that are commonly used to destroy microorganisms in health care settings. (p. 477)

    3.3 Outline the procedure for cleaning and disinfecting equipment in preparation for sterilization. (p. 478)

    3.4 Identify methods for cleaning and disinfecting equipment at home. (p. 478)

    3.5 Describe, using examples, two basic types of sterilants: Physical and chemical. (p. 478)

    3.6 Identify variables that determine the length of the sterilization process. (p. 479)

## TEACHING/LEARNING STRATEGIES

### Lecture/Discussion

Focus discussion on the nurse's responsibility in the practice of surgical asepsis.

### Written Exercise

Ask students to prepare a list of the similarities and differences that exist between medical and surgical aseptic practices. Ask them to share the information in class.

### Lecture/Discussion

Ask students to identify the reasons it would be important to observe sterile aseptic practices in the following: Surgical procedures, bladder catheterization, administration of injections and IV's, dressing changes, care of people with burns, and eye treatments.

### Lecture/Discussion

Discuss special precautions that should be taken when using various disinfecting agents.

Summarize the advantages and disadvantages of the various types of sterilization procedures.

### Clinical Laboratory Experience

Ask students to review the specific recommendations for cleaning and disinfecting procedures listed in their clinical facilities Infection Control Manual.

Arrange for students to visit the area in their clinical facility where reusable supplies are cleaned and disinfected or sterilized.

3.7 Discuss the function of sterilization
    indicators. (p. 479)

3.8 List and briefly describe the three
    types of sterilization indicators
    commonly used in hospitals. (p. 479)

3.9 Summarize basic methods of
    sterilization. Discuss the advantages
    and disadvantages of each approach.
    (p. 479)

3.10 List factors that indicate sterile
     equipment contamination. (p. 480)

3.11 Discuss the nurse's role in the
     disinfection and sterilization
     processes. (p. 480)

4.0 Explain and demonstrate how to set up a
    sterile field.

    4.1 Briefly describe a sterile field.
        (p. 480)

    4.2 Describe steps that must be taken to add
        supplies to an existing sterile field.
        (p. 480)

    4.3 Outline basic guidelines that the nurse
        should follow for the maintenance of a
        sterile field. (p. 481)

5.0 Demonstrate the procedure for donning and
    removing sterile gloves.

    5.1 Identify situations in which sterile
        gloves would be necessary or
        appropriate. (p. 484)

    5.2 List the steps involved in correctly
        donning sterile gloves. (p. 486)

    5.3 Outline steps in the procedure for
        removal of contaminated gloves. (p. 486)

6.0 List the basic principles of sterile
    technique and explain the rationale behind
    each principle.

    6.1 Describe the proper technique that the
        nurse should use when handling sterile
        supplies. (p. 482)

    6.2 Identify five precautions that should be
        taken by the nurse when handling sterile
        liquids. (p. 482)

    6.3 Identify the essential components of
        proper surgical attire. (p. 486)

7.0 Discuss the professional, psychosocial,
    legal, and financial implications of
    infection caused by careless technique when
    performing sterile procedures.

## Campus Laboratory Experience

Ask students to practice the following sterile
techniques with a classmate in the campus
laboratory setting: Establishing and maintaining
a sterile field; adding sterile supplies; handling
sterile supplies; surgical handwashing procedure;
and donning surgical gloves and other attire.

## Written Exercise

Have students outline the educational needs of a
person undergoing treatments requiring surgical
asepsis.

7.1 Discuss the nurse's role in the
infection control process. (p. 476)

8.0 Demonstrate the method for performing a
surgical scrub.

8.1 List general steps to be followed for a
surgical scrub. (p. 484)

**Campus Laboratory Experience**

Demonstrate the technique for performing a
surgical scrub. Allow students to practice the
procedure.

---

## MULTIPLE CHOICE QUESTIONS

1. Which of the following best describes the
concept of sterile asepsis?

    A. Activities designed to prevent infection
    in the sterile environment
    B. Measures used to render and maintain
    objects, areas, and body tissues free of
    all microorganisms
    C. Practices used to render and keep an
    environment free of microorganisms
    D. The absence of all disease-producing
    microorganisms in the environment

2. The nurse is not required to use sterile
technique when performing which of the
following procedures?

    A. Eye treatments
    B. Enemas
    C. Intramuscular injections
    D. Urinary catheterization

3. The boiling time for disinfecting an article
must be increased at elevations greater than
sea level because:

    A. Microorganisms are more resistant at
    higher elevations
    B. Normal boiling time may only render the
    article clean, not sterile
    C. Sterilization takes longer at higher
    elevations
    D. Water boils at a high temperature at sea
    level than it does at high elevations

4. When performing a sterile procedure, the
nurse should:

    A. Always check the sterilization indicator,
    as it assures sterility
    B. Always wear a mask
    C. Avoid the outer 1/2 inch of the sterile
    field, as it is considered contaminated
    D. Refrain from crossing over the sterile
    field

## CORRECT ANSWER AND RATIONALE

B   Sterile asepsis, or technique, is described as
those methods used to eliminate all microorganisms from objects, areas, and body
tissues. (p. 475)

B   Sterile technique is used during procedures in
which skin or mucous membranes are broken,
resulting in access to blood vessels. It is
also used when performing a procedure in or on
any sterile body part. (p. 475)

D   Altitude is an important factor that must be
considered by the nurse when boiling supplies
for disinfection purposes. Water boils at a
higher temperature at sea level than it does
at higher elevations. Boiling an article in
water may render it clean, but not sterile.
(p. 478)

D   When a non-sterile object is held above a
sterile object, gravity causes microorganisms
to fall onto the sterile field. (p. 481)

5. Why must the nurse keep all items above waist or table level when performing a sterile procedure?

    A. A larger percentage of microorganism are found below this level
    B. Items held lower are out of full view and cannot be guaranteed sterile
    C. Proximity to contaminated materials makes sterility doubtful
    D. The area below the waist is contaminated with microorganisms

B    Waist level and table level are considered margins of safety that can be uniformly enforced and that promote maximum visibility of objects. (p. 481)

6. Which of the following methods can be used to sterilize objects that are rubber, plastic, or heat sensitive?

    A. Autoclaving
    B. Ethylene oxide gas
    C. Quaternary ammonium compounds
    D. Radiation

B    Ethylene oxide gas is usually used to sterilize delicate plastic or rubber objects that cannot tolerate exposure to heat. Options C and D are methods of disinfection, not sterilization. (p. 479)

7. The nurse may add sterile items or liquids to a sterile field by:

    A. Applying clean gloves and then transferring the sterile item onto the sterile field
    B. Dropping the sterile item onto the field directly from its package
    C. Grasping the sterile item by an edge and then transferring it to the sterile field
    D. Picking up the sterile item with clean forceps and placing it carefully onto the sterile field

B    All items (gloves, forceps) must be sterile if they are to contact other sterile items. (p. 481)

8. When performing a surgical hand scrub, all of the following are correct <u>except</u>:

    A. Cleaning nails and cuticles with a plastic or orangewood stick
    B. Rinsing so that the water flows toward the hands
    C. Turning the hand-controlled faucets off with a sterile towel
    D. Scrubbing the hands for five minutes or more with an antimicrobial soap

B    The hands should be held higher than the elbows and away from the body during the scrub, so that the water flows toward the elbows. This allows the water to flow from the cleanest area to the least cleanest area. (p. 484)

9. When applying sterile gloves, which of the following would be <u>incorrect</u>?

    A. Grasping the first glove by the folded edge of the cuff
    B. Grasping the second glove by the top edge of the cuff
    C. Moving misplaced fingers into place after both gloves have been applied
    D. Maintaining sterility by allowing only sterile glove surfaces to touch

B    The second glove is donned by inserting the gloved, sterile hand underneath its cuff. Only the inside of the sterile cuff is to be touched. (p. 485)

# 27

# APPLYING EFFECTIVE BODY MECHANICS TO PREVENT INJURY

OBJECTIVES

1.0 Discuss basic principles of body mechanics as they relate to normal body alignment and body movement.

    1.1 Discuss the meaning of "correct body alignment." (p. 488)

    1.2 Enumerate the basic characteristics of an individual standing in a position of correct body alignment. (p. 488)

    1.3 Identify factors useful in assessing an individual's physical condition/energy expenditure. (p. 492)

    1.4 Discuss the importance of using a consistent approach in moving a person who needs assistance with body mechanic maneuvers. (p. 493)

    1.5 List basic nursing assessment guidelines that should be considered prior to moving other individuals. (p. 493)

    1.6 Describe the procedure for determining the amount that can be safely lifted by a health care provider. (p. 493)

2.0 Move effectively, efficiently, and safely.

    2.1 Outline guidelines that should be used to promote effective body movement. (p. 488)

3.0 List problems that can occur if effective body mechanics are not used while moving people.

    3.1 Identify care recipient problems that are caused by the improper use of body mechanics by the health care team. (p. 491)

    3.2 Identify and briefly describe care provider problems caused by the improper use of body mechanics: injury, pain, stress, and fatigue. (p. 492)

    3.3 Explore the nurse's legal responsibility/accountability for injuries caused an individual by the use of poor body mechanic techniques. (p. 492)

4.0 Avoid personal injury by using effective body mechanics while moving people.

TEACHING/LEARNING STRATEGIES

Lecture/Discussion

Have students outline basic guidelines used to promote effective body mechanics.

Campus Laboratory Experience

Ask a student to demonstrate a position of correct body posture.

Campus Laboratory Experience

Ask students to critique each others' performance of correct body mechanic techniques when practicing the skills listed in this chapter.

Lecture/Discussion

Focus discussion on the specific injuries that can be sustained by the nurse who uses poor body mechanics.

5.0 Apply the nursing process when moving people.

    5.1 Formulate appropriate nursing diagnoses for individuals with physical mobility problems. (p. 493)

    5.2 List basic nursing goals of care for individuals requiring assistance with basic body mechanic maneuvers. (p. 493)

    5.3 Identify criteria that can be used to evaluate the response of an individual to body mechanic maneuvers. (p. 494)

**Lecture/Discussion**

Ask students to identify ways in which each specific step of the nursing process is used to assure effective body mechanics and prevent injury when performing the skills in this chapter.

6.0 Perform emergency carries for helpless people.

    6.1 State the purpose for employing emergency carries. (p. 494)

    6.2 Identify basic contraindication/cautions the nurse should be aware of prior to moving a person with an emergency carry technique. (p. 494)

    6.3 Discuss activities of the nurse useful in preparing a person for an emergency carry. (p. 494)

    6.4 Outline the basic steps involved in moving a person in an emergency situation: Blanket carry, pack-strap carry, and swing carry. (p. 494)

**Campus Laboratory Experience**

Demonstrate emergency carry technique: Blanket-drag, pack-strap carry, and the swing-carry methods. Afterwards, divide students into small groups and allow them to practice each technique.

7.0 Move helpless people in bed and between bed and chair.

    7.1 Briefly state the reason for employing special techniques to move a helpless person in bed. (p. 497)

    7.2 Discuss the contraindications and precautions that should be considered when moving a helpless person in bed. (p. 497)

    7.3 Discuss the preliminary actions of the nurse who plans to move a helpless person in the bed. (p. 497)

    7.4 Identify steps the nurse should take to prepare a helpless person for a move in bed. (p. 497)

    7.5 State the steps involved in moving a helpless person up in bed and to the side of bed. (p. 500)

    7.6 State the definition and purpose of the procedure for transfer of a helpless person from bed to stretcher. (p. 501)

    7.7 Identify major contraindications and precautions related to transfer of a helpless person from bed to stretcher. (p. 501)

**Campus Laboratory Experience**

Demonstrate nursing procedures for moving a helpless person up in bed and moving a helpless person to the side of the bed. Allow students time to practice both techniques.

Demonstrate and then give students time to practice the technique used to assist a person with one-sided weakness in transferring from the bed to a chair or wheelchair.

In the campus laboratory facility, have a group of students demonstrate the procedure transferring a helpless person from the bed to the stretcher: Three-person carry and the draw sheet transfer methods. Have all other students practice the techniques when the demonstration is complete.

Provide a demonstration of the procedure used to transfer a person from the bed to a chair or wheelchair. Allow time to practice this skill.

Demonstrate the technique used to assist a person with one-sided weakness to sit on the side of the bed. Have students practice this skill.

Ask two students to demonstrate the procedure for assisting a person to dangle on the side of the bed. Instruct all students to practice this technique with a classmate.

7.8 Identify the teaching/learning needs of
a helpless person who is to be assisted
in moving from bed to stretcher.
(p. 501)

7.9 Describe preliminary nursing activities
used to prepare a helpless person for
transfer from bed to stretcher. (p. 501)

7.10 Outline the proper sequence of steps for
a three-person carry transfer of a helpless individual from bed to stretcher.
(p. 502)

7.11 Discuss nursing activities that must be
performed upon completion of the
transfer of a helpless individual from
bed to stretcher. (p. 505)

7.12 State the purpose of using a planned
technique to assist a person to sit on
the side of the bed. (p. 505)

7.13 Identify contraindications and cautions
the nurse should consider before
assisting a person to dangle on the side
of the bed. (p. 505)

7.14 Identify the educational needs of a
person who is to receive assistance in
dangling on the side of the bed.
(p. 505)

7.15 Describe the preliminary activities of
the nurse who plans to assist a person
to dangle on the side of the bed.
(p. 505)

7.16 Identify essential steps involved in
assisting a person to sit on the side of
the bed. (p. 505)

7.17 Identify important nursing
responsibilities that should be carried
out after assisting a person to dangle
on the side of the bed. (p. 507)

7.18 Describe the nursing procedure for
assisting people with one-sided weakness
to sit on the side of the bed. (p. 507)

7.19 Briefly describe the transfer of an
individual from bed to chair or
wheelchair. (p. 514)

7.20 Explore basic contraindications and
precautions the nurse should take into
consideration before assisting a person
from the bed to chair or wheelchair.
(p. 514)

7.21 Discuss preliminary activities the nurse
should perform in preparing to assist a
person in transfer from bed to chair or
wheelchair. (p. 514)

7.22 List the equipment needed by the nurse
to transfer a person from the bed to a
chair or wheelchair. (p. 514)

7.23 Outline the basic steps involved in
assisting a person from the bed into a
chair or wheelchair. (p. 515)

7.24 Describe the responsibilities of the nurse upon completion of a person transfer from bed to chair or wheelchair. (p. 516)

7.25 Outline the steps involved in a procedure designed to assist a person with one-sided weakness to transfer from the bed to a chair or wheelchair. (p. 517)

8.0 Use various mechanical lifts.

8.1 Briefly describe mechanical lifts that can be used to assist in an individual transfer: Hoyer mechanical lift and Surgilift. (pp. 509, 512)

8.2 Discuss various reasons for using mechanical lifts to assist in an individual transfer. (pp. 509, 512)

8.3 Describe contraindications and precautions the nurse should be aware of when using mechanical lifts to assist in person transfer. (pp. 509, 512)

8.4 Discuss the teaching/learning needs of individuals who are to be transferred using a mechanical lift. (pp. 509, 512)

8.5 Describe preliminary activities of a nurse who plans to move a person with a mechanical lift. (pp. 509, 512)

8.6 Identify the equipment that should be gathered by the nurse in order to transfer a person with a mechanical lift. (pp. 509, 512)

8.7 Discuss the final activities of a nurse who has transferred a person with a mechanical lift. (pp. 512-513)

9.0 Avoid personal injury when lifting objects from the floor.

9.1 Briefly discuss alternate methods a person can use to pick up objects from the floor. (p. 519)

9.2 Explore basic contraindications and cautions related to the procedure for picking up objects from the floor. (p. 519)

9.3 Identify the educational needs of a person who is being taught alternate methods for picking up objects from the floor. (p. 519)

9.4 List steps involved in alternate methods of picking up objects from the floor. (p. 519)

**Campus Laboratory Experience**

Have students view a demonstration of the techniques used to transfer individuals using Hoyer and Surgilift mechanical lifts. Allow students to practice this either in the clinical or campus laboratory.

**Campus Laboratory Experience**

Demonstrate alternate methods that the nurse can use to pick up objects from the floor. Provide time for practice of these skills.

1. Which of the following assessment data indicates poor body alignment in a person that is standing upright?

   A. Arms fall at side with the elbows slightly flexed
   B. Knees are slightly flexed
   C. Head is erect and slightly flexed
   D. Lower abdomen is pulled in and up

C    The head should appear erect, not leaning backward, or sideways. (p. 488)

2. When preparing to transfer a person from the bed to a stretcher, the nurse knows that all of the following basic body mechanic principles are true except:

   A. A wide base of support will give stability to the body
   B. More force is required to pull or push an object, than to lift it
   C. Objects placed near the lifter's center of gravity require less force to lift
   D. No movement will be possible if the load exceeds the force

B    It requires considerable more force to lift an object than it does to push or pull it. Lifting requires overcoming gravity. (p. 491)

3. Knowledge of good body mechanics will enable the nurse to:

   A. Avoid personal injury often sustained from poor lifting and moving techniques
   B. Move the person with minimal discomfort
   C. Properly explain the procedure to promote the individual's cooperation
   D. All of the above

D    All statements are correct. The use of proper body mechanics can eliminate numerous problems for both the person and the nurse. (p. 491)

4. Which of the following nurses is most likely to sustain a personal injury due to use of improper body mechanics? The nurse who:

   A. Lowers the head of the bed before attempting to move an individual up in bed
   B. Moves a slightly overweight individual up in bed without assistance
   C. Uses back muscles to lift and turn an individual
   D. Uses personal body weight to assist in lifting and turning

C    When lifting a person or object, the nurse should use the larger muscles of the legs and thighs rather than the smaller muscles of the back. This protects the intervertebral discs, which can be damaged when sudden or extreme force is exerted on them. (p. 490)

5. A nurse who weighs 140 pounds can safely lift:

   A. 49 pounds
   B. 70 pounds
   C. 75 pounds
   D. 140 pounds

A    It is recommended that a nurse not lift more than 35 per cent of the individual's body weight. In this situation, the amount is calculated as follows: 140 x 0.35 = 49 pounds. (p. 493)

SITUATION: A fire has erupted on your hospital unit. You are alone and must move all individuals in immediate danger to a place of safety. Questions 6 through 8 apply to this situation.

6. The most effective one-person carry technique in an emergency situation is the:

   A. Blanket drag
   B. Pack-strap carry
   C. Piggyback carry
   D. Shoulder carry

A    The blanket drag is the most efficient or useful one-person carry technique in an emergency situation. This method permits the transfer of individuals who are of heavier weight. It takes less energy to pull or slide a person than it does to lift them. (p. 494)

7. You are aware that you need assistance in moving all of the following individuals except:

A. A person using an artificial respirator
B. An extremely obese individual
C. A person with a recent spinal cord injury
D. A person who is paralyzed from a stroke

D    Emergency carry techniques are contraindicated in persons with spinal cord injuries or who are using respiratory aides. Several helpers may be required to move an extremely obese individual. (p. 494)

8. Other hospital personnel arrive to assist you, and soon all individuals on the unit have been moved to safety. What observations provide the basis for an objective observation of the your success?

A. All individuals were moved without injury
B. No complaints of discomfort were received during or following the moves
C. You experience no pain or discomfort during or following the moves
D. All of the above

D    All of the listed options should be used to evaluate the use of proper body mechanic techniques when transferring a person via one of the emergency carry techniques. (p. 494)

9. When planning to assist a person with moving, the nurse should first assess the person's:

A. Comfort level
B. Ability to follow directions
C. Physical size and reasons for the move
D. Tolerance of past moves

C    Upon entering the individual's room, the nurse should initially assess the person's size and the specific reason why they are being moved. Other data can be more efficiently gathered, once this information has been obtained. (p. 492)

10. When two nurses move a dependent person up in bed, the person's legs are flexed to:

A. Allow proper placement of the nurse's arms
B. Improve the person's center of gravity
C. Reduce friction on the bed during movement
D. Reduce the dragging effect of straight legs

D    The legs produce a dragging effect if left in a straight position when transferring a person up in bed. (p. 498)

11. Mr. Baker remains slightly sedated upon return from surgery. How many people will be needed to transfer this person from the stretcher into the bed using the lift and slide technique?

A. Two to three
B. Three
C. Three to four
D. Four

C    Three or four people are required to transfer a person via the lift and slide technique. (p. 501)

12. If a person experiences an extreme drop in blood pressure when changing from a lying to a sitting or standing position, it is called:

A. Hypotension
B. Orthopnea
C. Orthoptic hypotension
D. Postural hypotension

D    Postural hypotension occurs when a person moves from a lying position to a standing or sitting position. (p. 507)

13. The nurse can help minimize the effects of orthostatic hypotension by:

A. Advising gradual position changes
B. Encouraging leg exercises before getting out of bed
C. Remaining with the individual after assisting them to sit or stand
D. All of the above

D    All of the listed actions would help minimize the effects of orthostatic hypotension. (p. 507)

14. When assisting a person with left-sided weakness to transfer from the bed to a wheelchair, the nurse should place the wheelchair:

    A. At the head of the bed
    B. Behind the individual
    C. On the person's stronger side
    D. On the same side as the weakness

C  The wheelchair should be placed on the person's stronger side, as this allows them to pivot with the stronger leg. (p. 514)

# ASSESSING PULSE, RESPIRATION, AND BLOOD PRESSURE

## OBJECTIVES

1.0 Describe internal and external factors that influence vital signs.

    1.1 Describe the components of the cardiac cycle, asystole and diastole. (p. 528)

    1.2 Briefly discuss the homeostatic response of the heart to internal and external stressors. (p. 528)

    1.3 Explain the processes of internal and external respiration. (p. 534)

    1.4 List conditions that might cause a decreased level of oxygen in arterial blood. (p. 534)

    1.5 Identify factors that affect an individual's respiratory rate. (p. 535)

    1.6 Briefly explain the physiology of arterial blood pressure. (p. 538)

    1.7 Identify physiological factors that influence the level of arterial pressure. (p. 539)

2.0 State the normal values of pulse, respiration, and blood pressure, including the normal variations with age, sex, time of day, and activity.

    2.1 Briefly discuss two components of the normal heart beat, $S_1$ and $S_2$. (p. 531)

    2.2 Describe the influence of age and sex on the normal pulse rate. (p. 532)

    2.3 Outline changes that occur in the respiratory rate as a result of age. (p. 536)

    2.4 Discuss factors that influence normal variations in the average blood pressure reading: Genetic predisposition, sex, race, circadian rhythm, exercise, and position. (p. 539)

## TEACHING/LEARNING STRATEGIES

### Lecture/Discussion

Ask students to identify major factors that affect body pulse, respiration, and blood pressure.

### Class Activity

Ask students to monitor the pulse, respiration, and blood pressure of two different aged individuals. Have them discuss in class the differences in the values obtained.

### Group Activity

Ask students to pair into groups of two. Instruct one student to run in place for one full minute and the other student to take the pulse, respiration, and blood pressure before and after the exercise. Have students share their findings in class.

3.0 Perform the techniques of measuring vital signs accurately, including appropriate explanation to the individual and significant others.

3.1 Identify the two most common sites for routine pulse assessment in children and adults. (p. 528)

3.2 Identify the anatomical placement of various pulse sites: Radial, apical, temporal, carotid, femoral, popliteal, dorsalis pedis, and posterior tibial. (p. 528)

3.3 Describe the mechanism for obtaining the pulse rate in infants. (p. 528)

3.4 Explain the procedure for obtaining both apical and radial pulses. (p. 531)

3.5 Outline the procedure for measuring the pulse deficit. (p. 533)

3.6 Explain the procedure for assessing respirations. (p. 535)

3.7 List the standard equipment used when taking a blood pressure. (p. 540)

3.8 Describe two types of sphygmomanometers: Mercury manometer and aneroid manometer. (p. 540)

3.9 Outline guidelines that should be used in selection of proper blood pressure cuff sizes. (p. 541)

3.10 State the correct procedure for measuring an individual's blood pressure according to the following methods: Auscultory and palpatory. (p. 541)

3.11 State the correct procedure for obtaining blood pressure readings in the lower extremities. (p. 542)

3.12 Identify individuals who might require blood pressure measurement in the lower extremities. (p. 541)

3.13 Identify situations in which measurement of brachial pulses would be contraindicated. (p. 542)

3.14 State the correct procedure for assessing blood pressure in infants and children. (p. 544)

3.15 Discuss alternate methods of blood pressure measurement that may be used with children and infants: Doppler method and flush method. (p. 544)

3.16 Identify common sources of error that occur in blood pressure measurement. (p. 545)

## Lecture/Discussion

Focus discussion on the qualitative data used to assess the pulse: Rate, rhythm, force or quality; and elasticity of the vein wall.

Discuss the educational needs of an individual who is having their pulse, respiration, or blood pressure monitored.

## Campus Laboratory Experience

In the campus laboratory setting, ask students to identify common sites used to assess pulse.

Demonstrate the procedures for taking a person's pulse rate, respiration rate, and blood pressure. Ask students to practice this skill in the campus and clinical laboratory settings.

## Clinical Laboratory Experience

Have students monitor the vital signs of an assigned individual in clinical. Ask them to evaluate their findings in relation to the established norms for that age individual.

4.0 Distinguish normal from abnormal vital sign
data, considering individual characteristics
and the current physical and emotional state.

4.1 State the formula that should be used by
the nurse to determine accurate pulse
rates. (p. 532)

4.2 Define the terms, tachycardia and
bradycardia, and explain the
physiological mechanisms influencing the
development of each. (p. 533)

4.3 Identify common disorders/conditions
that cause tachycardia and bradycardia.
(p. 533)

4.4 Identify essential data to be considered
when obtaining/evaluating "routine"
vital signs. (p. 527)

4.5 Define the meaning of pulse deficit and
pulse quality. (p. 533)

4.6 Identify situations in which the nurse
might expect to find changes in the
normal pulse quality. (p. 534)

4.7 Discuss the physiological processes that
govern or control the act of respiration. (p. 535)

4.8 Briefly describe measures used to assess
the quality of an individual's
respirations. (p. 536)

4.9 Define dyspnea and describe data
indicative of this condition. (p. 536)

4.10 Describe four types of noisy
respirations: Stretor, stridor, wheeze,
and sigh. (p. 536)

4.11 Describe the character of specific
alterations in respiratory status:
Tachypnea, bradypnea, hypoventilation,
apnea, hyperpnea, and hyperventilation.
(p. 536)

4.12 Briefly describe abnormal patterns of
respiration: Cheyne-Stokes, Biot's,
Kussmaul's, and apneustic. (p. 537)

4.13 Briefly discuss assessment data
indicative of hypoxia. (p. 538)

4.14 Identify individuals who display a
greater risk or potential for the
development of abnormal blood pressure
levels. (p. 545)

4.15 Differentiate between hypotension and
hypertension. (p. 545)

4.16 List individual conditions that might
cause hypotension. (p. 545)

4.17 Identify individual conditions that
might produce hypertension. (p. 545)

## Lecture/Discussion

Discuss the qualitative data used to assess a
person's respiratory status: Rate and depth,
pattern of respiration, and significant physical
characteristics.

Explore the impact of a person's physical and
emotional state on the vital sign status.

## Written Exercise

Instruct students to outline the normal ranges for
pulse, respiration and blood pressure for
individuals throughout the developmental process.

5.0 Interpret data as they fit into each person's clinical picture, validating data when necessary, and communicating results to appropriate persons.

    5.1 Identify an individual's situations demanding routine assessment of all superficial pulses. (p. 528)

    5.2 List individual's situations in which it would be necessary to obtain an apical pulse, instead of a peripheral pulse. (p. 528)

    5.3 Briefly discuss instances in which the nurse might encounter pulse rhythm irregularities. (p. 533)

    5.4 Identify nursing responsibilities in relation to assessment/discovery of premature heart beats or irregularities. (p. 533)

    5.5 Briefly discuss the three-point scale used to document pulse quality. (p. 534)

    5.6 Identify individuals that would require continuous assessment of their respiratory status. (p. 535)

    5.7 Discuss the nurse's responsibility in communication and management of significant blood pressure readings. (p. 546)

    5.8 Demonstrate the ability to correctly record vital signs on the graphic sheet or narrative nursing record. (p. 547)

### Lecture/Discussion

Have students identify situations in which the pulse, respiratory status, and blood pressure should be monitored.

Have students identify the situations in which they would be required to report a person's vital signs to another health team member.

### Clinical Laboratory Experience

Provide an example of the different forms used in each clinical agency used by the students. Demonstrate the procedure for using each form correctly. Allow time for students to practice using the form for their specific clinical agency.

6.0 Use vital sign data in the assessment step of the nursing process, and plan appropriate intervention.

    6.1 Understand the importance of taking "routine" vital signs as an integral part of the nursing process. (p. 527)

    6.2 Explain the role of "routine" vital sign measurement in the assessment phase of the nursing process. (p. 527)

    6.3 Identify teaching/learning needs of an individual who will be required to monitor their blood pressure at home. (p. 542)

    6.4 Outline a teaching/learning program to instruct an individual in home monitoring of their blood pressure. (p. 543)

    6.5 Describe equipment that can be used to monitor the vital signs of critically ill individuals continuously and accurately: Cardiac monitor, doppler, ultrasonic flowmeter, arterial lines for direct BP measurement, and central venous pressure cathetors. (p. 546)

### Lecture/Discussion

Encourage a discussion of appropriate nursing measures that can be used when encountering a person with an altered vital sign status.

### Guest Speaker

Invite a person from the local chapter of the American Heart Association to speak in class on the role their agency assumes in the prevention of cardiovascular related diseases.

### Clinical Laboratory Experience

Ask students to incorporate vital sign activity into the assessment process for assigned individuals each week in the hospital.

1.  A person's vital signs should be monitored:

    A.  As often as their condition warrants
    B.  As ordered by the physician in the
        clinical record
    C.  Routinely every four hours
    D.  Upon admission and then every eight hours

A   Vital signs should be gathered by the nurse as
    often as deemed necessary.  (p. 527)

2.  When assessing Mr. Shaver's vital signs, you
    notice that his radial pulse is slightly
    irregular.  Which nursing action should you
    perform first?

    A.  Auscultate the apical pulse
    B.  Record your findings in the chart
    C.  Retake the radial pulse for one full
        minute
    D.  Notify the physician

C   The nurse should initially retake the radial
    pulse for one full minute, then use a
    stethoscope to auscultate the radial pulse.
    (p. 532)

3.  During cardiopulmonary resuscitation, the
    nurse can best assess the adequacy of blood
    perfusion by palpating the:

    A.  Brachial pulse
    B.  Carotid pulse
    C.  Femoral pulse
    D.  Radial pulse

C   The nurse can evaluate the circulation to the
    legs and the adequacy of perfusion during CPR
    by palpating the femoral pulse.  (p. 528)

4.  Which of the following statements related to
    the assessment of vital signs in an adult is
    false?

    A.  If the pulse or respiratory rate are
        abnormal, they should be counted for one
        full minute.
    B.  The pulse rate should be counted for 15
        seconds and multiplied times four.
    C.  The respiratory rate should be counted
        for 15 seconds and multiplied times four.
    D.  None of the above.

C   The respiratory rate is most accurately
    obtained by counting the rate for 30 seconds
    and multiplying times two.  (p. 535)

5.  Which condition stimulates the act of
    breathing in a healthy individual?

    A.  Anoxia
    B.  Hypercarbia
    C.  Hypoxemia
    D.  Acidosis

B   For most individuals, the normal stimulus to
    breathe is due to an increase of carbon
    dioxide in the blood, or hypercarbia.  (p. 535)

6.  Mr. Ford appears tired and anxious after a
    short walk in the hallway.  He tells the
    nurse that he "can't catch his breath."  This
    is correctly reported as:

    A.  Apnea
    B.  Dyspnea
    C.  Hyperpnea
    D.  Kussmaul's breathing

B   Dyspnea is defined as difficult, labored, or
    painful breathing.  (p. 536)

7.  A nurse might expect to see all of the
    following in an individual with hypoxia
    except:

    A.  Decreased blood pressure
    B.  Confusion and lethargy
    C.  Decreased pulse rates
    D.  Increased pulmonary ventilation

C   Hypoxemia is characterized by mental
    confusion, impaired motor function, increased
    pulse rates, increased respiratory rates, and
    an increased blood pressure.  Prolonged
    hypoxia may produce diaphoresis, loss of
    consciousness, and hypotension.  (p. 538)

8. When monitoring Mr. Hill's blood pressure, you are unsure of the point at which you heard the first sound. You should:

A. Deflate the cuff and attempt a measurement in the other arm.
B. Deflate the cuff to zero and immediately attempt to take the reading again.
C. Deflate the cuff to zero and wait 30 to 60 seconds before taking the BP again.
D. Reinflate the cuff and listen carefully for the first sound again.

C  The nurse should deflate the cuff to zero and wait 30 to 60 seconds before taking the reading again. (p. 543)

9. The nurse knows that hypertension is commonly seen in all of the following conditions except?

A. Acute myocardial infarction
B. Atherosclerosis
C. Kidney disease
D. Obesity

A  The blood pressure normal decreases in an individual experiencing an acute myocardial infarction in response to a decreased cardiac output. (p. 545)

10. When using a mercury manometer to measure a person's blood pressure, the nurse should do all of the following except:

A. Center the arrow marking on the cuff over the brachial artery
B. Palpate the radial artery and inflate the cuff to the point where the pulsation disappears
C. Release the cuff at an even rate of 2mmHg per heart beat
D. Wrap the cuff evenly around the arm, with the lower edge 2.5 to 5 cm above the brachial artery pulsation.

B  The cuff should be inflated 20 to 30mmHg above the point at which the radial pulsation disappears. If the cuff is not inflated high enough, the true systolic pressure may be missed. (p. 542)

# ASSESSING AND MAINTAINING BODY TEMPERATURE

OBJECTIVES

1.0 Convert the following temperature readings from one scale to the other: 34°C, 103°F, 110°F, 42°C.

    1.1 List two scales that are presently used to measure core body temperature. (p. 555)

    1.2 State the formula for converting/ obtaining Celsius and Fahrenheit equivalents. (p. 556)

2.0 Describe how the body normally produces and loses heat.

    2.1 Discuss the relationship between metabolism and heat production. (p. 552)

    2.2 Define metabolic rate. (p. 552)

    2.3 List five factors that increase the metabolic rate. (p. 552)

    2.4 Discuss, using examples, the four modes of thermolysis by which the body eliminates excess heat: Radiation, conduction, convention, and evaporation. (p. 552)

    2.5 Differentiate between a homeothermic and a poikilothermic animal. Give an example of each. (p. 553)

    2.6 Discuss the way in which the body exchanges heat to maintain a constant body temperature. (p. 552)

    2.7 Explain the way in which homeothermic animals regulate body temperature. (p. 554)

3.0 Cite internal and external variables that influence body temperature.

    3.1 Understand temperature regulation as a homeostatic body process. (p. 552)

    3.2 Identify variables that influence the effectiveness of body thermolysis. (p. 552)

    3.3 Discuss factors that affect normal body temperature (p. 555)

    3.4 Explain the effect of environmental temperature on body temperature (p. 555)

TEACHING/LEARNING STRATEGIES

Lecture/Discussion

Review the formulas used to convert temperature readings from Fahrenheit to Centigrade and Centigrade to Fahrenheit. Allow time for students to practice using each formula.

Written Exercise

Instruct students to write a brief summary of the body's thermoregulatory mechanisms and the mechanisms by which each operate.

Instruct students to outline the changes that occur in other body systems as a result of hypothermia and hyperthermia.

Lecture/Discussion

Facilitate a discussion of the factors that affect body temperature: Age, Circadian or diurnal rhythm, temperature variances of different body parts, hormonal effect, and stress.

Ask students to identify factors that can influence the development of abnormal body temperatures.

Class Activity

Ask students to compare their own body temperature at different times throughout the day.

3.5 Identify measures to promote temperature homeostasis in newborns. (p. 556)

3.6 Identify factors that cause higher body temperatures in infants and children. (p. 556)

3.7 Identify factors that cause lower body temperature in the elderly. (p. 556)

4.0 Describe the role of the hypothalamus in body temperature regulation.

5.0 Explain behavioral regulation of body temperature.

5.1 Explore the effects of circadian and diurnal rhythms on core body temperature (p. 556)

6.0 Cite the consequences of thermoregulatory breakdown.

6.1 Briefly explain the consequences of thermoregulatory failure. (p. 554)

7.0 Describe the nursing assessment of individuals with normal temperatures and of those with altered temperatures.

7.1 Define "normal" body temperature. (p. 555)

8.0 Explain the differences in the physiologic mechanisms leading to fever and those leading to heat-related disorders.

8.1 Identify factors that may cause abnormal elevations in body temperature. (p. 557)

8.2 List three heat related disorders that may cause abnormal elevations in body temperature. (p. 557)

8.3 Define malignant hypothermia and state its probable cause. (p. 557)

9.0 Discuss the etiology of fevers.

9.1 Differentiate between the following: Low-grade fever, high-grade fever, remittent fever, and fever of undetermined origin. (p. 557)

9.2 Briefly discuss the etiology of fever. (p. 558)

10.0 Describe the controversy underlying the treatment of fever.

## Lecture/Discussion

Ask students to identify individuals who are most at risk for problems with temperature maintenance.

## Lecture/Discussion

Focus discussion on the etiology and stages of fever. Emphasize assessment data that should be gathered when caring for a person throughout the stages of fever.

Have students identify ways in which fever can be described. Ask them to identify clinical examples of each.

11.0 Outline nursing intervention during the three stages of fever.

    11.1 Describe the natural course of fever in three stages: Onst, febrile, and defervescence. (p. 558)

    11.2 Identify nursing assessment data that should be gathered during each stage of fever. (p. 558)

    11.3 Describe basic nursing intervention useful in assisting persons with problems associated with fever elevation. (p. 559)

12.0 Discuss assessment and interventions for the following alterations in body temperature: (a) heat cramps, heat exhaustion, and heat stroke; (b) malignant hyperthermia; (c) hypothermia; and (d) frostbite

    12.1 Explain physiological changes induced by various heat-related disorders: Heat cramps, heat exhaustion, and heat stroke. (p. 560)

    12.2 Outline appropriate nursing intervention for individuals suffering from heat cramps, heat exhaustion, and heat stroke. (p. 560)

    12.3 Identify individuals who are at high risk for the development of a heat-related disorder. (p. 560)

    12.4 Discuss teaching/learning needs of individuals who possess a higher risk for the development of heat-related disorders. (p. 560)

    12.5 Describe the etiology of malignant hyperthermia (p. 561)

    12.6 Discuss the emergency care of an individual suffering from malignant hyperthermia. (p. 561)

    12.7 List the potential pathophysiology underlying hypothermia and give examples of each: Excessive heat loss, diminished heat production, and impaired thermoregulation. (p. 561)

    12.8 Differentiate between accidental, spontaneous and induced hypothermia. (p. 561)

    12.9 Identify clinical signs indicative of a hypothermic condition. (p. 562)

    12.10 List actions the nurse might take to assist a person who is experiencing hypothermia. (p. 562)

    12.11 List actions the nurse might take to assist a person who is experiencing hypothermia. (p. 562)

## Lecture/Discussion

Ask students to identify appropriate nursing measures for management of the person with a fever.

## Lecture/Discussion

Provide clinical examples of conditions that produce hypothermia/hyperthermia.

Explore nursing intervention measures useful in assisting individuals with heat-related disorders: Heat cramps, heat exhaustion, and heat stroke.

## Written Exercise

Ask students to identify data that should be included in the assessment of a person with an abnormally low body temperature. Have students plan appropriate nursing intervention for the person with hypothermia.

Have students list the clinical signs and symptoms of hypothermia and hyperthermia.

12.12 Briefly describe ways that health teaching can prevent hypothermia (p. 562)

12.13 Identify factors that may contribute to the development of frostbite. (p. 562)

12.14 Explain the physiological causes of frostbite. (p. 562)

12.15 List assessment data indicative of frostbite. (p. 562)

12.16 Plan appropriate nursing intervention for individuals experiencing frostbite. (p. 563)

12.17 Outline appropriate strategies for the prevention of frostbite. (p. 563)

13.0 Monitor oral, rectal, and axillary temperatures using mercury, electronic, and chemical dot disposable thermometer.

13.1 Identify equipment used to evaluate/ measure core body temperature. (p. 555)

13.2 Identify advantages and disadvantages of using a glass thermometer for temperature measurement. (p. 563)

13.3 Identify individuals in whom oral temperature measurement would be contraindicated. (p. 564)

13.4 Identify common thermal monitoring devices and describe the use of each. (p. 564)

13.5 Briefly describe the procedure for common temperature monitoring methods: Oral, rectal, and axillary. (p. 565)

13.6 Identify factors that influence the method of temperature measurement. (p. 565)

13.7 Describe alternate methods of temperature measurement. (p. 570)

13.8 Identify the recommended frequency for temperature monitoring (p. 570)

14.0 Recognize and document an abnormal temperature reading.

15.0 Recognize when a body temperature abnormality requires immediate intervention by the health care team.

## Campus Laboratory Experience

Ask students to pair into groups of two. Instruct students to monitor each other's temperatures after the ingestion of a cold beverage and a hot beverage.

Have students take their own oral temperature at different locations in the mouth. Ask them to report their findings in class.

## Clinical Laboratory Experience

As a part of a clinical experience, have students demonstrate the correct procedure for obtaining a person's temperature.

Demonstrate the techniques used to monitor temperature by each of the following methods: Oral, rectal, and axillary.

## Clinical Laboratory Experience

Ask students to review the graphic temperature records for a person in the clinical record. Encourage a discussion of why these values fluctuate.

1.  What is the Centigrade reading for an oral temperature of 100.4° Fahrenheit?

    A.  37°
    B.  36.6°
    C.  36°
    D.  None of the above

D   The formula for converting Fahrenheit temperatures to their respective Centigrade reading is as follows: $(5/9)(T_F - 32°)$. The correct answer for this situation is 38°C. (p. 556)

2.  A physician has ordered a hypothermic cooling blanket for a person with hyperthermia. This measure will promote heat loss via which of the following mechanisms?

    A.  Conduction
    B.  Convection
    C.  Evaporation
    D.  Radiation

B   Conduction of heat takes place between objects that are in direct contact with one another. (p. 553)

3.  Which of the following individuals would be least likely to experience hypothermia?

    A.  An alcoholic
    B.  An elderly individual
    C.  An obese person
    D.  A paralyzed person

C   The obese person would be least likely to experience hypothermia because of the insulating nature of fat. All other individuals would display an increased tendency for the development of hypothermia. (p. 552)

4.  If a person's oral temperature is 100.4°F., it is correctly referred to as a:

    A.  Fever
    B.  Low-grade fever
    C.  Recrudescent fever
    D.  None of the above

A   A fever is an elevation in body temperature beyond what is normal for the individual. This situation does not indicate how long the temperature has been elevated; therefore, it cannot be called a low-grade fever. (p. 557)

5.  During the first stage, or onset, of fever, the nurse might expect to see all of the following except:

    A.  Complaints of "feeling cold"
    B.  Flushing of the skin
    C.  Increased pulse rate
    D.  Shivering

B   Due to peripheral vasoconstriction during the first stage of fever, the skin could appear pale. (p. 558)

6.  John's oral temperature has suddenly risen to 103°F. Appropriate nursing actions at this time would include all of the following except:

    A.  Administering acetominophen
    B.  Alcohol sponge baths
    C.  Cool baths
    D.  Fanning

A   The nurse would need to obtain a physician's order to administer acetominophen. (p. 559)

7.  A family member experiences heat exhaustion. What should your initial nursing response be?

    A.  Have the person lie down and rest
    B.  Increase oral intake of fluid and salt
    C.  Immerse the person in an ice bath
    D.  Move the person to a cooler area

D   You should immediately move the person to a cooler location to prevent further elevation of body temperature. Options A and B should be instituted next. An ice bath is sometimes prescribed for an individual who has suffered a heat stroke. (p. 560)

8.  Mr. Phillips was recently admitted to the hospital for extensive burns received in an automobile accident. As a nurse, you are aware that Mr. Phillips may experience hypothermia in response to:

    A.  Diminished heat production
    B.  Excessive heat loss
    C.  Impaired thermoregulation
    D.  Ineffective temperature regulators

B   A person with extensive loss of skin surface due to burns will be unable to maintain body temperature because of excessive heat loss. (p. 561)

9.  Oral temperature measurement would be contraindicated in which of the following individuals? A person who is:

    A.  Receiving oxygen via a nasal cannula
    B.  Seizure prone
    C.  To have oral surgery in the A.M.
    D.  All of the above

B   Oral temperature is contraindicated in a person with a seizure disorder because of the increased risk of injury if a seizure occurred during the measurement. (p. 565)

10. The time required to obtain an accurate temperature varies according to the route of measurement. Which of the following time associations is incorrect?

    A.  Axillary - 11 minutes
    B.  Oral - 3 to 5 minutes
    C.  Rectal - 2 to 4 minutes
    D.  None of the above

B   Research has shown that the thermometer should be left in place for 9 to 10 minutes to accurately measure oral temperature. (p. 568)

# MEETING AWARENESS NEEDS

**OBJECTIVES**

1.0 Discuss the concept of "awareness" and its relationship to human function.

    1.1 Give examples of nursing diagnoses that focus on an individual's awareness needs. (p. 575)

    1.2 Describe the concept of awareness. (p. 576)

    1.3 Define the concept of stimulation. (p. 577)

    1.4 Describe the physiological stages of sensation. (p. 577)

    1.5 Identify seven different types of sensation. (p. 577)

2.0 Describe the behavior of people at the various levels of consciousness.

    2.1 Identify six levels of consciousness that may be used to describe a person's awareness of self, others, and environment. (p. 577)

3.0 Discuss the process of developing awareness from before birth through life.

    3.1 Identify internal and external variables that influence an individual's level of awareness. (p. 576)

    3.2 Discuss the development of awareness needs throughout the life cycle. (p. 577)

    3.3 Discuss the role of the reticular activating system in the management of environmental sensory stimulation. (p. 578)

4.0 Apply the nursing process in caring for people experiencing sensory deficit, sensory deprivation, and sensory overload.

    4.1 Identify common nursing goals related to a person experiencing awareness needs. (p. 576)

    4.2 State potential outcome criteria for evaluating the nursing intervention for individuals with actual or potential awareness problems. (p. 576)

**TEACHING/LEARNING STRATEGIES**

**Lecture/Discussion**

Discuss the effects of inadequate or excess sensory stimulation on human functioning.

**Lecture/Discussion**

Discuss the general procedure for determining a person's level of consciousness.

Have students identify factors useful in assessing a person's neurological status.

**Clinical Laboratory Experience**

Ask students to review the checklist used by their clinical facility to document a person's neurological status.

**Lecture/Discussion**

Ask students to share their feelings in times of sensory deprivation and overload.

Ask students to identify situations that can predispose persons to the development of sensory deprivation or sensory overload.

4.3 Discuss the essential awareness needs of hospitalized children: Sensory deprivation and overstimulation. (p. 577)

4.4 Outline nursing intervention to facilitate stimulation in the hospitalized child. (p. 577)

4.5 State four problems that may develop as a result of altered stimulation needs. (p. 578)

4.6 Identify examples of common sensory deficits. (p. 578)

4.7 Identify data indicative of a hearing deficit. (p. 578)

4.8 Differentiate between sensory deprivation and sensory deficit. (p. 578)

4.9 Identify essential data to obtain when assessing a person for a potential sight deficit. (p. 578)

4.10 Outline specific nursing measures for care of individuals with potential hearing or sight deficits. (p. 578)

4.11 List possible reasons for the development of sensory deprivation. (p. 578)

4.12 Identify subjective and objective data that may indicate sensory deprivation. (p. 578)

4.13 Discuss common nursing intervention measures used to prevent or decrease sensory deprivation. (p. 578)

4.14 Describe the concept of sensory overload. (p. 579)

4.15 Identify common causes of sensory overload. (p. 579)

4.16 Identify subjective and objective assessment data indicative of sensory overload. (p. 579)

4.17 Outline appropriate nursing intervention for individuals experiencing sensory overload. (p. 580)

5.0 Describe the concept of "intensive care unit psychosis."

5.1 Identify stimulation problems unique to individuals in the intensive care unit. (p. 580)

5.2 Discuss the etiology of intensive care psychoses. (p. 580)

Ask students to compare and contrast sensory deprivation with sensory overload.

Using the nursing process as a guide, ask students to describe the nursing care of a person who is experiencing sensory deprivation or sensory overload.

## Clinical Laboratory Experience

Have students identify individuals in their clinical agency who display a higher risk for the development of sensory deprivation.

## Lecture/Discussion

Briefly discuss the etiology of Intensive Care Psychoses.

6.0 Identify causes of disorganized thought and behavior patterns.

    6.1 Identify physiologic and psychosocial causes for unmet needs leading to disorganized thought processes and behavior patterns. (p. 580)

    6.2 Describe common manifestations of disorganized behavior and thought processes: Confusion, hallucinations, illusions, and delusional thinking. (p. 581)

7.0 Apply the nursing process in caring for people who are confused.

    7.1 Differentiate between confusion and delirium. (p. 581)

    7.2 Identify common causes of confusion. (p. 581)

    7.3 Identify characteristics that may be displayed by the confused person. (p. 581)

    7.4 List diagnostic information useful in the assessment of a confused person. (p. 581)

    7.5 List data that should be included when documenting the assessment of a confused person. (p. 582)

    7.6 Identify three major goals of care for confused people. (p. 582)

8.0 Describe the experiences of hallucination, illusion, and delusional thinking.

    8.1 Briefly describe other types of disorganized thought processes and behavior patterns: Hallucination, illusions, and delusional thinking. (p. 583)

    8.2 Briefly discuss causes for visual hallucinations. (p. 584)

## Written Exercise

Using the nursing process as a guide, ask students to formulate a plan of care to prevent or reduce confusion in a hospitalized individual.

## Lecture/Discussion

Have students explore the nurse's responsibility when caring for individuals experiencing hallucinations, illusions, or delusional thinking.

---

## MULTIPLE CHOICE QUESTIONS

1. A terminally ill person no longer responds to verbal stimuli, but moves spontaneously in response to physical stimuli. This behavior is representative of which level of consciousness?

    A. Coma
    B. Obtunded state
    C. Semicomatose
    D. Stuporous state

## CORRECT ANSWER AND RATIONALE

C  A person who is semicomatose will respond to physical stimuli (bright lights, light pin prick) with spontaneous reflex responses. (p. 577)

2. When planning care to meet the awareness needs of an individual, the nurse should understand that:

   A. A person's level of consciousness will directly affect their responses to external stimuli
   B. A person normally responds to several environmental stimuli at a time
   C. Responses to environmental stimuli are influenced by a person's level of growth and development
   D. All of the above

D   All listed options are true. (p. 576)

3. Which of the following individuals is most likely to develop sensory overload?

   A. A child hospitalized for the second time
   B. A hospitalized elderly person who usually lives alone
   C. A person who requires continuous 24 hour monitoring in the critical care unit
   D. A person who must share a hospital room with three other individuals

C   A person in the critical care unit is particularly prone to developing sensory overload. Many factors influence this increased susceptibility to sensory overload: Limited movement; presence of sights, sounds, smells, movement, and tactile stimulation that are unfamiliar; and an often frightening medical diagnosis. (p. 579)

4. A premature infant has been confined to an incubator for several months. The nurse knows that this infant is at risk for the development of sensory:

   A. Deficit
   B. Deprivation
   C. Distortion
   D. Overload

B   Sensory deprivation occurs when there is a limitation in the individual's ability to receive sensory stimuli. In this instance, the incubator serves as a barrier to the normal input of environmental stimuli. (p. 578)

5. A newly paralyzed individual tells their nurse that: "I can't tell where my legs are. It's as if they were asleep!" The nurse knows that this individual may be experiencing which type of sensory deficit?

   A. Cutaneous
   B. Kinesthetic
   C. Tactile
   D. Visceral

B   A person with a kinesthetic sensory deficit cannot tell the position of various body parts. (p. 577)

6. If a person with a hearing deficit cannot understand you, which of the following nursing actions would be most appropriate?

   A. Encouraging the person to have a hearing assessment test
   B. Giving the message to another significant other
   C. Restating the message, using nonverbal cues in addition to the spoken message
   D. Standing in front of the person and loudly repeating the message

C   Using both verbal and nonverbal messages would facilitate the communication process. The nurse should never resort to shouting or speaking loudly. (p. 579)

7. When caring for a person who is confused, the nurse should focus primarily on:

   A. Preventing further confusion
   B. Providing support and protection
   C. Maintaining reality orientation
   D. All of the above

D   There are three major nursing goals of care for the confused person: Preventing further confusion, support and protection, and reorientation to reality. (p. 582)

# 31
## MEETING MOBILITY NEEDS

OBJECTIVES

1.0 Define the different types of exercise.

    1.1 Discuss the advantages of aerobic exercise over other types of exercise. (p. 587)

    1.2 Describe the benefits of other types of exercise: Flexibility, strength-developing, and anaerobic exercise. (p. 588)

2.0 Document assessment of the individual before recommending an exercise program.

    2.1 Develop a physical fitness program designed to help an individual reach and maintain adequate physical fitness. (p. 588)

    2.2 List benefits of proper conditioning through exercise. (p. 588)

    2.3 Identify factors the nurse should consider before recommending a program of physical activity for an individual. (p. 588)

    2.4 Explore reasons for the development of an "addiction" to physical exercise. (p. 588)

    2.5 Outline essential physical assessment data that should be obtained before recommending a physical activity program. (p. 588)

    2.6 Identify psychosocial assessment data that must be considered when assisting a person to design an exercise program. (p. 588)

    2.7 State the formula used to calculate an individual's maximum heart rate. (p. 589)

    2.8 Briefly describe important information that the nurse should include when teaching an individual ways of minimizing the risks of exercise. (p. 589)

TEACHING/LEARNING STRATEGIES

Lecture/Discussion

Briefly describe types of physical fitness: Passive, muscular, flexibility, and endurance. (p. 587)

Class Activity

Conduct a survey of the exercise habits of class members.

Encourage each student to evaluate their own physical fitness status. Have them develop a plan for meeting any identified physical fitness needs.

Lecture/Discussion

Focus discussion on the factors that should be assessed by the nurse before recommending an exercise program for an individual.

Class Activity

Have students assess the motor functioning of a child, an adult, and an elderly person in the community. Ask them to compare and contrast their findings and share the results in class.

3.0 List the benefits of bedrest.

    3.1 Briefly describe five important benefits
        of bedrest. (p. 590)

Lecture/Discussion

Facilitate a discussion on the advantages and
disadvantages of bedrest.

Explore the effects of extended bedrest on a
person's daily functioning.

4.0 Describe the physiologic and psychosocial
    effects of immobility.

    4.1 Give examples of at least three nursing
        diagnoses related to immobility.
        (p. 586)

    4.2 Identify common nursing goals related to
        care of the immobilized individual.
        (p. 586)

    4.3 Describe criteria that might be used to
        evaluate nursing care for the
        immobilized person. (p. 586)

    4.4 Identify and briefly describe six common
        causes of immobility. (p. 589)

    4.5 Summarize major responses of the body to
        the stress of immobility. (p. 591)

    4.6 Identify and briefly describe four major
        musculoskeletal problems created by
        immobility. (p. 601)

    4.7 Identify assessment data useful in
        prevention of the musculoskeletal
        complications related to immobility.
        (p. 602)

    4.8 Plan appropriate nursing intervention to
        combat the development of backaches
        related to immobility. (p. 602)

    4.9 Identify complications that may occur as
        a result of osteoporosis. (p. 602)

    4.10 Describe nursing measures that can be
         used to prevent the development of
         contractures in an immobile person.
         (p. 602)

    4.11 Outline actions the nurse might take to
         prevent disuse osteoporosis. (p. 603)

    4.12 List and briefly describe four major
         effects of immobility on the
         cardiovascular system. (p. 605)

    4.13 Identify signs and symptoms of an
         inadequate blood supply to the lungs.
         (p. 610)

    4.14 Plan nursing intervention to prevent
         thrombus formation in an immobilized
         person. (p. 610)

    4.15 Summarize respiratory changes that occur
         in an immobilized person. (p. 610)

Lecture/Discussion

Ask students to state the definition of
immobility. Facilitate a discussion of the
various types of immobility.

Discuss the physical problems that can develop as
a result of immobility.

Written Exercise

Have students outline the effects immobility can
have on each body system.

4.16 Identify assessment data indicative of
venous thrombosis. (p. 610)

4.17 Enumerate the various factors that must
be considered in assessment of an
immobilized person's respiratory
functioning. (p. 610)

4.18 Describe nursing intervention strategies
effective in the prevention of
respiratory complications caused by
immobility. (p. 611)

4.19 Identify and briefly describe two ways
in which immobility can affect an
individual's metabolism and nutritional
status. (p. 611)

4.20 Identify ways in which the nurse can
assist an individual to counteract
changes in metabolic functioning that
are caused by immobility. (p. 611)

4.21 Plan appropriate nursing intervention to
prevent anorexia and malnutrition in an
immobilized person. (p. 611)

4.22 Identify factors that influence the
development of constipation in an
immobilized person. (p. 611)

4.23 List problems that may accompany the
constipation caused by immobility.
(p. 612)

4.24 Identify assessment data indicative of
constipation and fecal impaction.
(p. 612)

4.25 List actions the nurse might take to
prevent the development of constipation
and fecal impaction in an immobilized
person. (p. 612)

4.26 Give three reasons an immobilized person
may experience difficulty with
urination. (p. 612)

4.27 Discuss factors that influence the
development of urinary stasis in an
immobilized person. (p. 612)

4.28 Identify factors that influence the
development of urinary infections in an
immobilized person. (p. 612)

4.29 Specify assessment data that must be
included when assessing a person for
renal complications of immobility.
(p. 612)

4.30 Identify four major urinary problems
that may result as a consequence of
immobility. (p. 612)

4.31 Outline appropriate nursing intervention
measures useful in the prevention of
renal complications caused by
immobility. (p. 613)

4.32 Identify psychosocial problems that may be experienced by an individual with alterations in mobility. (p. 613)

5.0 Identify groups of people who are immobilized.

Clinical Laboratory Experience

Ask students to identify individuals in the clinical facility that are immobilized.

6.0 State the major therapies for the prevention and treatment of pressure sores.

**Lecture/Discussion**

Focus discussion on the various measures the nurse can utilize to prevent the occurrence of pressure sores in an immobilized individual.

6.1 List the major pressure point areas for an individual in a supine, side-lying, or prone position. (p. 590)

**Clinical Laboratory Experience**

Help students identify individuals in their clinical facility who display a high risk for the development of pressure sores.

6.2 List and briefly describe three major forces that play a role in the development of pressure sores. (p. 591)

6.3 Identify four stages used to classify the development or severity of a pressure sore. (p. 591)

Review the care of an individual in the clinical facility who is receiving treatment for a pressure sore.

6.4 Identify individuals who display a greater risk for the development of pressure sores. (p. 593)

6.5 Discuss data that should be included in the ongoing assessment of a person who has an increased risk for the development of pressure sores. (p. 593)

6.6 Identify appropriate nursing measures to prevent the development of pressure sores. (p. 593)

6.7 List and give examples of current therapies used in the treatment of pressure sores. (p. 596)

6.8 List information the nurse should include when evaluating the nursing care of an individual with a pressure sore. (p. 597)

7.0 Demonstrate positioning techniques to prevent the complications of immobility.

**Lecture/Discussion**

Assist students in identifying physiological and psychological data that can be used in assessing an immobile individual.

7.1 Define and identify the therapeutic purposes of placing an immobilized person in a prone position. (p. 597)

Ask students to identify nursing measures to maintain, promote and/or restore normal body alignment.

7.2 Identify contraindications and cautions the nurse should be aware of prior to placing an immobilized person in a prone position. (p. 597)

Discuss the use of supportive devices used to maintain correct body alignment.

7.3 Identify the teaching/learning needs of an immobilized individual who has been placed in a prone position. (p. 597)

**Campus Laboratory Experience**

7.4 List assessment data that should be gathered when planning to place an individual in a prone position. (p. 598)

Demonstrate procedures for positioning a person in bed. Allow time for students to practice each technique.

7.5 Identify the equipment and preparation procedures the nurse should utilize when placing an individual in the prone position. (p. 598)

7.6 Describe basic intervention techniques utilized by the nurse when placing an individual in the prone position. (p. 598)

7.7 List the information that should be included when documenting care of individuals who have been placed in a prone position. (p. 597)

7.8 Discuss final activities of the nurse upon placing an individual in a prone position. (p. 601)

8.0 Demonstrate range-of-motion exercises.

8.1 Define and identify the therapeutic purposes of passive range-of-motion exercises for an immobilized person. (p. 603)

8.2 List contraindications/cautions the nurse should take into consideration before providing passive range-of-motion exercises to an immobilized individual. (p. 603)

8.3 Briefly describe the educational needs of an individual receiving passive range-of-motion exercises. (p. 604)

8.4 Discuss preliminary assessment data that should be gathered by the nurse before providing passive range-of-motion exercises. (p. 604)

8.5 Outline measures used to prepare an individual for passive range-of-motion exercises. (p. 604)

8.6 Identify the equipment necessary for the provision of passive range-of-motion exercises. (p. 604)

8.7 Outline the appropriate steps the nurse should take to provide passive range-of-motion exercises. (p. 604)

8.8 Describe nursing actions that should be performed upon completion of passive range-of-motion exercises. (p. 605)

8.9 Define the following: Abduction, adduction, extension, flexion, internal rotation, external rotation, and hyperextension. (p. 605)

## Clinical Laboratory Experience

Arrange for students to observe the activities of the physical therapist in their clinical setting.

## Campus Laboratory Experience

Have students view a demonstration of a nurse performing range-of-motion exercises. Ask them to practice the skill with a classmate in the campus laboratory setting.

## Clinical Laboratory Experience

Ask students to identify individuals in their clinical setting that could benefit from the various range-of-motion activities. Upon demonstration of proficiency, allow students to perform ROM activities with selected individuals.

9.0 List the psychosocial problems encountered by
immobile people and describe nursing
intervention to alleviate these problems.

    9.1 List factors that may influence the
development of psychosocial problems in
an immobilized person. (p. 613)

    9.2 Discuss basic nursing intervention
useful in preventing or decreasing the
psychosocial problems resulting from
immobility. (p. 613)

    9.3 Identify general teaching/learning needs
of a person with alterations in
immobility. (p. 614)

## Lecture/Discussion

Explore nursing interventions that can be used to
assist a person to cope with the physiological
changes caused by immobility.

Ask students to identify the educational needs of
a person experiencing alterations in mobility.

---

## MULTIPLE CHOICE QUESTIONS

1. Mr. Chapman must perform isometric exercises
with his casted left leg. The nurse knows
that isometric exercises are designed to:

    A. Help maintain and increase muscle tone,
strength, and shape
    B. Help preserve muscle tone and strength
    C. Provide muscular contraction and
resistance through joint ROM
    D. Produce the stress necessary for bony
maintenance and growth

2. Which type of exercise would be
contraindicated in an individual with chronic
lung disease?

    A. Aerobic
    B. Anaerobic
    C. Flexibility
    D. Isometric

3. If a 30-year-old is to achieve maximum
benefit from a 20 minute aerobic exercise
period, the heart rate should be increased to
how many beats per minute?

    A. 133-152
    B. 154-176
    C. 130-150
    D. 125-152

SITUATION: Mrs. Conners, a 79-year-old woman, has
been confined to bed since suffering a stroke that
caused total right-sided paralysis. Since
hospitalization, she has become increasingly
confused, incontinent of urine, and now refuses to
eat. Questions 4 through 7 apply to this
situation.

4. Which of the following factors is least
likely to promote the development of skin
breakdown in Mrs. Conners?

    A. Age
    B. Decreased awareness of peripheral
circulation
    C. Refusal to eat
    D. Urinary incontinence

## CORRECT ANSWER AND RATIONALE

B  Isometric exercises contract muscles without
producing movement and therefore, assist only
in the maintenance of present muscle tone and
strength. (p. 602)

A  Aerobic exercises would be contraindicated in
a person with chronic lung disease because of
the increased amounts of stress it places on
the respiratory system. (p. 588)

A  The heart rate should reach 70 to 80% of its
maximum capacity during aerobic exercise. To
calculate the maximum heart rate in beats per
minute, the person's age should be subtracted
from 220. (p. 589)

C  Mrs. Conners' recent refusal to eat would be
the least significant factor at present. If
longstanding, however, malnourishment could
develop, causing an increased tendency for
skin breakdown due to inadequate protein and
vitamin intake. (p. 590)

5.  If left in a side-lying position for too long, Mrs. Conners will be especially prone to the development of pressure sores at which body areas?

    A.  Acromium process, ribs, greater tronchanter
    B.  Breast, acromium process, greater tronchanter
    C.  Cheek and ear, ribs, greater tronchanter
    D.  Ear, acromium process, and the malleolus

    D   The pressure points in a side-lying position are as follows: Ear, acromium process, ribs, greater tronchanter, medial and lateral condyles, and the malleolus. (p. 592)

6.  Despite preventive nursing measures, Mrs. Conners develops a shallow ulcer over the sacral area. The ulcer appears to extend into the subcutaneous fat. This is an example of which stage in the development of a decubitus ulcer?

    A.  Grade I
    B.  Grade II
    C.  Grade III
    D.  Grade IV

    B   A stage or grade II decubitus ulcer is shallow in appearance and extends into the subcutaneous fat. (p. 591)

7.  Measures to prevent further skin breakdown in Mrs. Conners should include:

    A.  Changing her position every hour
    B.  Ensuring a proper diet with sufficient protein, vitamins, and minerals
    C.  Using inflatable pressure rings on all bony prominences
    D.  All of the above

    B   A proper diet is needed to assist in tissue repair and growth. Option A is incorrect because it would not be necessary to turn the individual every hour; every two hours would be sufficient. Option C would be incorrect because inflatable donut rings tend to occlude the circulation around the body part that is being protected so, therefore, are contra-indicated. (p. 594)

8.  Which of the following topical agents would not be used to facilitate the healing process of a pressure sore?

    A.  Acetic Acid
    B.  Alcohol
    C.  Betadine
    D.  Hydrogen peroxide

    B   Alcohol should not be used when caring for a decubitus ulcer because of its extreme drying effect on the skin. (p. 596)

9.  To prevent disuse osteoporosis in an immobilized individual, the nurse should:

    A.  Begin weight-bearing activities as soon as possible
    B.  Increase calcium intake in the diet
    C.  Perform passive range-of-motion exercises
    D.  Teach the person isometric exercises

    A   To prevent disuse osteoporosis, the person must stand and bear weight as soon as possible. Simple range-of-motion activities will not be effective without resistance. A diet with adequate calcium is helpful, but will not prevent the osteoporosis. (p. 603)

10. Which of the following statements is incorrect?

    A.  A joint can become permanently fixed when ankylosed
    B.  All people possess similar range-of-motion capabilities
    C.  An immobilized joint will begin to exhibit connective tissue changes in as early as four days
    D.  Contractures are due to the atrophy of muscles

    B   A person's range-of-motion capabilities may vary for a variety of reasons which include: Physical structure, past exercise, and the presence of pathologic conditions. (p. 603)

11. When performing passive ROM, the nurse bends the arm at the elbow joint. This is an example of which type of ROM activity?

    A. Abduction
    B. Adduction
    C. Flexion
    D. Internal rotation

C   Flexion decreases the angle between two bones, or bends the joint. (p. 605)

12. The nurse is aware that continuous immobilization in a supine position:

    A. Can cause a decreased pulse rate and cardiac output.
    B. Decreases the work load of the heart.
    C. Predisposes the person to the development of orthostatic hypotension.
    D. Should be encouraged in a person whose heart needs rest.

C   After a period of immobility, a person may experience a sudden drop in blood pressure when assuming an erect position due to the failure of arteriolar vasoconstriction. Research has indicated that the supine position increases the workload of the heart. This results in an increased pulse rate, increased cardiac output, and increased stroke volume. Therefore, it is contraindicated in an individual whose heart needs rest. (p. 605)

13. All of the following measures would be effective in reducing the occurrence of the Valsalva maneuver in a bedridden individual except:

    A. Encouraging the individual to "bear down" while defecating
    B. Increasing bulk in the diet and encouraging fluids
    C. Instruct the individual to exhale while pulling up in bed
    D. Utilizing a sitting position for defecation when possible

A   The Valsalva maneuver may be elicited when a person strains upon defecation, which causes the person to exhale against a closed glottis. This traps air in the lungs and increases intrathoracic pressure. (p. 606)

14. Which of the following nursing actions would be useful in preventing the occurrence of thrombus formation in an immobilized individual?

    A. Coughing and deep breathing exercises
    B. Increasing fluid intake to decrease blood viscosity
    C. Massaging the lower extremities to aid in venous circulation
    D. Using the knee-gatch to promote venous return

B   Venous stasis, which predisposes a person to thrombus formation, is complicated by an increased viscosity of blood. Options A, C, and D would be contraindicated because: Rubbing the legs would dislodge a formed clot; the knee flexion position reduces venous return to the heart; and coughing and deep breathing exercises would be useful in preventing respiratory complications, but would not alter thrombus formation. (p. 610)

15. An individual with hypoxia may exhibit all of the following signs and symptoms except:

    A. Disorientation to surroundings
    B. Dyspnea
    C. Elevated pulse and temperature
    D. Fatigue and restlessness

C   Temperature elevation is an indication of a respiratory infection, not hypoxia. (p. 611)

16. Nursing intervention for the prevention of renal complications in an immobilized individual should routinely include all of the following except:

    A. Allowing the person to stand or use a bedside commode for elimination
    B. Encouraging a fluid intake of 2400 ml/day, unless contraindicated
    C. Instilling a urinary catheter to promote bladder emptying
    D. Providing privacy during elimination activities

C   A urinary catheterization is not routinely performed to prevent complications, but rather should be performed only when absolutely necessary. In addition, it requires a physician's order for insertion. (p. 613)

# PROVIDING PHYSICAL PROTECTION
# AND BODILY SUPPORT

OBJECTIVES

1.0  Assess a person's need for them.

2.0  Describe a basic understanding of their
     correct application and use.

   2.1  Identify devices used to assist a person
        with mobility.  Summarize the
        indications for use of each device.
        (p. 617)

   2.2  Identify three types of crutches and the
        indications for their use.  (p. 617)

   2.3  Describe the procedure used to ensure
        proper crutch fit.  (p. 618)

   2.4  Identify factors influencing the gait
        used in crutch walking.  (p. 618)

   2.5  Briefly describe the uses and techniques
        of the major crutch-walking gaits:
        Four-point alternating, three-point,
        two-point, swing-to-crutch, and
        swing-through-crutch gaits.  (p. 618)

   2.6  Identify two types of canes and the
        indications for the use of each.
        (p. 620)

   2.7  List factors that indicate proper cane
        length.  (p. 621)

   2.8  Describe the proper use of a cane.
        (p. 621)

   2.9  Briefly describe differences in a
        standard walker and a reciprocal
        walker.  (p. 621)

   2.10 Outline guidelines that may be used to
        assure proper walker height for
        individuals in your care.  (p. 621)

   2.11 Describe major differences in a traveler
        wheelchair and a universal wheelchair.
        (p. 621)

   2.12 List universal wheelchair variations and
        identify indications for the use of
        each.  (p. 621)

TEACHING/LEARNING STRATEGIES

Clinical Laboratory Experience

Have students identify individuals in the clinical
facility who could benefit from the use of various
protective/supportive devices.

Class Activity

Ask students to identify agencies in their
community who have as their primary focus suicide
prevention and crisis management.

Guest Speaker

Invite a physical therapist in each clinical
facility to a postconference period to demonstrate
the procedures used in selecting appropriate
mobility devices for an individual.  Ask them to
demonstrate the proper procedure for fitting an
individual with each of the following:  Canes,
crutches, and walkers.

Campus Laboratory Experience

Obtain various mobility devices for student
viewing in the campus or clinical laboratory:
Crutches, canes, walkers, wheelchairs, hydraulic
chairs, and elevator chairs.

Demonstrate the procedure for applying each type
of binder:  Chest, breast, straight, abdominal,
scultetus, and T-binders.

Demonstrate the procedure for applying various
types of restraints:  Wrist and ankle; chest and
waist; elbow; mitt; and body restraints.

Demonstrate the procedures for applying slings/arm
immobilizers.  Allow students to practice the
procedures in the campus laboratory setting.

Ask students to outline appropriate guidelines for
applying elastic bandages.  After a demonstration
of the procedure, allow students to practice the
technique.

Provide a demonstration of the correct procedure
for applying soft and hard cervical collars.

Clinical Laboratory Experience

Assist students in identifying individuals in
their clinical facility who could benefit from the
use of mobility devices.

2.13 Briefly describe additional wheelchair accessories that are currently available. (p. 622)

2.14 Discuss the function of a hydraulic chair for an immobilized individual. (p. 622)

2.15 Summarize ways in which movement devices facilitate the movement of immobilized individuals. (p. 622)

2.16 Briefly describe three types of mobility devices and indications for the use of each device: Back board, clam shell, and JED sled. (p. 623)

2.17 Describe various immobilization devices and the indications for their use: Binders, arm immobilizers, cervical collars, elastic bandages, and unna boots. (p. 623)

2.18 Outline general guidelines the nurse should use when applying or teaching a person about binders. (p. 623)

2.19 Describe the procedure for application of a straight abdominal binder. (p. 624)

2.20 List the steps the nurse should use to apply a scultetus binder. (p. 624)

2.21 Identify critical assessment data the nurse should gather after applying an abdominal binder (p. 625)

2.22 Describe the application procedure for a T-binder. (p. 625)

2.23 Outline the steps for correct application of slings and arm immobilizers. (p. 625)

2.24 Describe the correct method for application of a cervical collar. (p. 626)

2.25 Outline basic guidelines the nurse should use when applying cervical collars. (p. 627)

2.26 Explain the procedure for application of unna boots. (p. 628)

2.27 Specify assessment data that should be gathered by the nurse after the application of unna boots. (p. 628)

2.28 Briefly describe positioning devices that can be used to prevent contractures in an immobilized person: Footboards, trochanter rolls, hip abduction pillows, sandbags, bed cradles, and hand rolls. (p. 628)

Assist students in identifying individuals in their clinical facility who could benefit from the use of: Pad and artificial sheepskins; rings and cushions; and heel and elbow protectors.

Arrange for students to observe individuals in their clinical facility who are using specialized frames, mattresses and beds for the prevention of pressure sores.

Ask students to review the established suicide precautions used in their clinical facility.

2.29 Briefly describe various protective
devices that can be used to prevent
pressure sores, and the possible
indications for the use of each: Beds,
frames, mattresses, and other protective
devices. (p. 629)

2.30 Describe the procedure for turning an
individual on a Stryker frame. (p. 630)

2.31 List the advantages of using a Stryker
wedge frame to turn an immobilized
person as opposed to a regular Stryker
frame. (p. 631)

2.32 Identify essential assessment data that
should be gathered when turning a person
on the CircOlectric bed. (p. 631)

2.33 Explain the procedure for the use of a
CircOlectric bed. (p. 631)

2.34 Describe the proper use of a kinetic
treatment table. (p. 631)

2.35 Describe precautions the nurse should
take when using an air or fluid-filled
mattress to promote circulation in an
immobilized individual. (p. 634)

2.36 Articulate the nurse's responsibility
with regard to the use of the
following: Pad or "artificial"
sheepskins, rings or cushions, and heel
or elbow protectors. (p. 635)

2.37 Describe the physiological mechanisms by
which antiembolism stockings prevent
thrombophlebitis. (p. 635)

2.38 Identify individuals who might benefit
from the application of antiembolism
stockings. (p. 635)

2.39 Discuss nursing responsibilities in
relation to individuals with
antiembolism stockings. (p. 636)

2.40 Discuss important factors that the nurse
must consider when using restraints.
(p. 636)

2.41 Describe the mechanism for applying
restraints on severely agitated or
combative individuals. (p. 637)

2.42 Outline measures the nurse can utilize
to facilitate easy removal of restraints
during emergencies. (p. 638)

2.43 Describe the safest position to place an
individual in who has physical
restraints. (p. 639)

2.44 Briefly discuss the nurse's role in the
care of restrained individuals. (p. 639)

2.45 List data that should be documented in the clinical record of a person requiring physical restraints. (p. 639)

2.46 Briefly describe various types of restraints, and identify the indication for their use: Wrist and limb, chest or waist, elbow, mitt, and body restraints. (p. 639)

2.47 Identify guidelines the nurse should utilize when applying wrist or ankle restraints. (p. 639)

2.48 Identify important factors the nurse should remember when applying chest and waist restraints. (p. 640)

2.49 Describe the procedure for application of a total body restraint. (p. 641)

2.50 Describe measures that may be instituted to provide an environment that is free of hazards. (p. 641)

2.51 Define the meaning of "suicide precautions." (p. 643)

2.52 List important guidelines that must be followed when providing care to individuals with "suicide precautions." (p. 643)

3.0 Assess individual reactions to them.

### Values Clarification

Ask students to share their personal feelings with regard to the use of restraints.

### Communication Activity

Encourage students to interview individuals in community who require long-term wheelchair use. Encourage them to elicit information regarding lifestyle changes that have been necessary as a result of the individual's mobility needs.

4.0 Assist individuals and significant others to adjust to their use.

### Class Activity

Ask two students to volunteer to use either a wheelchair or crutches for an entire day. Have them discuss the experience the next day in class.

5.0 Assess and prevent complications associated with them.

  5.1 Identify major complications that may result from the use of chest binders. (p. 624)

  5.2 Identify possible complications that may arise as a result of abdominal binders. (p. 624)

  5.3 Identify complications that are often associated with sling use. (p. 626)

### Lecture/Discussion

Summarize the complications that can occur with use of the various devices for bodily protection and support.

5.4 State four major complications
associated with the use of cervical
collars. (p. 627)

5.5 Discuss hazards associated with the use
of restraints. (p. 637)

6.0 Discuss legal ramifications of their
inappropriate use.

7.0 Plan and implement ways of helping the
individual and significant others learn about
them.

7.1 Identify factors that should be
considered by the nurse before teaching
an individual to crutch-walk. (p. 619)

7.2 Outline the steps used to teach an
individual to crutch-walk. (p. 619)

7.3 Discuss the procedure for teaching an
individual to learn advanced
crutch-walking maneuvers: Standing from
a sitting position, sitting from a
standing position, stair climbing, and
descending stairs. (p. 619)

7.4 Identify other important points that
should be included when teaching a
person to crutch-walk. (p. 619)

7.5 Identify safety factors the nurse should
be aware of before operating or teaching
others about the operation of a wheelchair. (p. 622)

7.6 Describe specific teaching/learning
needs of an individual who has either a
chest or breast binder prescribed for
home use. (p. 624)

7.7 Identify important points that should be
emphasized when teaching an individual
about the use of a sling. (p. 626)

7.8 Enumerate teaching/learning needs of an
individual requiring a cervical collar.
(p. 627)

7.9 Identify essential learning/teaching
needs of an individual with an elastic
bandage. (p. 627)

7.10 State the teaching/learning needs of
individuals who have had unna boots
applied. (p. 628)

7.11 Identify educational needs of
individuals using antiembolism
stockings. (p. 636)

## Lecture/Discussion

Explore the legal ramifications of restraint
application. (p. 639)

## Group Activity

Ask students to divide into small groups. Have
each group prepare a teaching/learning plan for
individuals requiring the use of one of the
following: Crutches, wheelchair, binder, and
cervical collar. Allow time for a brief oral
presentation in class.

8.0 Document nursing intervention about them.

    8.1 List information that should be documented by the nurse when teaching a person to crutch-walk. (p. 620)

    8.2 Describe data that should be included when documenting the care of individuals requiring cervical collar application. (p. 627)

    8.3 List data that should be included when documenting the application and use of elastic bandages. (p. 627)

    8.4 Identify information that should be included in documentation of the care of individuals requiring antiembolism stockings. (p. 636)

    8.5 Discuss specific information that should be addressed in the clinical record of individuals using protective or supportive devices. (p. 636)

    8.6 Identify data that should be included in the nursing record of individuals who are secluded for therapeutic purposes. (p. 642)

    8.7 Identify information that should be included when documenting the care of a person with "suicide precautions." (p. 643)

9.0 Evaluate nursing intervention about them.

## Lecture/Discussion

Ask students to identify the data that should be documented in the chart of a person requiring restraint use.

Impress upon students the necessity of properly documenting cervical collar applications.

Discuss the information that the nurse should document in the clinical record of a person who is on suicide precautions.

---

## MULTIPLE CHOICE QUESTIONS

1. To assure proper crutch fit, the nurse should measure:

    A. From the axillary fold to the heel of the foot
    B. From the axilla to a diagonal point on the heel two inches away from the body
    C. From the axilla to a point on 6 to 8 inches behind the heel
    D. The person's height and subtract 16 inches

2. The crutch gait that most resembles normal walking is the:

    A. Four-point alternating gait
    B. Orthopedic gait
    C. Three-point gait
    D. Two-point gait

3. Mr. Burns can bear full weight on his right leg, but has been instructed to bear no weight on his casted left leg. Which gait will he need to use when crutch walking?

    A. Four-point alternating
    B. Swing-to-crutch
    C. Three-point
    D. Two-point

## CORRECT ANSWER AND RATIONALE

D  Measurements for crutches may be made in several ways. Option D is the only correct way listed to assure correct crutch fit. For other techniques, see page 628 in the text. (p. 618)

A  The four-point gait technique is a relatively safe, slow gait desirable for older, less stable people. An examination of the techniques used in the four-point gait technique reveals that it is the closest to normal walking. (p. 618)

C  The three-point, or orthopedic gait, is used when complete weight bearing is allowed on one foot and partial or no weight bearing on the other foot. (p. 617)

4.  When teaching a person with crutches to stand from a sitting position, you should instruct them to place the crutches together on which side of the body?

    A.  Either side
    B.  The affected side
    C.  The unaffected side
    D.  The stronger side

B   When standing from a sitting position, the person should place both crutches together on the affected side. This provides a firm support, as they push down with the other hand against a chair to push themselves up. (p. 619)

5.  Which of the following criteria could not be used to evaluate the proper use of a walker by an individual?

    A.  The elbows are flexed about 30 degrees
    B.  The feet are apart to provide a wide base of support
    C.  The walker is moved forward and when stable, the person walks into it
    D.  The walker height is adjusted to just above waist level

D   Walker height is adjusted so that the user's elbows are flexed at an angle of 30 degrees while grasping the handgrips with the wrists extended. This places the height of the walker just below waist level. (p. 621)

6.  Which of the following movement devices cannot be used to carry a person?

    A.  Back board
    B.  Clam shell
    C.  JED sled
    D.  Stretcher

C   The JED sled is composed of several lightweight, but rigid, plastic "boards" and a plastic bar. It is used to move a person toward you, and cannot be used to carry an individual. (p. 623)

7.  A nurse might use a binder for which of the following reasons?

    A.  Keep dressings in place
    B.  Reduce breast engorgment in a non-nursing mother
    C.  Reduce tension on wounds and suture lines
    D.  All of the above

D   All listed options are common uses of the binder. (p. 624)

8.  All of the following would be appropriate when applying a cervical collar in an emergency situation for a person with a suspected cervical spine injury except:

    A.  Moving the head to an erect position to apply the collar
    B.  Placing the person on a back board after the collar application
    C.  Taping the person's head to a back board before transport
    D.  Using head traction to facilitate collar application

A   If a cervical spine injury is suspected, the collar should be applied to the neck in the position in which the neck was found. Further cervical spine damage can occur if the neck is manipulated during collar placement. (p. 627)

9.  Which of the following would be contraindicated when applying an ace bandage to an extremity?

    A.  Applying the bandage in a proximal to distal direction
    B.  Holding the bandage close to the body part being bandaged
    C.  Using a figure-of-eight pattern to bandage around joints
    D.  Using a herringbone pattern to bandage arms and legs

A   The dressing should be applied in a distal to proximal direction, or following the direction of circulation. This minimizes venous congestion, stasis, and edema. (p. 627)

10. A nurse wishes to minimize the occurrence of postural hypotension in a paralyzed individual. Which of the following devices could be used to assist in the attainment of this goal?

   A. CircOlectric bed
   B. Clinitron bed
   C. Roto Rest table
   D. Stryker Frame

A  The CircOlectric bed may be moved to many positions, not just supine and prone, thus improving vascular tone. (p. 631)

SITUATION: Mr. Higgins appears extremely confused and disoriented. As you near his bed, he swears and attempts to hit you with his fist. Question 11 through 13 relate to this situation.

11. Your best initial response to this situation would be to:

   A. Ask another nurse to stay with him, while you telephone the physician
   B. Obtain an order to restrain him, the next time the physician makes rounds
   C. Obtain assistance and then restrain him temporarily until the physician can be contacted
   D. Restrain him temporarily, then attempt to contact the physician for an order

C  The nurse should never leave a person alone to contact the physician for a restraint order. Assistance should be obtained (to prevent injury to the nurse), and then restraints applied temporarily until a physician's order can be obtained. (p. 637)

12. Which nursing action is appropriate when caring for Mr. Higgins?

   A. Assessing him daily for complications associated with the use of restraints
   B. Changing his position at least every two hours
   C. Always restraining him in a supine position
   D. Removing all restraints once a day

B  The individual who is restrained should undergo frequent position changes. Since Mr. Higgins is combative, the nurse should never remove all restraints at once. To prevent aspiration he should be placed in a three-quarter supine position. Ongoing assessment throughout the day is important to prevent any complications associated with the use of restraints. (p. 637)

13. Later in the day, Mr. Higgins asks the nurse why he has been restrained. The nurse's best response would be:

   A. "Don't you remember, you tried to hit me this morning."
   B. "The restraints are just to keep you from falling out of bed."
   C. "The restraints were applied to prevent you from hurting yourself."
   D. "You get confused sometimes and try to hurt other people."

C  The individual should be told that the restraints were applied to prevent him from injuring himself. Other responses would be inappropriate. The person in restraints needs to know that they aren't being punished. (p. 639)

14. To provide safe and effective care for an individual with "suicide precautions," the nurse should:

   A. Allow the person to keep only personal hygiene items
   B. Apply soft restraints if necessary
   C. Assess the person every hour
   D. Lock potentially dangerous medical supplies away

D  Options A, B, and C are incorrect because: The individual should be checked every thirty minutes; only locking restraints should be used; and all items (including personal hygiene items) that could be hazardous should be removed from the person's environment. (p. 643)

# MEETING HYGIENE AND PHYSICAL
# COMFORT NEEDS

OBJECTIVES

1.0 Understand common principles and personal
variations in the satisfaction of hygiene and
physical comfort needs.

    1.1 Explore the influence of personal values
on an individual's hygienic practices.
(p. 644)

    1.2 Briefly describe the basic structure and
function of the skin. (p. 661)

    1.3 Identify basic principles underlying
care of the skin. (p. 662)

    1.4 Outline data that should be obtained in
a nursing assessment of the skin.
(p. 662)

    1.5 Give examples of nursing diagnoses
related to impaired skin integrity.
(p. 663)

    1.6 Explore factors that may influence an
individual's bathing habits and use of
skin care preparations. (p. 663)

2.0 Apply the nursing process to the satisfaction
of hygiene and physical comfort needs.

    2.1 Explore ways in which the nurse can
communicate respect for an individual's
"personal space." (p. 646)

    2.2 Identify common nursing goals of care
related to hygienic needs. (p. 646)

    2.3 Identify factors that determine nursing
priorities of care when planning
activities to meet hygienic needs.
(p. 646)

    2.4 Briefly describe various types of
hygienic care: Complete morning care,
partial morning care, early morning
care, and hour of sleep care. (p. 646)

    2.5 Identify criteria used in the evaluation
of skin care. (p. 663)

TEACHING/LEARNING STRATEGIES

Lecture/Discussion

Facilitate a discussion of the personal variables
that influence a person's personal hygiene
practices.

Ask students to describe the appearance of a
well-groomed professional nurse.

Discuss ways in which the nurse's professional
appearance can affect the creation of a
therapeutic nurse-client relationship.

Review the basic structure and function of the
integumentary system.

Ask students to identify normal and abnormal data
that should be obtained during examination of the
skin: Color, skin temperature, suppleness,
intactness and lesions, sensation, and cleanliness.

Clinical Laboratory Experience

Ask students to review the dress code formulated
for nurses in their clinical facility. Have them
compare it with the dress code used by their
program in nursing.

Ask students to identify individuals in their
clinical facility with potential impaired skin
integrity.

Lecture/Discussion

Ask students to identify procedures other than
bathing that can be used to assist an individual
with their total hygienic needs.

Have students compare the similarities and
differences in the different types of baths:
Shower or bathtub bathing; bedbaths; century tub
baths; and towel baths. Ask them to identify
situations appropriate for the use of each.

Have students review the common principles
applicable to all types of bathing that are listed
on page 663 in the text.

Campus Laboratory Experience

Demonstrate the procedure for giving a complete
bedbath. After the demonstration, have each
student practice the technique by practicing it on
another student.

2.6  Briefly describe the responsibilities of
     the nurse when assisting an individual
     with a shower or bathtub bath.  (p. 664)

2.7  Identify problems that may be
     experienced by an individual during
     bathing.  (p. 665)

2.8  Discuss safety measures that can be used
     to reduce injuries associated with
     showering.  (p. 665)

2.9  Identify individuals who may require a
     bedbath.  (p. 665)

2.10 Identify assessment data that can be
     obtained while administering a bedbath.
     (p. 665)

2.11 Briefly describe four methods of bedbath
     delivery:  Complete bedbath, towel bath,
     partial bedbath, and self-help bath.
     (p. 666)

2.12 Define and state the purpose of a
     complete bedbath.  (p. 666)

2.13 Identify contraindications/cautions the
     nurse should be aware of when
     administering a complete bedbath.
     (p. 666)

2.14 Explain preliminary activities of the
     nurse administering a complete bedbath.
     (p. 666)

2.15 List the equipment needed to administer
     a complete bedbath.  (p. 666)

2.16 Describe the essential steps of a
     complete bedbath.  (p. 666)

2.17 Outline activities of the nurse upon
     completion of a complete bedbath.
     (p. 670)

2.18 List data that should be documented in
     the record of an individual who has
     received a complete bedbath.  (p. 670)

2.19 Discuss the advantages and disadvantages
     of using a towel bath, as opposed to the
     more traditional bathing techniques.
     (p. 670)

2.20 List two major uses of the towel bath.
     (p. 670)

2.21 Identify supplies and cleaning agents
     used to administer a towel bath.
     (p. 670)

2.22 Describe the appropriate steps that
     should be taken by the nurse
     administering a towel bath.  (p. 671)

3.0 Identify and plan ways to meet
learning/teaching needs about personal
hygiene.

    3.1 Identify basic guidelines that should be
utilized by the nurse when planning
teaching/learning activities. (p. 647)

    3.2 Explore ways in which health teaching
can be used to promote good hygienic
practices and enhance skin integrity.
(p. 664)

    3.3 Describe the teaching/learning needs of
an individual who requires a complete
bedbath. (p. 666)

4.0 Assist a person to use a bedpan and urinal.

    4.1 List four ways the nurse can best assist
a hospitalized individual to meet
elimination needs. (p. 648)

    4.2 Outline essential data that should be
included in a nursing assessment and
plan of care to promote an individual's
elimination health. (p. 648)

    4.3 Differentiate between the various types
of bedpans, and give indications for the
use of each: Standard, pediatric, and
fracture. (p. 649)

    4.4 Describe the steps for placement and
removal of a bedpan without individual's
assistance. (p. 649)

    4.5 Identify ways in which the nurse can
assist a male or female individual to
use a urinal. (p. 650)

    4.6 List nursing actions that should be
carried out for a person using a bedside
commode for elimination. (p. 650)

    4.7 Discuss ways in which the nurse can
assist a hospitalized individual with
handwashing. (p. 651)

5.0 Describe alterations of the oral cavity.

    5.1 Identify specific problems a person may
experience as a result of poor oral
health care. (p. 651)

    5.2 List factor that may influence the
practice of inadequate oral hygiene.
(p. 651)

    5.3 Identify reasons the nurse may neglect
an individual's oral care, and related
teaching, needs. (p. 651)

    5.4 Discuss factors the nurse must consider
when assessing the oral hygiene needs of
an individual with dentures. (p. 652)

    5.5 Discuss factors that determine the
frequency and type of oral hygiene care
needed by an individual. (p. 652)

## Clinical Laboratory Experience

Assist students in developing a teaching/learning
plan to assist a person to prevent major oral
cavity alterations: Dental caries and periodontal
disease.

## Campus Laboratory Experience

After demonstration, ask students to practice the
techniques used in assisting individuals with
bedpans and urinals.

## Clinical Laboratory Experience

Upon demonstration of proficiency, allow students
to assist individuals in the clinical setting with
bedpans and urinals.

## Lecture/Discussion

Ask students to identify factors that influence
the development of oral cavity alterations:
Dental caries, periodontal disease, and the
problems that occur as a result of compromised
health.

## Written Exercise

Instruct students to outline the data that should
be used to assess an individual's oral health care
status. Ask them to use this information to
assess the oral health care of a classmate.

## Campus Laboratory Experience

Demonstrate the procedure for administering oral
health care to comatose individuals.

5.6 Identify data that should be gathered when assessing an individual's oral health status. (p. 653)

5.7 Identify basic equipment needed during an oral examination. (p. 652)

5.8 Outline the steps in an oral examination. (p. 652)

5.9 Briefly describe the two major oral health care problems: Dental caries and periodontal disease. (p. 654)

5.10 Discuss important factors to be considered when planning nursing care for an individual with dental caries or periodontal disease. (p. 654)

5.11 Identify oral health care problems that may develop in an individual with a compromised general condition. (p. 654)

5.12 List information that should be included in a daily nursing examination of individuals who display a greater risk for the development of oral health care problems. (p. 655)

5.13 Give examples of nursing diagnoses related to oral health care needs. (p. 655)

5.14 Identify common goals of care that can be utilized to guide the nursing care of individuals with oral health care needs. (p. 655)

5.15 List the equipment needed to provide oral care to a bedridden individual. (p. 656)

5.16 Describe the procedure for brushing and flossing natural teeth. (p. 656)

5.17 Identify special devices that may be used to assist a person who cannot brush their teeth normally. (p. 656)

5.18 Identify essential aspects of oral care for individuals with dentures. (p. 657)

5.19 Describe the oral nursing care measures that may be implemented for individuals with excessive dryness or irritation of the oral mucosa. (p. 657)

5.20 Describe the nursing procedure for giving oral care to a comatose or helpless person. (p. 658)

5.21 Identify criteria the nurse may use to evaluate the effectiveness of oral hygiene care. (p. 658)

6.0 Assist people with hearing aids and contact lenses.

6.1 Identify essential data to be included in an assessment of the eyes. (p. 658)

Have students bring their own oral care products to a campus laboratory experience. Ask them to take turns administering oral care to a classmate. Allow time for them to describe their feelings during the experience.

Clinical Laboratory Experience

Ask students to use the nursing process, to plan and implement oral health care for an individual in their clinical facility.

Lecture/Discussion

Ask students in the class to describe their own personal practices with regard to the use of glasses or contact lenses. Have them compare their practices with those described in the text.

6.2 Identify the basic steps involved in hygienic care of the eyes. (p. 658)

6.3 Discuss the special eye care needs of comatose individuals. (p. 658)

6.4 List basic steps used to care for eyeglasses. (p. 659)

6.5 Describe nursing measures to assist a person in the cleansing of a prosthetic eye. (p. 659)

6.6 Outline essential guidelines to be followed when assisting a person with the care of contact lenses. (p. 659)

6.7 List the kinds of data that should be included in an assessment of an individual's ears. (p. 660)

6.8 Identify and briefly describe four basic types of hearing aids. (p. 660)

6.9 Briefly describe proper care of external hearing aid devices. (p. 660)

6.10 List the four basic parts of a hearing aid. (p. 660)

6.11 Identify criteria that can be used to evaluate the effectiveness of nursing care related to eye, ear, and nasal hygiene. (p. 661)

6.12 Describe nursing measures used to promote good nasal hygiene. (p. 661)

6.13 Explain the steps involved in insertion of a hearing aid device. (p. 661)

Ask students to identify the assessment data that should be gathered when performing hygienic care to the eyes, ears, and nose.

Instruct students to include care of the eyes, ears, and nose when assisting individuals with hygienic needs.

Briefly discuss the types of hearing aid devices that are used by people who have difficulty hearing. Ask students to describe special care involved in the use of each device.

Have students describe the factors that should be considered to assure correct hearing aid insertion.

7.0 Identify agents used in skin care.

7.1 List three factors that influence the selection of agents used to clean and protect the skin. (p. 663)

7.2 List skin care options that are available for individuals with normally dry skin. (p. 664)

7.3 List six major purposes of medicated baths. (p. 672)

8.0 Compare principles used for bathing infants with those for bathing adults.

8.1 Identify seven major benefits of bathing. (p. 663)

8.2 Outline basic principles of care that are applicable to all types of bathing. (p. 663)

8.3 List safety factors the nurse should take into consideration before bathing an infant. (p. 672)

8.4 Identify basic guidelines to be followed when giving an infant a bath. (p. 672)

## Class Activity

Ask students to identify the personal hygiene products that are available in a local drug store. Have them compare their findings in class.

## Clinical Laboratory Experience

Ask students to identify the agents used in their clinical facility to clean and protect the skin.

## Campus Laboratory Experience

Discuss the guidelines that should be used by the nurse to bathe an infant. Ask students to compare the commonalities and differences between this technique and the techniques used for bathing an adult.

9.0 Plan special care required for perineum, hair, and feet.

    9.1 State three purposes of perineal care and identify indications for it's use. (p. 672)

    9.2 Review the anatomy and physiology of the male and female perineal areas. (p. 673)

    9.3 Discuss the underlying principles influencing perineal care. (p. 674)

    9.4 Identify nursing assessment data that may indicate the need for perineal care. (p. 674)

    9.5 List three major nursing goals of perineal care. (p. 674)

    9.6 Describe basic nursing intervention useful in assisting a person with perineal care. (p. 674)

    9.7 Identify individuals who might require special perineal care. (p. 675)

    9.8 List criteria used to evaluate the effectiveness of perineal care. (p. 675)

    9.9 Identify five major goals of nail and foot care. (p. 676)

    9.10 List assessment data that should be gathered during the general bath, that would assist the nurse in determining the need for basic nail and foot care. (p. 676)

    9.11 Briefly describe basic hygienic care of the nails and feet. (p. 676)

    9.12 List criteria that can be used to evaluate care of the nails and feet. (p. 677)

    9.13 Summarize the basic structure and function of the hair. (p. 683)

    9.14 Identify appropriate nursing goals for care of the hair. (p. 683)

    9.15 List information that should be included in a general assessment of the hair. (p. 683)

    9.16 Identify data that might indicate the need for hair care assistance. (p. 683)

    9.17 Outline appropriate nursing measures used in the provision of basic daily hair care. (p. 684)

    9.18 Describe special hair care considerations that may be required as a result of hair texture, curliness, or individual style preference. (p. 684)

    9.19 Discuss the nurse's responsibility with regard to the care of individuals using wigs or hair pieces. (p. 685)

## Lecture/Discussion

Ask student to discuss measures used to provide effective nail and foot care.

Ask students to describe nursing measures that can be used to assist a person with special hair care needs: Tangled or matted hair and pediculosis.

## Clinical Laboratory Experience

After demonstrating the correct procedure, ask students to assist individuals in the clinical area with perineal care.

Using the nursing process as a guide, ask students to plan and implement hair care techniques for assigned individuals in the clinical agency.

9.20 Plan appropriate nursing intervention for people with special hair care problems: Tangled or matted hair and pediculosis. (p. 685)

9.21 Describe the procedure for shampooing a person's hair in a sitting position, on a stretcher, and in bed. (p. 685)

9.22 List equipment and supplies needed when performing a shampoo. (p. 686)

9.23 Describe nursing measures related to care of a mustache or beard. (p. 686)

9.24 Enumerate reasons for shaving a hospitalized individual's hair. (p. 687)

9.25 Identify basic guidelines that should be followed when shaving another individual. (p. 687)

9.26 Describe criteria used to evaluate care of the hair. (p. 687)

10.0 Practice methods of therapeutic massage of back, hands, and feet.

10.1 Identify at least three reasons the professional nurse might perform a massage. (p. 677)

10.2 Identify areas of the body that should not be massaged without a specific physician's order. (p. 677)

10.3 Briefly describe the procedure used to provide hand, foot, and body massage. (p. 677)

10.4 Describe criteria that should be included in an evaluation of the effectiveness of a massage. (p. 683)

11.0 Maintain a comfortable and therapeutic bed for a person confined to bed.

11.1 List, and briefly describe, items commonly found in a basic hospital unit. (p. 647)

11.2 Describe three types of beds that are commonly used in health care facilities: Manually-operated, hydraulic, and electric. (p. 647)

11.3 Identify criteria that can be used to evaluate the need for linen change. (p. 687)

11.4 Describe various types of bed linens and the indications for their use: Full sheet, draw sheet, mattress pad, blanket, bedspread, and pillow case. (p. 688)

11.5 List potential individual problems that may be caused by bed linens. (p. 688)

11.6 Discuss the major functions and purposes of bed siderails. (p. 688)

## Campus Laboratory Experience

Have students practice performing hand, foot, and body massage on a classmate.

## Lecture/Discussion

Ask students to briefly discuss additional bed equipment that can be used to facilitate the hospitalized individual's comfort.

## Campus Laboratory Experience

Demonstrate the procedure for making occupied and unoccupied beds. Ask each student to practice each technique in the campus laboratory setting.

## Clinical Laboratory Experience

Ask students to identify the components of a basic hospital unit. Have them identify the items that are used in their clinical facility.

Ask students to identify individuals in their clinical facility that could benefit from the use of other additional bed equipment: Footboards, trapeze and traction, overbed cradles, alternating pressure mattresses, eggcrate mattresses, sheepskins, and chux.

11.7 Discuss responsibilities of the nurse prior to attempting bed position changes. (p. 688)

11.8 Describe the two common bed positions: Contour and Fowler's position. (p. 688)

11.9 Understand basic concepts, principles, and activities associated with bed making: Asepsis, body mechanics, work organization, individuality, and safety. (p. 689)

11.10 List contraindications and precautions the nurse should consider when making an occupied bed. (p. 689)

11.11 Explore the educational needs of a person who requires an occupied bed linen change. (p. 689)

11.12 List equipment needed to perform an occupied bed linen change. (p. 690)

11.13 Describe the steps involved in changing the linens on an occupied bed. (p. 690)

11.14 Discuss responsibilities of the nurse upon completion of an occupied bed linen change. (p. 694)

11.15 Describe modifications in the bed making procedure that result from the use of additional bed equipment: bed boards, footboards, trapeze, protective bed items, overbed cradle, alternating-pressure pad, eggcrate mattress, "sheepskins," and chux. (p. 694)

---

## MULTIPLE CHOICE QUESTIONS

1. Which of the following should occur when placing an immobilized person on a bedpan?

   A. After placement, slightly raising the head of the bed
   B. Asking the person to turn toward you for bedpan placement
   C. Raising the bed to a comfortable working height, and lowering both siderails
   D. Using good aseptic technique throughout the procedure

2. The nurse can decrease Mrs. Lane's embarrassment and discomfort when receiving perineal care by:

   A. Maintaining a professional attitude and approach
   B. Pulling the curtain around her and closing the door to the room
   C. Avoiding unnecessary exposure
   D. All of the above

## CORRECT ANSWER AND RATIONALE

D    Due to the increased number of bacteria present in the perineal area, the nurse should always use good aseptic technique when providing elimination care. (p. 649)

D    Each of the listed actions would assist in decreasing the individual's discomfort and embarrassment when receiving perineal care. (p. 649)

3.  After placing a person on a bedpan, the nurse should elevate the head of the bed to a near sitting position to:

    A.  Assimilate a normal elimination posture
    B.  Prevent undue pressure on the soft tissue of the buttocks
    C.  Promote the individual's comfort
    D.  Reduce the individual's risk of soiling the bed linens

A   The bed is raised to a mid- or high-Fowler's position because this position most resembles normal elimination posture.

    This position allows for gravity to aid in the defecation process. (p. 649)

4.  When performing an oral examination, which of the following findings would suggest poor oral hygiene practices?

    A.  Inflammation of the palate
    B.  Red, shiny, edematous gingival tissue
    C.  Red tongue coloring
    D.  Scanty salivation

B   Options A, C, and D are rarely if ever caused by poor oral hygiene. For a summary of the significant assessment findings and their potential causes, see page 653 in the text. (p. 653)

5.  The primary goal of nursing care when providing oral hygiene is to:

    A.  Achieve effective oral hygiene
    B.  Achieve oral comfort and cleanliness
    C.  Maintain integrity of the teeth and oral mucous membranes
    D.  Prevent any infections from occurring in the oral cavity

C   Option C is the overall goal of oral care. Other options are subgoals of care. (p. 655)

6.  Which of the following is a correct statement?

    A.  A slightly abrasive toothbrush should be used to properly clean the teeth
    B.  Proper brushing technique should remove all dental plaque and debris from around the teeth
    C.  The toothbrush should be held at a 45 degree angle when cleaning the inside surface of the back teeth
    D.  Waxed floss is recommended because it is more absorbent

C   The toothbrush should be held at a 45 degree angle when cleaning the inside and outside surfaces of the back teeth. (p. 656)

7.  All of the following measures are appropriate when providing routine eye care to a comatose person except:

    A.  Cleaning from the inner to the outer canthus
    B.  Taping the eyes shut if the corneal reflex is absent
    C.  Using a separate corner of the washcloth for each eye
    D.  Using a warm water or saline compress to remove any crusted secretions

B   If the eyes of a comatose person remain open, they should be closed and covered with a protective shield. They should never be taped shut. (p. 658)

8.  When providing basic hygienic care, you notice several pinpoint red spots on Mrs. Carter's upper extremities. This is correctly called:

    A.  Ecchymosis
    B.  Erythema
    C.  Petechiae
    D.  Purpura

C   Petechiae are pinpoint sized reddish spots. (p. 662)

9.  The nurse should plan to perform routine bath activities:

    A.  According to individual preference
    B.  Early each morning
    C.  Just prior to bedtime
    D.  Whenever soiling occurs

A   A person's bathing habits and the skin care products are strongly influenced by their cultural background. Whenever appropriate, the nurse should take the individual's preferences into consideration. (p. 663)

SITUATION: Mr. Jacobs, a 79-year-old nursing home resident, has been admitted to the hospital for pneumonia. Upon admission his vital signs are: T-102.8; P-98; R-24; and BP-90/64. Due to the normal aging process, Mr. Jacobs requires the use of a hearing aid and eyeglasses. The physician has placed him on complete bedrest. Questions 10 through 15 apply to this situation.

10. Mr. Jacobs perspires throughout the evening. To promote his comfort, the nurse frequently washes his face, neck, hands, axillae, and perineum. This type of hygienic care is called:

    A. Assisted bedbath
    B. Complete bedbath
    C. Partial bedbath
    D. Therapeutic bath

C   When providing a partial bedbath, the nurse washes the face, hands, and other areas of the body that have the most secretions. (p. 666)

11. When giving Mr. Jacobs's bath, which of the following should occur first?

    A. Covering Mr. Jacobs with a bath blanket
    B. Gathering the necessary hygienic aids and equipment
    C. Offering the bedpan or urinal
    D. Removing the top bed linens

C   Before beginning hygienic care, the nurse should provide an opportunity for the individual to urinate or defecate. This helps the individual to feel more relaxed and comfortable, and prevents interruption during hygienic practice. (p. 649)

12. Which of the following measures is appropriate when caring for Mr. Jacobs's external hearing aid?

    A. After cleansing, blowing excess moisture from the tubing
    B. Immersing the entire device in water to cleanse it
    C. Soaking the earmold in a mild alcohol solution once a week
    D. Using a pipecleaner to remove wax and other debris from the tubing

A   The nurse should dry the device thoroughly after cleansing, blowing excess moisture from the tubing. A pipecleaner or other sharp device should never be used because it can poke a hole through the tuning. (p. 660)

13. The nurse uses long, firm strokes toward the heart when cleansing the lower extremities for all of the following reasons except:

    A. Decrease "tingling" sensations
    B. Facilitate removal of microorganisms
    C. Increase arterial blood return
    D. Stimulate venous circulation

C   The nurse can achieve options A, B, and D when using long, firm strokes to clean and dry a person's lower extremities. (p. 670)

14. To promote Mr. Jacobs's safety during an occupied linen change, the nurse should:

    A. Assess Mr. Jacobs for any movement limitations
    B. Keep both siderails raised during the procedure
    C. Place the bed in the lowest possible position when beginning the procedure
    D. All of the above

A   Option A is the only appropriate measure listed that will enhance the individual's safety during an occupied bed linen change. The nurse would be using poor body mechanic techniques if options B and C were used, and would increase both injury to herself/himself if performed. (p. 694)

15. Upon completion of an occupied linen change, the nurse should do all of the following except:

    A. Evaluate the individual's response to the procedure
    B. Replace the call signal within the person's easy reach
    C. Return the bed to a low position and raise both siderails
    D. Return unused linens to the linen closet

D  Unused linens should never be returned to the linen cart or closet, as they are considered contaminated. (p. 694)

# 34
# MEETING REST AND SLEEP NEEDS

## OBJECTIVES

1.0 Define rest and sleep in functional terms.

    1.1 Discuss factors that might influence an individual's definition of rest. (p. 698)

    1.2 Explore the role of rest in health and illness. (p. 698)

    1.3 Summarize three major prerequisites necessary for rest and relaxation. (p. 699)

    1.4 Define the concept of sleep. (p. 699)

    1.5 Describe the necessary elements of optimal sleep. (p. 702)

2.0 Discuss the nature of sleep, identifying sleep stages and the order in which they normally appear in the sleep cycle.

    2.1 Briefly describe two distinct types of sleep activity: REM and non-REM sleep. (p. 699)

    2.2 Describe the four stages of non-REM sleep. (p. 700)

    2.3 Compare and contrast the physiological body changes that occur in REM and NREM sleep. (p. 700)

    2.4 Diagram the normal sleep stage cycle. (p. 701)

    2.5 Describe the concept of circadian rhythm. (p. 701)

    2.6 Explain the relationship of the circadian rhythm to the rest-activity cycle. (p. 701)

3.0 Describe the three major categories of sleep disorders, i.e., insomnias, hypersomnias, and sleep apneas.

    3.1 Describe three major categories of sleep disturbances: insomnia, hypersomnia, and sleep apnea. (p. 702)

    3.2 Discuss alterations in the sleep stage cycle that are experienced by an individual with a sleep disorder. (p. 702)

## TEACHING/LEARNING STRATEGIES

### Written Exercise

Ask students to write their own personal definitions of rest and sleep. Have them compare their definitions with those listed on pages 698-699 in the text.

### Lecture/Discussion

Explore the impact that the circadian rhythm has on the sleep process.

Facilitate a discussion of the factors influencing the amount of sleep an individual requires to maintain health and well-being.

### Class Activity

Ask students to observe an individual during the initial stages of sleep. Have their observations in class.

### Group Activity

Divide students into groups. Ask each group to prepare a brief oral presentation on the effects of sleep for one of the stages in the life cycle.

### Lecture/Discussion

Focus discussion on the major sleep disorders: insomnia, hypersomnias, and sleep apnea. Ask students to identify the physical and psychosocial effects of each.

3.3 Outline common interventions effective in the treatment of common sleep disorders. (p. 702)

3.4 Explore the influence of the sleep stage cycle on the development of sleep apneas. (p. 703)

3.5 Describe the physiological manifestations of central and obstructive sleep apneas. (p. 703)

4.0 Identify major factors that can cause sleep disruption for people in health care facilities.

4.1 Discuss the etiology of common sleep problems often experienced by hospitalized individuals: Circadian desynchronization, sleep deprivation, sleep fragmentation, and REM/NREM rebound. (p. 703)

5.0 Assess the person's sleep patterns by talking with the individual and/or significant others.

5.1 Identify common factors that contribute to the development of problems related to sleep. (p. 705)

5.2 List information that should be included in an assessment of an individual's normal sleep habits. (p. 705)

6.0 Describe the effect various medications have on sleep patterns.

6.1 Explore the impact of various pharmacologic agents on the sleep activity cycle. (p. 705)

7.0 Apply the nursing process to minimize sleep disruption for people in health care facilities.

7.1 Describe basic nursing intervention useful in assisting a person to minimize disruption of the sleep-activity cycle. (p. 706)

7.2 Identify appropriate goals of care for nursing intervention to promote sleep. (p. 706)

## Lecture/Discussion

Ask students to discuss their own experiences with sleep deprivation.

## Clinical Laboratory Experience

Arrange for students to visit the critical care unit in their clinical facility. Ask them to identify factors in this environment that could influence the development of sleep pattern disturbances.

## Written Exercise

Before reading the chapter material, ask students to outline the data that they feel should be included in the assessment of a person's rest and sleep status. Upon completion of the material in the chapter, ask students to review the outline for its completeness. Have them share the results in class.

Instruct students to keep a diary of their rest and sleep patterns for one week. Afterwards, encourage them to assess whether or not these patterns are adequate for meeting the body's basic need for rest and sleep.

## Campus Laboratory Experience

Ask students to perform a sleep assessment on another classmate. Have them share the problems they identified in class.

## Lecture/Discussion

Ask students to describe the effects of hypnotics, amphetamines, and alcohol on sleep. Assist them in identifying the physiological reasons promoting each effect.

## Clinical Laboratory Experience

Ask students to identify individuals in the clinical area who are most prone to the development of sleep pattern disturbances.

7.3 Describe criteria that can be used to
    evaluate nursing intervention designed
    to promote effective sleep. (p. 707)

8.0 Implement physical and psychologic interven-
    tions to promote rest and sleep.

    8.1 State examples of nursing diagnoses that
        focus on rest and sleep needs. (p. 697)

    8.2 Identify potential goals of nursing care
        for rest and sleep needs. (p. 698)

    8.3 List general criteria that can be used
        to evaluate nursing intervention related
        to rest and sleep needs. (p. 698)

## Clinical Laboratory Experience

Have students formulate an appropriate plan of
care for the individual experiencing a sleep
disturbance.

Have students formulate a plan of care to minimize
or alleviate rest and sleep disturbances that they
have identified for individuals in their care.

---

## MULTIPLE CHOICE QUESTIONS

1.  Which of the following individuals would
    experience the most difficulty in attaining
    rest and relaxation? The individual whose
    nurse:

    A. Answers the call light promptly
    B. Encourages expression of feelings
    C. Provides information about an upcoming
       diagnostic test after being asked
    D. Spends time listening to the individual's
       personal concerns

2.  Physiological behaviors exhibited during the
    REM stage of sleep include all of the
    following except:

    A. Apnea
    B. Decreased cerebral metabolic activity
    C. Increased gastric secretion rates
    D. Increased respiratory rates

3.  Mr. Perry has been unable to sleep since
    being admitted to the intensive care unit.
    The nurse is aware that continued deprivation
    of REM sleep may cause:

    A. Altered sensory perception
    B. A state of mental confusion
    C. Paranoid behavior
    D. All of the above

4.  When caring for a person following a period
    of sleep deprivation, the nurse knows that
    all of the following are correct except:

    A. Dream activity may occur during stage IV
       NREM and REM sleep
    B. Most REM activity will occur during the
       second half of a night's sleep
    C. The average length of the sleep activity
       cycle is 90 minutes
    D. When both stage IV NREM and REM sleep are
       deprived, REM rebound will predominate

## CORRECT ANSWER AND RATIONALE

C   The nurse should provide explanations about
    upcoming diagnostic tests and procedures
    before being asked by the individual. The
    individual may have lost considerable rest
    before getting the courage to question the
    nurse. (p. 698)

B   Cerebral metabolic activity is generally
    increased during the REM stage of sleep. It
    is theorized that information is processed and
    reviewed during this stage of sleep. (p. 700)

D   Research has shown that REM sleep deprivation
    may precipitate disrupted perceptions that are
    manifested by disorientation, delusions, and
    even hallucinations. (p. 700)

B   Following deprivation of stage IV NREM and REM
    sleep, rebounds, or consistent quantitative
    increases in these sleep stages, occur during
    the bulk periods that follow. (p. 704)

5. Mr. Whitman recently suffered a myocardial infarction. The nurse knows that it is important to prevent sleep deprivation in this individual because:

   A. Proper rest is necessary for healing of cardiac tissue
   B. REM rebound periods can be too stressful, initiating another MI
   C. It can increase the incidence of disorientation in this individual
   D. Sedatives are contraindicated in individuals who have suffered a heart attack

B   Because sympathetic nervous system discharge is pronounced during REM sleep, excessive myocardial stimulation can lead to ischemia and/or infarction during sleep periods in which REM sleep occurs more frequently and for longer periods such as in rebound. (p. 704)

6. Arrange the stages of the normal sleep cycle in their appropriate order.

   A. Stages 1, 2, 3, 4, REM
   B. Stages 1, 2, 3, 4, 3, 2, REM
   C. Stages 1, 2, 3, 4, 3, 2, 1, REM
   D. Stages 1, 2, 3, 4, 3, 2, 1

B   The normal sleep cycle is composed of the following cycle: Stages 1, 2, 3, 4, 3, 2, REM. (p. 701)

7. Mr. Dowell frequently experiences brief, irresistible periods of sleep. This is called:

   A. Cataplexy
   B. Sleep paralysis
   C. Hypersomnia
   D. Narcolepsy

D   The person who suffers from narcolepsy experiences excessive daytime sleepiness and irresistible, relatively brief attacks of sleep. (p. 702)

8. Since her husband's death five weeks ago, Mrs. Barker has needed to take a hypnotic agent to facilitate sleep. If this medication is abruptly discontinued which of the following may occur?

   A. REM rebound
   B. Heightened sensory perceptual awareness
   C. Increased emotional stability
   D. All of the above

A   Many commonly used sedative and hypnotic agents alter sleep by suppressing REM activity. The development of these REM debts sets the stage for perceptual and emotional disturbances and for potentially dangerous rebounds. (p. 705)

9. Assessment data indicative of a potential sleep pattern disturbance include all of the following except:

   A. Is in unusual sleep environment
   B. Has been taking chloral hydrate at home to assist with sleep
   C. Is frequently awakened throughout the night for nursing rounds
   D. Frequently naps for short intervals throughout the day

B   Chloral hydrate is an effective sedative that causes minimal or no disruption in the sleep stage cycles. Options A, C, and D are all significant findings that may indicate a potential sleep pattern alteration. (p. 705)

10. Mr. Ball, a night supervisor for a local factory, has been admitted to the hospital for minor surgery. Which of the following would be least effective in meeting his rest and sleep needs?

    A. Provide a warm glass of milk before bedtime
    B. Encourage him to retire at 10 pm each evening
    C. Give him a backrub
    D. Provide light diversional activity before bedtime

B   The nurse should attempt to assimilate Mr. Ball's normal sleeping patterns. Since he works nights at a local factory, he probably sleeps primarily during the daytime hours. (p. 706)

# 35

## FACILITATING RELIEF FROM PAIN

OBJECTIVES

1.0 Describe the psychologic and physical phenomenon of pain.

   1.1 Identify factors influencing the unique nature of pain (p. 711)

   1.2 Describe the concept of pain tolerance. (p. 712)

   1.3 Briefly describe the function of pain as it relates to body defenses against injury. (p. 713)

   1.4 Explore the relationship of the body's three major lines of defense against injury: Withdrawal reflexes, visceral reflexes, and voluntary responses. (p. 713)

   1.5 Discuss the three components of pain sensation: Reception, perception, and reaction. (p. 713)

   1.6 Explore the influence of physiological and emotional factors on the perception of pain. (p. 714)

   1.7 List factors that can influence the perception and meaning of pain for an individual. (p. 714)

   1.8 Define the concept of pain threshold. (p. 714)

   1.9 Discuss the difference in pain threshold and pain tolerance. (p. 714)

   1.10 Identify the relationship of pain sensation and pain reaction to the pain experience. (p. 714)

   1.11 Discuss the role of the cerebral cortex in the pain experience. (p. 714)

   1.12 Identify two factors that influence the brain's ability to localize pain. (p. 714)

   1.13 Discuss sociocultural factors that determine an individual's definition of pain. (p. 715)

   1.14 Identify factors that contribute to the anxiety of a person experiencing pain. (p. 716)

TEACHING/LEARNING STRATEGIES

Lecture/Discussion

Focus discussion on the body's various defenses against pain: Withdrawal reflexes, visceral reflexes, and voluntary responses.

Have students discuss pain in terms of its "component parts:" Reception, perception, and reaction.

Focus discussion on the body's mechanism for localizing pain in the body.

Ask students to describe the process for transmission and perception of painful stimuli.

Ask students to identify variables that may alter a person's perception and response to pain.

1.15 Explore the impact of an individual's
     ethnic affiliation on the attitude of
     pain.  (p. 716)

1.16 Identify factors useful in assessing the
     meaning that pain may hold for an
     individual.  (p. 716)

1.17 Compare and contrast the experience of
     psychogenic pain to that of pain
     produced by organic disease.  (p. 717)

1.18 List general factors that contribute to
     the "nature" of various types of pain.
     (p. 717)

1.19 Identify common pathophysiological
     causes of pain.  (p. 719)

1.20 Identify observable signs and symptoms
     of pain that are elicited by the
     autonomic nervous system.  (p. 720)

1.21 Compare and contrast sympathetic and
     parasympathetic responses to pain.
     (p. 720)

1.22 Discuss variables that may influence a
     person's ability to accurately describe
     the pain experience.  (p. 720)

1.23 Explore the impact anxiety can have on a
     person's pain experience.  (p. 722)

1.24 Identify factors that influence the
     development of a person's behavioral
     response to pain.  (p. 726)

2.0 List and differentiate between facts and
    fallacies about pain.

## Class Activity

Ask students to identify some of the common
misconceptions that an individual may have about
pain.  Have them elicit and evaluate a family
member's beliefs related to each fallacy.

3.0 Discuss various ways of defining pain.

## Lecture/Discussion

3.1 Explore various definitions of pain.
    (p. 712)

Ask students to list terms describing the worst
pain that they have ever experienced.

3.2 Briefly describe two distinct types of
    pain in relation to duration:  Acute and
    chronic.  (p. 712)

Provide clinical examples of each type of pain:
Acute, limited, intermittent, persistent, and
intractable.

3.3 Differentiate between the following
    types of pain:  Limited, intermittent,
    persistent, and intractable.  (p. 712)

3.4 Identify terminology frequently used by
    an individual to describe the experience
    of pain.  (p. 717)

4.0 Apply the nursing process to a person
    experiencing pain.

## Written Exercise

4.1 Give examples of nursing diagnoses that
    focus on the needs of individuals with
    pain.  (p. 709)

Ask students to list criteria that would be useful
in evaluating the effectiveness of pain control
measures.  Have them compare their responses to
those of another student in the class.

4.2 Identify common nursing goals of care for individuals with pain. (p. 710)

4.3 Discuss behavioral outcomes that may be used to evaluate the effectiveness of nursing intervention related to pain. (p. 710)

4.4 Identify factors that influence the nurse's attitude toward pain. (p. 715)

4.5 Identify ways in which the nurse can promote accurate descriptions of the pain experience. (p. 720)

4.6 List essential knowledge the nurse must possess to perform effective intervention for individuals experiencing pain. (p. 721)

4.7 Discuss the meaning of the statement, "A nurse both produces and relieves pain." (p. 721)

4.8 Discuss ways in which the nurse can use preoperative teaching to reduce postoperative pain and discomfort. (p. 726)

5.0 Plan effective nursing care for people experiencing pain, including psychologic, physical, and pharmacologic aspects of care.

5.1 Discuss the variety of traditional Eastern and Western methods of pain control that are currently in use today. (p. 710)

5.2 Discuss the role of documentation in the diagnosis, treatment, and care of individuals experiencing pain. (p. 718)

5.3 Identify data that the nurse should obtain when assessing the nature of an individual's pain. (p. 718)

5.4 Discuss the importance of ongoing assessment when caring for individuals experiencing pain. (p. 719)

5.5 Identify characteristics by which psychogenic pain can be assessed. (p. 719)

5.6 List factors the nurse should consider when planning nursing care for the relief of pain. (p. 722)

5.7 Identify self-directed, noninvasive measures a person can use to facilitate relief from pain. (p. 722)

5.8 Identify the essentials of teaching an individual to utilize self-directive, noninvasive pain relief measures. (p. 722)

Clinical Laboratory Experience

Assist students in applying appropriate pain assessment techniques to a person in the clinical area.

Lecture/Discussion

Have students identify the factors that should be considered when selecting appropriate nursing intervention for the person who is experiencing pain.

5.9 Briefly describe various self-directed, noninvasive pain relief measures: Relaxation techniques: distraction; guided imagery; cutaneous stimulation; exercise; hypnosis; and family, group, or individual therapy. (p. 723)

5.10 Identify techniques the nurse can use to diminish a person's pain-related anxiety. (p. 723)

5.11 Describe ways in which the nurse can reduce an individual's fear of pain. (p. 723)

5.12 Discuss a variety of diversional activities that can be utilized to decrease a person's focus on pain. (p. 725)

5.13 Outline the role of the nurse in combating a person's anticipatory fear of pain. (p. 726)

5.14 Describe the advantages of a "patient-controlled analgesia system." (p. 727)

5.15 Outline essential physical aspects of care that the nurse can utilize to increase a person's tolerance of pain. (p. 727)

5.16 List three reasons the application of heat or cold reduces or relieves pain. (p. 728)

5.17 Outline guidelines for administering analgesic medications. (p. 728)

5.18 Briefly discuss the nurse's responsibility with regard to the administration of analgesics. (p. 729)

5.19 List important factors the nurse should know in order to make informed decisions about analgesic medication administration. (p. 729)

6.0 Discuss specific components of care for people experiencing chronic intractable pain.

6.1 List nursing actions that can be carried out to decrease the suffering of individuals with chronic intractable pain. (p. 730)

6.2 Discuss concerns related to the management of severe chronic pain of nonmalignant origin with analgesic medication. (p. 730)

6.3 List examples of nondrug interventions that can be used to battle chronic pain of malignant origin. (p. 731)

6.4 Compare and contrast the management of progressive pain of malignant origin to that of severe chronic pain of non-malignant origin. (p. 731)

## Lecture/Discussion

Ask students to compare and contrast the approaches used to treat chronic pain and terminal pain.

6.5 Identify variables that influence the pain associated with an individual who has disseminated cancer. (p. 731)

6.6 Explain the rationale for administering narcotic analgesics on a regularly scheduled basis to individuals with progressive pain of malignant origin. (p. 731)

6.7 Identify other drugs that are frequently used in conjunction with narcotic analgesics to facilitate the control of pain of malignant origin. (p. 731)

6.8 Give examples of alternate therapies that may be used to decrease pain associated with malignant disease. (p. 732)

7.0 Discuss the problems of people unable to experience pain.

7.1 Identify factors the nurse must consider in order to prevent injury in an individual who lacks the ability to experience the sensation of pain. (p. 732)

## Lecture/Discussion

Assist students in identifying appropriate safety measures that should be used for the person who cannot experience pain.

Have students identify clinical examples of individuals who are unable to experience pain.

---

## MULTIPLE CHOICE QUESTIONS

1. An individual has intractable pain. This is best described as pain that:

   A. Cannot be tolerated
   B. Induced by internal irritants
   C. Lasts longer than six months
   D. Occurs with neoplastic disease

2. Mrs. Moore experiences persistent, chronic pain of the lower back. An assessment of the person with chronic pain might reveal all of the following except:

   A. Narrowed range of interests
   B. Depression and anger
   C. Increased BP and diaphoresis
   D. Increased medication for pain control

3. Which of the following statements is incorrect?

   A. The intensity, duration, and rhythmicity of pain varies according to the organ involved.

   B. Pain is present only when there is demonstrable injury, disease, or noxious stimulation.
   C. Individuals vary in the intensity and duration of pain that they are willing to endure.
   D. Pain is difficult to assess because of its subjective nature.

## CORRECT ANSWER AND RATIONALE

A   Intractable pain is pain that cannot be controlled, relieved, or cured. It does occur commonly with neoplastic diseases, but can occur for other reasons. (p. 712)

C   The person who suffers from chronic pain rarely, if ever, exhibits any of the clinical signs of pain, such as: increased BP, increased pulse rate, increased respiratory rate, and diaphoresis. (p. 713)

B   Pain may be present in the absence of any demonstrable injury, disease, or noxious stimulation. An example is the phantom limb pain that occurs in a person who has had an amputation. (p. 712)

4.  In order to provide therapeutic care for the person who is experiencing pain, the nurse should first examine:

    A.  Personal feelings toward the person experiencing pain
    B.  Personal attitudes toward pain and suffering
    C.  Cultural values influencing the person's pain experience
    D.  All of the above

D   If the nurse is to deliver therapeutic care for the person with pain, all of the listed options must first be closely examined. (p. 714)

5.  When assessing a person in pain the nurse is aware that all of the following are true except:

    A.  Pain that originates in body organs is usually poorly localized.
    B.  Pain receptors are most prevalent in the skin and surface tissues.
    C.  Long-term pain often results in an increased sympathetic response.
    D.  Pain duration and severity significantly influence a person's physiological response.

C   People with chronic pain usually adapt to it so that they show no behavioral or physiologic signs. (p. 712)

6.  As a result of his cultural influences, Mr. Banks quietly accepts intense post-operative pain. To promote this individual's comfort, the nurse should:

    A.  Advise the individual that he will recover sooner if he accepts treatment for the pain
    B.  Administer medication for pain around every four hours for the next two days
    C.  Base effective nursing intervention on the nonverbal cues that are elicited
    D.  Continue offering medication for pain several times a day

C   The nurse can gather data about the severity of Mr. Banks's pain by observing nonverbal expressions of pain. (p. 715)

7.  Which of the following individual's pain tolerance will be least affected by other contributing factors? A person who:

    A.  Is all alone in a room at night
    B.  Is engaged in conversation with a significant other
    C.  Is immobilized and must depend on others for all needs
    D.  Slept poorly throughout the previous night

B   The individuals in options A, B, and C are likely to have a reduced tolerance for pain because of other contributing factors. Numerous factors, joined together, contribute to the "nature" of various pains. The individual in option B may effectively increase their tolerance to pain by engaging in diversionary activities. (p. 717)

8.  A person who is experiencing pain is asked by the nurse to rate their pain as slight, moderate, or severe. This information will help the nurse to determine the:

    A.  Character of the pain
    B.  Intensity of the pain
    C.  Periodicity of the pain
    D.  Reaction to the pain

B   Because of variable individual psychophysiologic factors, it is often difficult to assess the intensity of pain. Some idea of the intensity of pain can be gathered by encouraging the individual to rate their pain on any one of a number of scales. (p. 718)

9.  Which of the following is not a typical sympathetic response to pain?

    A.  Pupil dilation
    B.  Pallor
    C.  Increased BP
    D.  Fainting/unconsciousness

D   Sympathetic responses to pain are elicited in as the body attempts to maintain homeostasis. They are designed to prepare the body for a fight or flight response. (p. 720)

10. A small child, who is experiencing pain, is given a toy with which to play. This technique is used to alter pain:

   A. Interpretation
   B. Perception
   C. Reaction
   D. Reception

B   Techniques that distract a person's attention away from the pain experience, alter the perception of pain. (p. 723)

11. Mrs. Lawrence, who was admitted to the hospital with a severe kidney infection, tells her nurse that she is "extremely uncomfortable this morning." The nurse should:

   A. Assume that she is in pain
   B. Administer an analgesic to relieve the pain
   C. Perform a more detailed assessment of her pain
   D. Attempt to determine the source of the discomfort

D   The nurse should clarify what Mrs. Lawrence means by "uncomfortable." The nurse should never assume that an individual is in "pain," but should always perform a more detailed assessment before taking any action. (p. 720)

12. John recently had a cast applied for a compound fracture of the tibia. Nursing measures to reduce the incidence of pain in this individual would include all of the following except:

   A. Applying heat to the casted limb
   B. Administering analgesic medications ordered by the physician
   C. Elevating the extremity on pillows
   D. Immobilizing the extremity initially

A   Options C and D would promote the individual's comfort by reducing the incidence of swelling and local pressure. Option B would assist in altering the perception of pain. Application of heat would be contraindicated, since its primary function would be to reduce fluid accumulation in the already edematous extremity. (p. 727)

13. The nurse can promote the comfort of a person with chronic, intractable pain by:

   A. Ensuring that their feelings are understood
   B. Promoting productive, meaningful activity throughout the day
   C. Providing prompt assistance when needed
   D. All of the above

D   All of the listed options would facilitate comfort in the person with chronic, intractable pain. For a complete listing of appropriate intervention, see pages 729-730 in text. (p. 729)

# 36

# MEETING BASIC NUTRITIONAL NEEDS

## OBJECTIVES

1.0  Define the basic functions of the major nutrients, vitamins, and minerals.

    1.1  State the basic definition of the term nutrition.  (p. 736)

    1.2  Identify the relationship of proper nutritional support to the basic functioning of living organisms. (p. 736)

    1.3  Define specific terms related to basic nutrition:  calorie, kilocalorie, basal energy requirement, and ideal body weight.  (p. 737)

    1.4  Describe the method used to determine adult basal metabolic rates.  (p. 737)

    1.5  Identify factors influencing a person's total energy requirements.  (p. 737)

    1.6  Discuss the basic energy-yielding nutrients and their caloric values. (p. 737)

    1.7  Explain the significance of caloric intake to maintenance of ideal body weight.  (p. 738)

    1.8  Describe the five essential groups of nutrients required by the body for adequate nutrition.  Include in this discussion:  purposes and functions in the body; methods of absorption, digestion, metabolism, and storage by the body; and specific dietary sources of each.  (pp. 738-743)

    1.9  Describe the term glycemic index and the effect it has on body functioning. (p. 739)

2.0  Evaluate a person's dietary intake and nutritional status.

    2.1  Identify the recommended daily allowances and dietary examples of the basic four food groups as outlined by the Food and Nutrition Board of the National Academy of Sciences.  (p. 736)

    2.2  State the definition of recommended dietary allowances as described by the Food and Nutrition Board.  (p. 736)

## TEACHING/LEARNING STRATEGIES

### Group Activity

Divide the class into five groups.  Ask each group to prepare a classroom presentation of one of the five essential groups of nutrients:  carbohydrates; fats; proteins; vitamins and minerals; and fluids. This discussion should include the purpose and function of the nutrient in the body; methods of absorption, digestion, metabolism, and storage by the body; and specific dietary sources of each.

### Communication Activity

Ask students to assess a community individual's knowledge of the basic principles of nutrition. Discuss findings in class.

### Lecture/Discussion

Summarize the role of the "recommended dietary allowances" in meeting the nutritional requirements of healthy individuals.

### Group Activity

Divide students into small groups.  Ask one-half of the groups to plan a balanced vegetarian meal, the other half to plan a balanced non-vegetarian meal.  In class, have each group discuss the rationale for their food choices.

2.3 Analyze the value of using the RDA as a standard of reference for assessing the dietary adequacy of diseased individuals. (p. 737)

2.4 Briefly discuss advantages and disadvantages of strict adherence to a vegetarian diet. (p. 746)

2.5 Identify responsibilities of the health care professional engaged in nutritional counseling with individuals or groups. (p. 748)

2.6 Identify essential data to be obtained when assessing an individual's nutritional status. (p. 748)

2.7 Identify the specific purposes and types of data obtained from food records or food diaries. (p. 752)

2.8 Outline the clinical signs and symptoms of malnutrition. (p. 753)

2.9 Relate the significance of anthropometric measurements to nutritional status. (p. 754)

2.10 Identify specific biochemical tests used in the assessment of nutritional status and discuss the advantages of their use. (p. 754)

3.0 Discuss the impact of pregnancy, lactation, illness, and injury on dietary needs.

3.1 Briefly discuss popular beliefs related to the use of food additives, organic foods, and nutritional supplements. (p. 743)

3.2 Discuss ways in which nursing knowledge can be utilized to confront situations of "good fadism." (p. 744)

3.3 Identify the purpose of food additives and potential health problems they may cause. (p. 744)

3.4 Discuss the pro's and con's of using organically grown foods and supplemental foods in the diet. (p. 744)

3.5 Describe the positive and negative effects that vitamin and mineral supplements can have on an individual's health. (p. 745)

3.6 Identify preventive and therapeutic roles of "special foods" in the diet. (p. 746)

4.0 Describe in what ways social factors such as culture, financial status, religion, social circumstances, and activity patterns affect dietary choices and requirements.

Divide students into small groups of four or five. Instruct each group to plan a nutritionally balanced meal for a family of four, costing no more than $5.00. Ask each group to prepare a brief presentation of the nutritional value of the meal according to RDA requirements.

### Class Activity

Instruct students to keep a record of their food and fluid intake for twenty-four hours. Evaluate in terms of RDA requirements, basic four food groups, and caloric intake. Identify potential excesses and deficits in dietary intake. Discuss findings in class.

### Guest Speaker

Invite a nutritionist from a local hospital to discuss the techniques used to evaluate an individual's nutritional status, and the methods of intervention used to alleviate identified problems.

### Class Activity

Have students examine the list of ingredients for 15 food items in their home. Ask them to keep a list of the products that contain food additives, such as, vitamin and mineral supplements or preservatives. Discuss the results in class.

Ask students to interview personnel in a local health food store regarding the superiority of organic or "natural" goods over processed foods. Report findings in class.

4.1 Identify factors that influence a person's food intake, dietary patterns, and nutritional status. (p. 748)

4.2 List factors involved in the regulation of appetite and possible problems that may occur if these homeostatic mechanisms malfunction. (p. 748)

4.3 Describe ways in which the financial position of an individual may affect nutritional status. (p. 749)

4.4 Discuss the impact of geographic location on food consumption. Identify cultural factors that may influence eating habits. (p. 749)

4.5 Provide examples of religious practices that may influence dietary intake. (p. 749)

4.6 Discuss the impact social events and conditions may have on nutritional status. (p. 749)

4.7 Identify variations in nutritional needs according to age. (p. 750)

4.8 Identify ways in which food preferences and nutritional requirements may influence an individual's dietary intake. (p. 750)

4.9 Describe physiological responses and other reactions an individual may have to certain foods or food groups. (p. 750)

4.10 List actions the nurse might utilize when assisting persons requiring dietary modifications. (p. 750)

4.11 Summarize alterations in nutritional status that often accompany pregnancy and lactation. (p. 750)

4.12 Discuss the impact media has had on dietary intake and food related behaviors. (p. 750)

4.13 Identify the nutritional implications of consistent drug and alcohol abuse. (p. 750)

4.14 Describe potential problems and the possible nursing implications for people experiencing illness and injury. (p. 750)

4.15 Provide examples of how variations in activity patterns can influence nutritional status. (p. 750)

## Clinical Laboratory Experience

Instruct students to gather a dietary history from an individual in the hospital or an individual at a local health department. Ask them to evaluate the data in terms of potential nutritional problems and factors that are influential in the individual's dietary choices.

| MULTIPLE CHOICE QUESTIONS | CORRECT ANSWER AND RATIONALE |
|---|---|

MULTIPLE CHOICE QUESTIONS

1. Which of the following statements are correct?

   A. An individual's nutritional needs remain the same throughout life.
   B. Nutrition is the sum of processes by which a living organism ingests, digests, absorbs, transports, and uses nutrients.
   C. Many of the nutrients needed by the body must be obtained through medication.
   D. Nutritional needs are the same for all states of health.

2. In order to provide effective nursing care for individuals experiencing nutritional problems, the nurse needs to be aware of:

   A. Basic concepts of good nutrition
   B. Emotional attitudes toward food
   C. Individual food preferences
   D. All of the above

3. The Recommended Dietary Allowances formulated by the Food and Nutrition Board:

   A. Illustrate minimal nutritional requirements of all healthy individuals
   B. Can always be used as a standard of reference for assessing nutritional status
   C. Outline adequate daily requirements of specific nutrients for almost every healthy person
   D. Make allowances for nutritional needs in any state of health

4. The daily basal energy requirements for a 50-year-old male with an ideal body weight of 150 lbs. is approximately:

   A. 1350 kcal
   B. 1500 kcal
   C. 1650 kcal
   D. 2000 kcal

5. How many kilocalories will an individual receive if a meal provides 325Gm of carbohydrate, 24Gm of protein, and 10Gm of fat?

   A. 314 kcal
   B. 468 kcal
   C. 516 kcal
   D. 544 kcal

6. A kilocalorie is best described as:

   A. The amount of heat required to increase one gram of water by one degree Celsius
   B. The amount of heat required to increase ten grams of water by ten degrees Fahrenheit
   C. The amount of heat required to increase one gram of water by one degree Fahrenheit
   D. The amount of heat required to increase one kilogram of water by one degree Celsius

CORRECT ANSWER AND RATIONALE

B   Response B is a correct statement of a definition of the concept of/for nutrition. Studies have indicated that the nutritional needs of people are altered by age, disease, activity, and stress. All nutrients required by the body for growth and function can be obtained by using a variety of food combinations. (pp. 736-737)

D   The nurse providing nutritional support for individuals must be knowledgeable of the basic principles of nutrition and food composition, and sensitive to the role food plays in the lives of individuals and groups. (pp. 736-737)

C   Recommended Dietary Allowances are levels of intake of essential nutrients considered to be adequate in meeting the known nutritional needs of almost every healthy person. The RDA, as a standard of reference, may be of limited value if the person under considera- tion is distinctly different from the average, healthy person. (pp. 736-739)

B   The basal energy needs of persons over 45 years of age can be estimated by multiplying ideal body weight by 9 kcal for women and by 10 kcal for men. (pp. 737)

A   The basic energy yielding nutrients supply calories in the following amounts: Fat - 9 kcal/Gm; Carbohydrates - 4 kcal/Gm; and Protein - 4 kcal/Gm. (pp. 736)

D   A calorie is the amount of heat needed to raise the temperature of one gram of water one degree Celsius; therefore, a kilocalorie is the amount of heat needed to increase one kilogram of water one degree Celsius. (pp. 736-739)

7. Which of the following individuals has the greatest total energy requirements?

   A. A teenager playing competitive tennis
   B. A hospitalized individual who is confined to bed
   C. A hospitalized individual engaged in ambulation activities
   D. A woman cleaning house

A   The total energy needs of an individual increase proportionately with physical activity. (p. 736)

8. Carbohydrates are necessary in the diet because they:

   A. Assist in the maintenance and repair of body tissues
   B. Provide the body with the most concentrated source of energy
   C. Provide the body with an unlimited storage form of energy
   D. Are the most readily available source of energy

D   Glucose, an end-product of di- and poly-saccharide digestion, is the major source of energy for the body. Glycogen, the stored form of glucose found in the liver and muscles, is used by the body for energy before fats and proteins. Fats provide the body with the most concentrated form of energy, producing 9 kcal/Gm ingested. After depleting circulating blood glucose and stored glycogen, the body begins to breakdown fats and proteins for energy. (p. 738)

9. All of the following statements about proteins are true except:

   A. Incomplete proteins are found in meat, milk, cheese, and eggs.
   B. Proteins play a major role in the manufacture of enzymes and hormones.
   C. The primary function of dietary protein is to provide amino acids for growth and maintenance of body tissues.
   D. All body cells contain amino acids, the structural building unit of proteins.

A   Statements B, C, D are all correct statements related to proteins. Meat, milk, cheese, and eggs are all examples of complete proteins. (p. 741)

10. Fats serve all of the following functions in the body except:

   A. Assists in the absorption of water soluble vitamins: C and B-Complex group
   B. Provides almost unlimited stores of energy in the form of adipose tissue
   C. Protects the vital organs in the form of subcutaneous fat
   D. Supplies the body with cholesterol, a precursor of the sex and adrenal hormones

A   Fats enable the transport of the fat-soluble vitamins A, D, E, and K. Major functions of fat include: acts as insulator for the body, and supplies cholesterol for the synthesis of sex hormones and adrenal corticoids. (pp. 739-740)

11. Which of the following nutrients is not important for the growth of skin and mucous membranes?

   A. Vitamin A
   B. Niacin
   C. Proteins
   D. Vitamin D

D   Vitamin D enhances the growth and development of bones. (p. 743)

12. Which of the following foods should the nurse recommend for an individual with Vitamin K deficiencies?

   A. Citrus fruits
   B. Liver
   C. Whole milk
   D. Enriched cereals

B   Dietary sources of Vitamin K include: green leafy vegetables, cheese, egg yolks, and liver. (p. 743)

13. The nurse is aware that the potential risk
    for vitamin and mineral deficiencies is
    greatest in which of the following
    individuals:

    A. Joe, who drinks heavily on occasion
    B. Sue, who is on a 1500 calorie reducing
       diet
    C. Don, who suffers from numerous food
       allergies
    D. Carey, a breastfed infant

C   Individuals with numerous food allergies or
    intolerances may suffer from vitamin and
    mineral deficiencies due to their limited food
    choices and preferences. (pp. 736-742)

14. Additives were traditionally used to:

    A. Promote aesthetic value of food
    B. Assist in long-term preservation of food
    C. Improve the color and consistency of food
    D. Enhance the palatability of food

B   Additives have traditionally been used to help
    preserve food for future use. (p. 743)

15. In counseling an individual with a Vitamin A
    deficiency, which foods should be encouraged?

    A. Green and yellow vegetables and fruits
    B. Liver, egg yolks, and whole milk
    C. Green vegetables, vegetable oils
    D. Liver, egg yolks, and whole grain breads

B   Dietary sources of Vitamin A include: liver,
    egg yolks, cream, butter, or fortified
    margarine and whole milk. (p. 743)

16. Common fallacies related to the nutritive
    value of "health" foods include all of the
    following except:

    A. Organically grown foods are nutritionally
       superior
    B. Unprocessed or natural foods are more
       healthful
    C. Natural vitamins do not contain synthetic
       ingredients
    D. Vitamin megadoses sometimes produce toxic
       effects

D   Many people tend to support the misconception
    that vitamins taken in large doses have a
    greater health benefit, unaware of the
    potential toxic effects. (pp. 745-746)

17. The strict vegetarian will experience the
    greatest difficulty in acquiring which
    nutrient in their diet?

    A. B-Complex vitamins
    B. Complete proteins
    C. Fat-Soluble vitamins
    D. Incomplete proteins

B   Complete proteins contain all of the essential
    amino acids in quantities and ratios needed by
    the body. They are derived from animal
    sources; therefore, the strict vegetarian will
    have to include an appropriate combination of
    incomplete proteins in their diet, in order to
    provide a balanced ratio of essential amino
    acids. (pp. 741-748)

SITUATION: Mrs. Chang, a 35-year-old Oriental female, has been admitted to the hospital for malnutrition. When gathering the nursing history, Mrs. Chang tells you that her husband died two years ago, leaving her alone to support four small children. Existing on a very limited budget, she has found it increasingly difficult to meet her family's nutritional needs. Questions 18 through 22 apply to this situation.

18. Based on the above data, the nurse might make the following diagnosis for Mrs. Chang:

A. Nutrition, Alterations in; Less than body requirements related to malnutrition
B. Malnutrition related to inadequate food intake
C. Nutrition, Alterations in; Less than body requirements related to difficulty procuring food
D. Nutrition, Alterations in: Less than body requirements related to cultural practices

C  The nurse should avoid the use of medical diagnoses in statements of nursing diagnoses. (p. 754)

19. Mrs. Chang's current nutritional habits are most significantly influenced at this time by which of the following factors?

A. Culture
B. Age
C. Financial status
D. Social circumstances

C  The limited amount of money available to low- or fixed-income groups is often inadequate to buy enough food to prevent hunger, let alone promote good health. Therefore, low-income persons commonly have difficulty meeting their nutritional needs. (p. 749)

20. The nurse carefully examines Mrs. Chang for physical signs associated with malnutrition. All of the following assessment data is abnormal except:

A. Heart rate 110 beats/minute, blood pressure 130/80
B. Tongue-rough/deep red in appearance
C. Areas of skin depigmentation
D. Pale conjunctivae

B  The tongue is normally deep red in appearance, not swollen or smooth. Malnourished individuals often display rapid heart rates above 100 beats/minute, skin color loss, and pale eye membranes. (p. 753)

21. When discharged from the hospital, the dietician suggests that Mrs. Chang be requested to keep a careful record of the types and amounts of foods consumed for a period of seven days. The nurse is aware that potential benefits of this dietary record include all of the following except:

A. Assist in the individualization of dietary modifications
B. Can be used as an absolute indication of adequate nutrition
C. Provides presumptive evidence of specific dietary inadequacies
D. Provides information useful in assessing the need for further evaluation

A  The food record cannot be used as an absolute indication of adequate nutrition, but it is widely used to obtain presumptive evidence of dietary inadequacies or excesses. (p. 752)

22. The nurse recognizes that Mrs. Chang's cultural background may influence her nutritional practices. Which actions by the nurse are most likely to be helpful in teaching her about nutrition?

   A. Gather information pertaining to the food habits and customs of Oriental people
   B. Identify cultural practices that are potentially harmful
   C. Support every positive aspect of the chosen cultural food pattern
   D. All of the above

D   All of the listed actions are necessary if the nurse is to promote needed dietary changes related to cultural dietary customs. (p. 749)

23. Scurvy results from a deficiency in:

   A. Vitamin A
   B. Vitamin B6
   C. Vitamin D
   D. Vitamin C

D   Scurvy results from a severe deficiency of foods containing the essential nutrient, Vitamin C. (p. 744)

# 37

# MEETING SPECIAL NUTRITIONAL NEEDS

## OBJECTIVES

1.0 Describe special nutritional needs during each stage of the life cycle.

    1.1 Describe variables influencing nutritional needs of infancy. (p. 758)

    1.2 Briefly discuss the advantages of breast feeding vs. bottle feeding during infancy. (p. 758)

    1.3 Identify essential components the nurse should be prepared to include in a teaching program for the mother who chooses to breastfeed. (p. 759)

    1.4 Outline specific data the nurse should include when counseling parents who elect to bottle feed their infant. (p. 759)

    1.5 Discuss specific nutritional problems that may be encountered by the preterm infant. (p. 759)

    1.6 Summarize ways in which developmental needs may influence the nutritional status of the preschool child. (p. 759)

    1.7 Explain the role various nutrients may play in meeting the increased metabolic demands of adolescence: overeating, anorexia nervosa, and bulemia. (p. 760)

    1.8 Outline the nutritional needs of the average adult. (p. 762)

    1.9 Briefly discuss the altered nutritional needs imposed on the individual during pregnancy. (p. 762)

    1.10 List and briefly describe women who may exhibit a greater risk for the development of nutritional problems during pregnancy. (p. 762)

    1.11 Identify the unique nutritional needs of the lactating woman. (p. 762)

    1.12 Describe the nutritional requirements and problems encountered during later maturity. (p. 762)

2.0 Describe four standard dietary regimens.

    2.1 Briefly discuss two primary objectives of diet therapy. (p. 763)

## TEACHING/LEARNING STRATEGIES

### Group Activity

Divide students into small groups. Ask each group to summarize the physiological body changes and the resulting nutritional needs for one stage in the life cycle. Discuss findings in class.

### Class Activity

Instruct students to gather a dietary history for a person in the community. Ask them to develop a nutritional plan for maintenance or weight control of this individual throughout the life cycle.

2.2 Summarize the purpose of a general
hospital diet. (p. 763)

2.3 Describe basic modifications of the
general hospital diet: clear liquid,
full liquid, and soft diets. (p. 763)

2.4 Identify common health problems that
would require the use of a modified
general hospital diet. (p. 763)

2.5 Discuss specific nutritional needs of an
individual during the preoperative,
intraoperative, and postoperative
periods of surgery. (p. 763)

3.0 Define basic dietary approaches to various
pathophysiologic conditions:

a. Errors in metabolism: diabetes
mellitus, hypoglycemia, phenylketonuria,
gout.

3.1 Briefly describe and state the etiology
of: gout, diabetes mellitus, and
hypoglycemia. (p. 763)

3.2 Identify nursing goals of care and
possible modes of intervention for the
individual with selected metabolic and
endocrine diseases: gout, diabetes
mellitus, and hypoglycemia. (p. 763)

3.3 Briefly discuss the nature and etiology
of the disease phenylketonuria and
outline specific dietary measures used
in its management. (p. 764)

b. Gastrointestinal disorders: duodenal
and gastric ulcers, diverticulosis,
enteritis, and ulcerative colitis.

3.4 Discuss the role of the GI System in the
digestive process. (p. 768)

3.5 Identify specific nutritional problems
associated with GI disease and state
possible modes of dietary intervention.
(p. 769)

c. Liver and Gallbladder disorders:
hepatitis, cirrhosis, cholelithiasis
(gallstones).

3.6 Briefly discuss major functions of the
Liver and Gallbladder. (p. 769)

3.7 List and briefly describe diseases
affecting the Liver and Gallbladder that
may require special nutritional
precautions: hepatitis, cirrhosis, and
cholelithiasis. (p. 769)

## Group Activity

Divide students into small groups. Ask each group
to identify the types of foods that would be
allowed/contraindicated for one of the four
standard dietary regimens: General, soft, full
liquid, and clear liquid.

## Written Exercise

Ask students to prepare a nutritional plan of care
for a hospitalized individual receiving a standard
or modified standard hospital diet. Include in
this plan the rationale for food selections and
amounts according to the basic RDA requirements.

## Clinical Laboratory Experience

Have students review the dietary manual in their
clinical facility. Ask them to identify the diets
that are available for individuals with specific
disease disorders.

## Class Activity

Ask students to visit a local supermarket and
perform a survey of the types of foods that are
available for people with special nutritional
needs. Ask them to share their findings in class.

## Group Activity

Divide students into small groups. Assign each
group to develop a nursing plan of care for
meeting the nutritional needs for one of the
following: Diabetes, diverticulosis, cirrhosis,
hypertension, kidney failure, and lactose allergy.

## Written Exercise

Using the nursing process as a guide, request
students to develop a written nutritional plan to
meet the needs of an individual with one of the
following conditions: Diabetes mellitus, gout, or
hypoglycemia.

3.8 Outline clinical signs and symptoms
indicative of: hepatitis, cirrhosis,
and cholelithiasis. (p. 769)

3.9 Identify essential dietary measures to
be included when planning nutritional
care for the individual with: liver
disease and gallbladder disease.
(p. 769)

d. Cardiovascular disorders: atherosclerosis, congestive heart failure,
hypertension.

3.10 Identify and give a brief description of
three cardiovascular disorders requiring
dietary modifications: atherosclerosis,
congestive heart failure, and hypertension. (p. 770)

3.11 Explore the physiological effects of
various cardiovascular diseases:
atherosclerosis, congestive heart
failure, and hypertension. (p. 771)

3.12 Identify risk factors that may
contribute to the development of:
atherosclerosis, congestive heart
failure, and hypertension. (p. 770)

3.13 Briefly discuss measures that can be
utilized to reduce dietary intake of
cholesterol in the individual with
atherosclerosis. (p. 771)

3.14 Outline appropriate dietary
modifications for the person with
congestive heart failure and
hypertension. (p. 772)

e. Kidney disorders: glomerulonephritis,
nephrotic syndrome, kidney failure.

3.15 Discuss alterations in kidney functioning produced by various inflammatory and
degenerative diseases: acute glomerulonephritis, nephrotic syndrome, and
chronic renal failure. (p. 770)

3.16 Describe clinical features indicative of
acute glomerulonephritis, nephrotic
syndrome, and chronic renal failure.
(p. 770)

3.17 Summarize the dietary recommendations
for management of various kidney
disorders: acute glomerulonephritis,
nephrotic syndrome, and chronic renal
failure. (p. 770)

f. Immune disorders: allergies.

3.18 State the difference between a food
allergy and a food intolerance. (p. 774)

3.19 Identify clinical symptoms that may be
manifested in individuals with food
allergies or food intolerances. (p. 774)

3.20 Discuss actions the nurse might take to
help meet an individual's food sensi-
tivity needs. (p. 775)

4.0 Identify some important factors in the control of obesity and anorexia nervosa.

   4.1 State the definition of the term obesity. (p. 765)

   4.2 Identify common health problems that are frequently associated with obesity. (p. 765)

   4.3 Describe two standard forms of measurement often used to evaluate an individual's appropriate body weight: average weight and body mass index. (p. 765)

   4.4 Briefly discuss five popular theories related to the cause of obesity. (p. 765)

   4.5 Describe various treatment strategies effective in the treatment of obesity. (p. 765)

   4.6 Enumerate the various factors that must be considered when planning a weight reduction program for the obese individual. (p. 765)

   4.7 Describe the underweight individual and explore the etiology. (p. 768)

   4.8 Discuss nursing goals of care and possible interventions that will assist the underweight individual to produce a positive caloric balance. (p. 768)

5.0 Define the options in feeding when standard oral meals cannot be tolerated.

   5.1 Identify and discuss alternate feeding methods that can be utilized to meet the nutritional needs of the individual who cannot ingest sufficient nutrients: enteral nutrition and parenteral nutrition. (p. 775)

   5.2 Outline nursing responsibilities associated with the provision of parenteral nutrition and enteral nutrition. (p. 775)

6.0 Describe the role of the nurse in ensuring that a specific diet meets the needs of the individual.

   6.1 Discuss the role of dietary and nutritional factors in the development of cancer. (p. 773)

   6.2 Identify potential nutritional problems encountered by the cancer individual and possible modes of intervention. (p. 773)

   6.3 Explore the psychologic and sociologic impact dietary management may have on the individual. (p. 775)

**Lecture/Discussion**

Ask students to share the advice they would give to a person who wishes to lose weight.

**Class Activity**

Ask a volunteer to visit a local chapter of the American Anorexia Association. Have them identify the agency's role in assisting an individual with this disorder. Allow them to share their findings in class.

Have students examine the dietary literature available in a local bookstore for individuals wishing to reduce their weight. Ask them to report on the number and types of books available.

Ask students to identify the weight loss programs that are available for individuals in their community. Elicit volunteers to visit several of the programs. Ask them to obtain information on the following: Advantages and disadvantages of the program; services offered; cost of the program; and the ability of the program to meet the needs of individuals at all ages in life. Have them share their findings in class.

**Guest Speaker**

Invite a pharmacist in each clinical facility to speak briefly in a post-conference period on the concept of total parenteral nutrition.

**Lecture/Discussion**

Ask students to identify the role of the student nurse in assisting an individual with special nutritional needs.

**Guest Speaker**

Invite a dietician in each clinical facility to a post-conference period to discuss the types of services they offer for individuals with special nutritional needs.

6.4  List nursing actions that can be
     utilized to maintain or promote an
     individual's appetite.  (p. 775)

6.5  Identify general nursing
     responsibilities that should be
     considered when serving food to the
     hospitalized or institutionalized
     individual.  (p. 776)

6.6  Outline appropriate nursing measures for
     the individual experiencing nutritional
     problems related to:  nausea/vomiting
     and dysphagia.  (p. 776)

7.0  Identify community resources for nutritional
     and diet therapy.

     7.1  Identify educational needs of the
          individual requiring a special diet.
          (p. 776)

     7.2  Describe appropriate nursing measures
          that can be instituted for the
          individual being discharged from the
          hospital with a special diet.  (p. 777)

## Lecture/Discussion

Ask students to identify the community resources
they would recommend for individuals with each of
the different types of special nutritional needs.

## Class Activity

When eating in a local restaurant, ask students to
identify the foods that could be consumed by
individuals with special nutritional needs.  Have
them discuss their findings in class.

---

## MULTIPLE CHOICE QUESTIONS

1.  Which of the following suggestions would not
    be appropriate when counseling a new mother
    regarding the nutritional needs of her infant?

    A.  Introducing textured foods when the
        infant is four to six months of age
    B.  Slowly increasing the volume of food
        ingested
    C.  Use fresh homogenized milk to increase
        the infant's protein intake
    D.  Use only prepared formulas sufficient in
        calories, iron, and vitamins D/C

2.  Which of the following statements is false?

    A.  A decreased interest in food during the
        pre-school years can promote dietary
        deficiencies.
    B.  Good food habits are formed during the
        childhood years.
    C.  Nutritional requirements during the
        preschool years are similar to those of
        adulthood.
    D.  The environment in which a child lives
        determines their nutritional status.

3.  Which of the following nutrients are
    especially important during the period of
    adolescence?

    A.  Calcium
    B.  Iron
    C.  Vitamins A and C
    D.  All of the above

## CORRECT ANSWER AND RATIONALE

C  The increased protein content in homogenized
   milk can facilitate the occurrence of
   intestinal bleeding and iron deficiency anemia
   if given to an infant in the first six to
   twelve months of life.  (p. 759)

C  Because of continued growth and development,
   nutritional requirements are considerably
   higher in the preschool child than in the
   adult.  (pp. 761-762)

D  During adolescence, calcium is important for
   the support of long bone calcification, and
   iron is critical for maintaining increased red
   blood cell mass.  Vitamins A and C are also
   important at this stage in growth and
   development.  (p. 760)

4. Which of the following factors influence the development of eating disorders during adolescence?

   A. Feelings of inferiority
   B. Increased awareness of body image
   C. Need to control one aspect of life
   D. All of the above

   **D** Numerous factors promote the development of eating disorders during the stage of adolescence. The adolescent may overeat to overcome feelings of inferiority. An increased awareness of body image may promote compulsive dieting. In addition, an adolescent who suffers from anorexia nervosa may be attempting to gain control over one aspect of their life. All three conditions are more prevalent in the adolescent female. (p. 760)

5. All of the following individuals are at risk for the development of malnutrition during pregnancy except:

   A. An adolescent
   B. A woman with a chronic disease
   C. A woman who is pregnant for the first time
   D. A woman who is the mother of a two-month-old infant

   **C** Women who display a higher risk for malnutrition during pregnancy include: Adolescents, women with previous pregnancy difficulties, women after a short interconceptual period, women of low socioeconomic levels, and women with heart disease, diabetes, or other chronic diseases. (p. 762)

6. If a female required 2000 kcal per day at age 25, she will require approximately how many calories at age 75?

   A. 1200
   B. 1300
   C. 1500
   D. 1550

   **B** As a rule, daily caloric requirements decrease by seven per cent with each decade after the age of 25. This individual's requirements would be approximately 35 per cent less than at age 25 and would, therefore, need to be reduced by 700 kcal. (p. 762)

7. The physician has ordered a clear liquid diet for Mrs. Gaines. Which of the following items would be prohibited on this diet?

   A. Clear broth
   B. Cranberry juice
   C. Popsicles
   D. Tomato juice

   **D** A clear liquid diet includes tea, broth, gelatin dessert, and other "clear" liquid items. (p. 763)

8. Food is withheld during the immediate preoperative period primarily because it may:

   A. Be vomited and aspirated during anesthesia
   B. Increase the occurrence of postoperative gastric distention
   C. Interfere with the surgical procedure itself
   D. All of the above

   **A** Food is primarily withheld in the immediate preoperative period because it may be vomited and aspirated during anesthesia or recovery from anesthesia. Additional secondary reasons include options B and C. (p. 763)

9. Which of the following obese individuals is most likely to achieve successful weight loss? The individual who:

   A. Has been told that obesity is hazardous to their health
   B. Has many other obese friends
   C. Is of a low socioeconomic status
   D. Is recording their daily food consumption

   **D** The person who maintains a daily record of food intake is more aware of their food consumption and, therefore, tends to eat less. Obese individuals are rarely motivated to lose weight because of potential health problems. They also require encouragement and support from their significant others. Last of all, a person of low socioeconomic status may be unable to purchase the types of foods promoted on most reducing diets. (p. 765)

10. You have been asked to care for a 27-year-old female with ulcerative colitis. You are aware that dietary intervention for this disease would include all of the following except:

    A. Increased caloric intake
    B. Increased amounts of protein
    C. Two to three large meals per day
    D. Vitamin and mineral supplements

    **C** Frequent small feedings are advised for the person with ulcerative colitis. (p. 769)

11. Mr. Clark has a severe case of liver cirrhosis. As a result of the disease, he has developed both abdominal ascites and esophageal varices. Which of the following dietary measures would be contraindicated in this individual?

A. Increased carbohydrate intake
B. Increased protein intake
C. Sodium restriction
D. Soft, smooth textured foods

B   A low-protein diet is advocated when liver damage is severe. This is primarily because the liver plays a major role in protein metabolism. (p. 770)

12. A mild low sodium diet would restrict which of the following foods?

A. Cottage cheese
B. Kosher foods
C. Popcorn
D. Roast beef

B   Kosher foods are restricted because of the higher salt content used during their preparation. (p. 772)

# 38

# MEETING THE NEED FOR FLUID AND ELECTROLYTE BALANCE

## OBJECTIVES

After studying this chapter, you will be able to discuss the following concepts:

1.0  The percentage of water in the adult human body.

    1.1  List eight primary functions of water in living beings. (p. 782)

    1.2  Identify factors that affect an individual's total body water. (p. 782)

    1.3  Summarize the percentage of body weight that body water constitutes. (p. 782)

    1.4  Discuss the nursing implications related to percentage of body water during infancy and in late adulthood. (p. 782)

2.0  Water distribution through the body's fluid compartments.

    2.1  Briefly discuss water distribution between: The intracellular and extracellular components, and the vascular and interstitial components. (p. 782)

    2.2  Identify factors that influence body water balance. (p. 782)

    2.3  Describe the role of baroreceptors in the regulation of body fluid volume. (p. 791)

    2.4  Explain, using an example, the mechanisms by which body fluid is regulated. (p. 791)

3.0  The composition of the body fluids in each of these fluid compartments.

    3.1  Describe the terms: Electrolyte and non-electrolyte. (p. 784)

    3.2  Identify important cations and anions necessary in body fluid metabolism. (p. 784)

    3.3  Describe the chemical nature of electrolytes. (p. 784)

    3.4  Discuss the relationship between cations and anions in body fluid metabolism. (p. 784)

## TEACHING/LEARNING STRATEGIES

### Written Exercise

Ask students to diagram the composition of body fluids in intracellular and extracellular fluid compartments.

Ask students to outline the route that fluids take from the time they are ingested until they are absorbed or excreted from the body.

### Lecture/Discussion

Ask students to identify the major ways in which body fluids are delivered to and from body fluid compartments.

3.5 List four major physiologic functions of electrolytes. (p. 784)

3.6 Briefly discuss units of measurement used to describe body fluids and electrolytes: Liter, milliliter, cubic centimeter, gram, milligram, and milliequivalent. (p. 784)

3.7 Outline the major electrolytes present in the body's extracellular and intracellular fluid compartments. (p. 786)

3.8 List the normal ranges/laboratory values for plasma, electrolytes, and proteins in an adult: Sodium, potassium, chloride, bicarbonate, and colloids. (p. 786)

3.9 Discuss the role of the hypothalamus in the regulation of body fluids and electrolytes. (p. 792)

3.10 Identify factors that stimulate/inhibit the body's thirst mechanism. (p. 793)

4.0 Semipermeable membranes and their role in control of body water distribution.

4.1 Briefly describe the concepts of osmolality and active transport. (p. 786)

4.2 Discuss the roles osmolality and active transport in the regulation of fluid and electrolytes, between the intracellular and extracellular body compartments. (p. 787)

4.3 Outline the process of fluid transport between the vascular compartment and the interstitial fluid compartment. (p. 788)

4.4 Briefly discuss three major factors involved in the maintenance of blood volume and in the prevention of edema: Blood hydrostatic pressure, colloid osmotic pressure, and filtration pressure. (p. 788)

4.5 Explain the role of the lymphatic system in the transportation of fluid between the plasma and interstitial fluid compartments. (p. 788)

4.6 List and describe the major factors influencing blood hydrostatic pressure. (p. 789)

4.7 Discuss the effect of osmolality on ADH release. (p. 790)

5.0 The role of proteins n the plasma and in cell protoplasm.

### Lecture/Discussion

Assist students in understanding the movement of fluid and electrolytes within the body.

Describe the mechanism by which semipermeable membranes control body water distribution.

### Lecture/Discussion

Help students to understand the role of proteins in the plasma and in the cell protoplasm.

5.1 Define the terms proteinate and colloid
in relation to fluid and electrolyte
metabolism. (p. 784)

5.2 Describe the chemical nature of plasma
proteins. (p. 784)

5.3 Identify important plasma proteins
necessary for fluid and electrolyte
metabolism in the body. (p. 784)

6.0 The role of the kidney in maintaining fluid
and electrolyte balance.

6.1 Outline and briefly describe the major
functions of the kidney in the homeostatic process. (p. 794)

6.2 Identify ways in which the kidneys
assist the body in maintenance of
hydrogen ion balance. (p. 796)

6.3 Discuss the role of hydrogen ions in
acid-base balance. (p. 795)

7.0 The important hormones involved in the
maintenance of fluid and electrolyte balance.

7.1 List the neuroendocrine hormones
involved in the homeostatic balance of
fluid and electrolytes within the body.
(p. 790)

7.2 Briefly discuss the role of the antidiuretic hormone in the regulation of
body fluids and electrolytes. (p. 790)

7.3 Identify conditions that stimulate the
production of antidiuretic hormone and
consequently cause water conservation.
(p. 790)

7.4 Identify factors that suppress the
release of ADH. (p. 790)

7.5 Summarize the role of aldosterone in the
regulation of body fluids and electrolytes. (p. 790)

7.6 Summarize factors that stimulate and
inhibit the release of ADH. (p. 791)

7.7 Identify the primary functions of
thyroid and parathyroid hormones in
fluid and electrolyte balance. (p. 793)

7.8 List the mechanisms by which the parathyroid gland controls the metabolism of
calcium and phosphate. (p. 793)

7.9 Discuss the function of the
renin-angiotensin system in aldosterone
secretion. (p. 791)

Lecture/Discussion

Ask students to identify the body hormones that
assist in the body maintenance of fluid and
electrolyte balance. Have them discuss the
mechanism by which each works.

In the clinical situation you should be able to:

1.0 Identify those individuals assigned to you who are at risk for developing an imbalance.

### Lecture/Discussion

Ask students to summarize the role of major body systems in the maintenance of fluid and electrolyte balance: Lungs, kidneys, circulatory, endocrine, nervous system, and the gastrointestinal tract.

Discuss the role of the acid-base system in maintenance of body homeostasis.

### Clinical Laboratory Experience

Assist students in identifying individuals in the clinical area who display a greater risk for the development of fluid and electrolyte disorders.

2.0 Prevent imbalances from developing in these individuals.

### Written Exercise

Ask students to outline nursing measures to prevent fluid and electrolyte imbalances for the individuals in their care.

2.1 Identify dietary nutrients that must be consumed daily by an individual to maintain normal electrolyte balance. (p. 786)

2.2 Summarize the normal intake and output necessary to maintain body water balance in an adult for a 24-hour period. (p. 783)

2.3 Outline the minimal fluid intake that an average person requires daily in order to meet body fluid requirements. (p. 783)

2.4 Compare and contrast the fluid requirements necessary for normal balance with those necessary for basal functioning. (p. 783)

2.5 Identify factors that increase an individual's fluid requirement levels. (p. 783)

2.6 Identify major factors that influence the development of edema. (p. 789)

2.7 Explore the consequences that can occur as a result of an obstruction of the lymphatic system. (p. 789)

2.8 Summarize the causes and effects of increased aldosterone secretion. (p. 792)

2.9 Identify disease conditions that may precipitate an impairment in renal functioning. (p. 794)

2.10 Discuss the etiology of fluid and electrolyte imbalances related to saline deficits and excesses in the body. (p. 797)

2.11 Identify factors that influence the development of hypokalemia and hyperkalemia. (p. 798)

2.12 Identify major factors influencing the
development of calcium fluid and electrolyte imbalances. (p. 798)

2.13 Identify factors that influence magnesium fluid and electrolyte imbalances.
(p. 798)

2.14 Explain the etiology of protein induced
fluid and electrolyte imbalances.
(p. 799)

2.15 Identify basic and specific causes for
the development of: Metabolic acidosis,
metabolic alkalosis, respiratory acidosis, and respiratory alkalosis.
(p. 799)

2.16 Identify individuals at risk for the
development of fluid and electrolyte
imbalances. (p. 801)

2.17 Identify specific conditions that may
indicate the need for tube feedings.
(p. 808)

2.18 Identify situations necessitating the
administration of intravenous
infusions. (p. 808)

3.0 Assess for the early signs of imbalance and
report them accurately.

4.0 Assess an individual's fluid and electrolyte
status.

4.1 Summarize the function of the gastrointestinal system in the maintenance of
fluid and electrolyte balance. (p. 794)

4.2 Describe the purpose of obtaining a
urine specific gravity. (p. 794)

4.3 Identify the normal pH ranges for various body fluids: Blood, intracellular
fluid, urine, cerebrospinal fluid,
gastric juice, and bile. (p. 795)

4.4 Outline common physiological problems
that result from abnormal blood pH.
(p. 795)

4.5 Identify four regulatory systems that
control pH balance in the body. (p. 795)

4.6 Summarize the role of the buffer system
in regulation of hydrogen ion balance.
(p. 795)

4.7 Briefly discuss the mechanisms by which
the respiratory system controls and
regulates hydrogen ion balance in the
body. (p. 796)

## LEARNING ACTIVITIES

### Lecture/Discussion

Summarize the basic functions of body
electrolytes: Sodium, potassium, calcium,
magnesium, hydrogen ions, and proteins.

Discuss the major homeostatic regulators
controlling sodium, potassium, calcium, magnesium,
hydrogen ion, and proteins in the body.

Identify body systems that serve as the major
homeostatic regulators of fluid and electrolyte
balance.

Identify and describe three major categories of
fluid and electrolyte imbalances.

Briefly describe indices used to assess and
diagnose individuals with suspected fluid and
electrolyte imbalances.

### Clinical Laboratory Experience

Arrange for students to visit the laboratory
setting in their clinical facility. Afterwards,
have them identify the major laboratory studies
used to evaluate an individual's fluid and
electrolyte status.

Have students identify potential or actual fluid
and electrolyte disturbances for individuals in
their care. Ask them to formulate a plan of care
to assist the individual with these needs.

4.8 Identify mechanisms involved in cellular regulation of hydrogen ion balance. (p. 796)

4.9 Define and discuss two major types of imbalances that result from the failure of the body to regulate hydrogen ion: Acidosis and alkalosis. (p. 796)

4.10 Differentiate between metabolic and respiratory acid-base imbalances. (p. 796)

4.11 Explain the relationship of bicarbonate to carbonic acid that is necessary in the blood to maintain normal acid-base balance. (p. 796)

4.12 Identify factors influencing the development of fluid and electrolyte imbalances due to water deficit or water excess. (p. 797)

4.13 Identify assessment data indicative of body water deficits and excesses. (p. 797)

4.14 List assessment data indicative of a saline deficit or excess. (p. 797)

4.15 Identify clinical signs and symptoms of a potassium deficit or excess. (p. 798)

4.16 Identify the physiological manifestations of hypocalcemia and hypercalcemia. (p. 798)

4.17 List assessment data indicative of a magnesium deficit or excess. (p. 798)

4.18 Identify criteria used to assess protein fluid and electrolyte imbalances. (p. 799)

4.19 Identify the clinical signs and symptoms of: Metabolic acidosis, metabolic alkalosis, respiratory acidosis, and respiratory alkalosis. (p. 799)

4.20 Summarize normal laboratory values for blood counts: Hemoglobin, red blood cells, hematocrit, reticulocytes, white blood cells, and the differential count. (p. 806)

4.21 Identify normal ranges for plasma chemical constituents in a healthy individual: $Na+$, $K+$, $Ca++$, $Mg++$, $HCO_3-$, $HPO_4-$, Protein, and pH. (p. 806)

4.22 List and briefly describe laboratory tests used to measure saline and osmolality balance. Include normal values for each test. (p. 807)

4.23 Identify normal arterial blood gas values. (p. 807)

4.24 Differentiate between pH values present in acid-base balance and acid-base imbalance. (p. 807)

4.25 Identify data that should be assessed when caring for an individual receiving parenteral hyperalimentation. (p. 811)

4.26 Identify criteria that the nurse should monitor when administering IV infusions. (p. 810)

5.0 Intervene knowledgeably to prevent and to treat fluid and electrolyte imbalances.

5.1 Describe basic nursing intervention useful in assisting an individual who is experiencing a water deficit or excess. (p. 797)

5.2 Identify ways in which the nurse can assist a person who is experiencing a deficit or excess in body saline. (p. 797)

5.3 Discuss essential nursing measures for care of an individual experiencing potassium fluid and electrolyte imbalances. (p. 798)

5.4 List nursing actions that can be carried out for an individual experiencing a calcium fluid and electrolyte imbalance. (p. 798)

5.5 Identify appropriate nursing interventions useful in assisting an individual with magnesium related fluid and electrolyte imbalance. (p. 798)

5.6 Outline appropriate nursing measures for care of an individual with a protein deficit. (p. 799)

5.7 Identify interventions that are used to counteract problems related to: Metabolic acidosis, metabolic alkalosis, respiratory acidosis, and respiratory alkalosis. (p. 799)

5.8 Identify appropriate nursing goals for individuals needing fluid replacement or limitation. (p. 806)

5.9 Outlines guidelines for treating individuals with fluid and electrolyte imbalance. (p. 806)

5.10 Identify factors influencing the type of IV solutions that may be ordered for an individual. (p. 808)

5.11 List five essential elements that should be included in every IV infusion order. (p. 808)

5.12 List and briefly describe commonly used intravenous solutions. (p. 809)

## Lecture/Discussion

Have students identify factors that may interfere with the satisfaction of an individual's fluid and electrolyte needs.

Have students review anatomy and physiology related to chapter content.

Facilitate a discussion on the effect unmet fluid needs can have on the satisfaction of other basic human needs.

Discuss the medical therapies that are prescribed for specific fluid and electrolyte deficits.

## Guest Speaker

Invite a pharmacist from each clinical facility to a post-conference period to discuss the various drug preparations that are available to assist individuals with altered fluid and electrolyte status.

5.13 State mathematical formulas used to calculate IV infusion flow rates. (p. 809)

5.14 Identify drop factors for common IV apparatus sets. (p. 810)

5.15 Identify two alternate ways for maintaining correct IV flow rates. (p. 810)

5.16 List two major reasons for administering blood transfusions. (p. 810)

5.17 Identify specific purposes for the administration of parenteral hyperalimentation. (p. 810)

5.18 Briefly describe three major complications of parenteral hyperalimentation. (p. 811)

---

## MULTIPLE CHOICE QUESTIONS

## CORRECT ANSWER AND RATIONALE

1. Which of the following statements is correct?

   A. The percentage of fluid present in the body increases with age
   B. Total body weight is 45 to 60% water in an average adult
   C. Water is excreted from the body by the kidneys, lungs, and gastrointestinal tract
   D. Water is the single largest constituent of the human body

   B   The percentage of fluid present in the body varies proportionately with age. The average adult's total body weight is 45-60% water. The percentage of body fluid present in the body decreases with age. Water is excreted from the body via the kidneys, lungs, skin, and gastrointestinal tract. (p. 782)

2. All of the following statements about body fluid compartments are false, except:

   A. The major cation of the intracellular fluid is sodium
   B. The composition of intracellular fluid is not as critical to the body as that of the extracellular fluid
   C. The distribution of water between the intracellular and extracellular compartments is governed by osmosis
   D. Electrolytes move from one fluid compartment to another by diffusion and filtration

   C   The distribution of water between the intracellular and extracellular compartments is governed by osmosis. The movement of water between the vascular and interstitial spaces is controlled by the process of filtration. (p. 782)

3. Which of the following best describes an electrolyte?

   A. Positive or negative charged particles, often called ions
   B. Substances that disassociate in solution into electrically charged particles, ions
   C. A substance capable of breaking into ions
   D. Positive or negative charged substances

   B   Option B is the most complete definition of an electrolyte. (p. 784)

4. Electrolytes in the body's intracellular and extracellular fluid compartments are:

A. The same, but vary in their concentrations
B. Similar in concentration only
C. Vary in both type and amount
D. Different in type, but of similar weight

A  Extracellular fluids and intracellular fluids contain the same electrolytes, but in different amounts. (p. 786)

5. Which of the following associations is incorrect?

A. Sodium -- 135-145mEqL
B. Potassium -- 3.0-5.5mEqL
C. Chloride -- 98-106mEqL
D. Bicarbonate -- 25-29mEqL

B  The normal range for plasma potassium is 3.5-5.0mEqL in an adult. (p. 786)

6. Which of the following individuals would display the greatest potential for the development of a fluid and electrolyte imbalance?

A. An infant with moderate diarrhea
B. An elderly individual
C. An individual working outside in a hot climate
D. All of the above

A  Children, because of their relatively small body water content and greater metabolic rate, are particularly vulnerable to dehydration and other electrolyte imbalances. (p. 783)

7. A unit of measurement used to describe the chemical activity of an electrolyte is:

A. Milligram
B. Cubic Centimeter
C. Millivolt
D. Milliequivalent

D  A milliequivalent (mEq) is the measure of the chemical activity or chemical combining power of an ion. It is the measure of the power of a cation to combine with an anion, thus making a molecule. (p. 786)

8. As a nurse, you should be aware that an individual's water output is principally regulated by the:

A. Amount of water consumed daily
B. Kidneys and gastrointestinal tract
C. Antidiuretic hormone
D. Kidneys, GI tract, and antidiuretic hormone

D  Water loss is controlled by the antidiuretic hormone, the kidneys, and the gastrointestinal tract. (p. 787)

9. The nurse knows that thirst may occur as a result of:

A. Decreased osmotic pressure
B. Decreased extracellular fluid volume
C. Increased extracellular fluid volume
D. Decreased sodium intake

B  Thirst may be stimulated by hyperosmolality, decreased extracellular fluid volume, dry mucous membranes in the mouth, low water intake, excessive water loss, excessive sodium intake, and excessive intake of isotonic or hypotonic intravenous solutions. (p. 793)

10. The body has four regulatory mechanisms that maintain normal balance. Arrange them in the order that they are activated.

A. Lungs, cells, kidneys, and buffer systems
B. Kidneys, lungs, cells, and buffer systems
C. Buffer systems, lungs, cells, and kidneys
D. Buffer systems, kidneys, lungs, and cells

C  The four regulatory systems (listed in order of activation) are: the buffer systems, the lungs, the cells, and the kidneys. (p. 795)

SITUATION: Mr. Cox has been diagnosed with pulmonary emphysema. This disease interferes with pulmonary gas exchange and causes a retention of carbonic acid in the blood.

Questions 11 and 12 relate to this situation.

11. As a result of the increased carbonic acid, Mr. Cox's blood pH will:

   A. Become less acidic
   B. Become more acidic
   C. Become more alkaline
   D. Remain the same

B   The pH of Mr. Cox's blood will become more acidic than normal, due to the increase in carbonic acid in the blood. (p. 800)

12. As a nurse, you are aware that Mr. Cox has a great potential for the development of:

   A. Metabolic acidosis
   B. Metabolic alkalosis
   C. Respiratory acidosis
   D. Respiratory alkalosis

C   Respiratory abnormalities that result in failure to excrete CO2 adequately cause an increase in hydrogen ion content in the blood. This may result in respiratory acidosis. (p. 800)

13. Which of the following assessment data would be indicative of respiratory alkalosis?

   A. Abnormally slow respirations, urine pH of 7.2, plasma pH of 7.5
   B. Abnormally increased respirations, blood gas carbon dioxide of 40
   C. Urine pH of 7.1, plasma pH of 7.55, and pCO2 of 30
   D. Muscle twitches, unconsciousness, and decreased respirations

C   Assessment data indicative of respiratory alkalosis are: abnormally rapid respirations, lightheadedness, muscle twitch, tetany, generalized convulsions, and unconsciousness. Lab findings may include: urine pH above 7; plasma pH above 7.45; plasma bicarbonate depressed below 25 mEqL in adults and 20 mEqL in children; blood gas carbon dioxide drops below 35 mm Hg. (p. 800)

14. Nursing intervention for an individual with metabolic acidosis may include all of the following except:

   A. Oral and parenteral fluids to correct dehydration
   B. High proteins, high calorie, high carbohydrate diet
   C. Daily measurement of intake and output
   D. Daily weight

B   A low-protein, high-calorie, high-carbohydrate diet can be used to treat an individual with metabolic acidosis. (p. 799)

15. In assessing an individual for a potential fluid and electrolyte imbalance, the nurse is aware that factors associated with an increased risk include:

   A. Receipt of IV fluids
   B. No oral intake
   C. Excessive loss of body secretions
   D. All of the above

D   Imbalances may be caused by any factor that results in a deficit or excess of body water and electrolytes. (p. 801)

16. Which assessment data may indicate a potential fluid and electrolyte imbalance:

   A. Intake and output imbalances
   B. Changes in mental alertness
   C. Alterations in cardiac rate and rhythm
   D. All of the above

D   All options may be indicative of fluid and electrolyte imbalance. For a complete list of pertinent assessment data, see page 803-804 in text. (pp. 803-804)

17. Assessment of an individual with hyperkalcemia might include which of the following data:

A. Increased intestinal motility, malaise, and weakness
B. Serum potassium of 6.0mEqL, oliguria, and bradycardia
C. Elevated serum potassium levels, shallow respirations, and tachycardia
D. Shallow respirations, diarrhea, and anuria

B   An excess of serum potassium might cause: Diarrhea, intestinal colic, oliguria progressing to anuria, and bradycardia progressing to cardiac arrest. Laboratory findings would reveal an elevated serum potassium above 5.5mEqL. (p. 798)

18. Laboratory tests used to measure saline and osmolality balance would include all of the following except:

A. Serum sodium
B. Blood urea nitrogen
C. Hemoglobin
D. Urine specific gravity

C   Laboratory tests useful in determining saline and osmolality balance include: Serum osmolality, serum sodium, blood urea nitrogen, hematocrit, urine specific gravity, and urine osmolality. (p. 807)

19. A physician orders 1000ml of 5% dextrose/water to be infused intravenously over 12 hours. If the nurse uses an administration set with a 15gtt/ml drop factor, the IV flow rate will be:

A. 25gtt/min
B. 22gtt/min
C. 21gtt/min
D. 31gtt/min

C   The flow rate for the ordered IV can be mathematically calculated as follows: (p. 809)

$$\frac{1000ml \times 15gtt/ml}{60min/hr \times 12\ hr} =$$

$$\frac{15,000\ gtt}{720\ min} = 21\ gtt/min$$

20. Risks of parenteral hyperalimentation include all of the following except:

A. Dehydration
B. Glucose overload
C. Hypoglycemia
D. Fluid overload

C   Major complications of parenteral hyperalimentation include: Sepsis, catheter dislocation, and osmotic diuresis. Both dehydration and glucose overload occur in conjunction with osmotic diuresis. The administration of any IV infusion may result in a fluid overload. Since parenteral hyperalimentation solutions are intended to provide total nutritional needs, rarely would they result in hypoglycemia. (p. 811)

# MEETING URINARY ELIMINATION NEEDS

OBJECTIVES

TEACHING/LEARNING STRATEGIES

1.0 Discuss normal anatomy and physiology of the urinary tract.

1.1 List and briefly describe the function of the urinary tract. (pp. 813-814)

1.2 Briefly discuss the mechanism by which urine is produced by the urinary system. (p. 814)

Lecture/Discussion

Ask students to review the normal anatomy and physiology of the urinary tract system: Kidneys, ureters, urinary bladder, and the urethra.

2.0 Describe the act of micturation and factors that influence it.

2.1 Describe the voluntary and involuntary processes of micturation. (p. 815)

2.2 Briefly explore psychological factors influencing the process of micturation. (p. 815)

2.3 Identify personal factors that are responsible to an individual's voiding pattern. (p. 815)

2.4 Identify specific reasons for enuresis. (p. 815)

2.5 Explore the impact of culture on the voiding process. (p. 815)

2.6 Discuss the impact that fluid and dietary intake have on an individual's normal micturation process. (p. 815)

2.7 Describe the affect of diuretics, cholinergics, analgesics, and tranquilizers on the micturation process. (p. 815)

2.8 Discuss other factors that may influence the micturation process: Hormonal changes, pregnancy, prosthetic hypertrophy, and age. (p. 816)

Lecture/Discussion

Facilitate a discussion of the variables that influence the process of micturation.

Have students discuss the normal body processes or urine production and excretion.

3.0 List data needed to assess a person's urinary status.

3.1 Discuss normal and abnormal characteristics of urine. (p. 817)

Lecture/Discussion

Ask students to differentiate between the normal and abnormal characteristics of urine.

Class Activity

Instruct students to keep a record of their own fluid intake and output for a period of twenty-four hours.

3.2 Enumerate the various factors that must
be considered when assessing urinary
specimens: Frequency, amount, pH, color,
opacity, odor, and specific gravity.
(p. 817)

Written Exercise

Ask students to list the data that is required to
adequately assess an individual's urinary elimination status.

## Clinical Laboratory Experience

Ask students to monitor the fluid intake and output for an assigned individual in the clinical
area.

4.0 Demonstrate the collection of urine specimens:
clean-catch midstream samples, double-void
samples, and 24-hour urine specimens.

## Lecture/Discussion

Ask students to describe the procedure for collecting sterile and clean-catch midstream urine
specimens.

4.1 List four specific ways of collecting
urine specimens for diagnostic study.
(p. 816)

4.2 Discuss the purpose of collecting a
clean-catch urine specimen. (p. 816)

4.3 Describe the steps taken to obtain a
clean-catch urine specimen. (p. 816)

4.4 Discuss the advantages and disadvantages
of obtaining a urine specimen by catheterization. (p. 817)

4.5 Identify the purpose and describe the
essential steps for obtaining timed-
collection urinary specimens. (p. 817)

4.6 Discuss the purpose of double-voided
urinary specimens. (p. 817)

4.7 Outline the guidelines for obtaining a
double-voided urinary specimen (p. 817)

4.8 Describe specific urinary color changes
that are induced by the consumption of
medication. (p. 818)

4.9 Describe basic diagnostic tests the nurse
frequently performs on urine: Dipstick
tests, glucose and ketone testing, and
specific gravity determination. (p. 818)

5.0 Describe how to perform selected diagnostic
tests on urine.

## Lecture/Discussion

Discuss the role of the nurse in assisting an
individual who is to have a diagnostic procedure
performed to evaluate urinary system functioning.

5.1 Explore potential problems that may
result from performance of diagnostic
tests. (p. 816)

## Campus Laboratory Experience

Have students obtain their own urine specimen in
the campus laboratory setting. Ask them to perform tests for specific gravity and determination
of glucose on the specimen.

5.2 Identify and briefly discuss common
diagnostic tests performed in assessment
of the urinary tract: Intravenous
pyelogram, excretory urogram, and
cystoscopy. (p. 819)

5.3 Describe basic nursing intervention useful in assisting a person who has undergone an intravenous pyelogram, excretory urogram, or cystoscopy. (p. 820)

6.0 Discuss nursing interventions to aid individuals in maintaining a normal urinary elimination.

6.1 Outline nursing intervention measures that can be carried out to assist a person in maintaining normal urinary tract functioning. (p. 820)

6.2 Briefly describe ways that health teaching can help prevent urinary elimination problems. (p. 821)

7.0 Describe the following nursing diagnoses and their management: urinary retention, urinary incontinence, urinary tract infection, urinary tract stones, urinary diversion, and inadequate renal function.

7.1 Identify common problems and selected nursing diagnoses related to people with urinary elimination problems. (p. 813)

7.2 State appropriate nursing goals related to the care of individuals with urinary elimination needs. (p. 813)

7.3 Identify outcome criteria that can be used to evaluate the nursing care of individuals with problems related to urinary elimination. (p. 813)

7.4 Outline common micturation problems related to muscle tone. (p. 815)

7.5 Identify common urinary problems that may be experienced by a post-surgical individual. (p. 816)

7.6 Discuss potential urinary problems that may result from disturbances in sensory and motor abilities. (p. 816)

7.7 Describe nursing intervention strategies that would be useful in assisting a person experiencing alterations in urinary elimination due to urinary retention. (p. 821)

7.8 Identify essential nursing measures for care of a person with alterations in urinary elimination due to retention with overflow. (p. 822)

7.9 Discuss nursing care of individuals with alterations in urinary elimination due to incontinence. (p. 822)

7.10 List and briefly describe common causes of urinary incontinence. (p. 822)

## Clinical Laboratory Experience

Arrange for students to visit the radiology department in their clinical facility to view the performance of a common urinary diagnostic procedure.

## Written Exercise

Instruct students to develop a nursing plan of care to prevent the occurrence of urinary elimination problems.

## Clinical Laboratory

Assist students in identifying individuals in the clinical area that are more prone to the development of urinary elimination problems.

## Group Activity

Divide students into small groups. Ask each group to develop a plan of care to meet the needs of an individual with one of the common urinary elimination problems: Urinary retention, incontinence, urinary tract infections, and renal failure.

## Campus Laboratory Experience

Provide an example of the form that is used in each clinical facility for documenting fluid intake and urinary output. Allow students to practice using the form for their clinical facility.

## Clinical Laboratory Experience

Ask students to perform a urinary assessment on an assigned individual in the clinical area. Assist them in formulating an appropriate plan of care to assist the individual with any identified urinary system disturbances.

7.11 Differentiate between major types of
    urinary incontinence:  Stress inconti-
    nence, urge incontinence, and enuresis.
    (p. 822)

7.12 Identify specific medical measures that
    are frequently employed to manage the
    problem of urinary incontinence.
    (p. 823)

7.13 Outline skin care measures the nurse
    should institute for a person experienc-
    ing urinary incontinence. (p. 823)

7.14 Discuss general nursing care appropriate
    for individuals with external urinary
    drainage systems. (p. 823)

7.15 List and discuss important factors
    involved in the care of a person with
    alterations in urinary elimination due
    to a urinary tract infection. (p. 824)

7.16 Discuss the role of the nurse in the
    care of an individual with alterations
    in urinary elimination due to urinary
    tract stones. (p. 824)

7.17 List and discuss important factors
    involved in the care of individuals with
    alterations in urinary elimination due
    to urinary diversion. (p. 825)

7.18 Explain the process of nursing inter-
    vention for a person with alterations in
    urinary elimination due to inadequate
    renal function. (p. 825)

8.0 Describe the major components of a
    bladder-training program.

    8.1 Describe the nurse's role in a bladder
        training program for an individual with
        urinary incontinence. (p. 823)

---

## MULTIPLE CHOICE QUESTIONS

I.  Which of the following statements related to
    the anatomy and physiology of the kidneys is
    incorrect?

    A.  The kidneys play a significant role in
        the maintenance of body homeostasis
    B.  The process of glomerular filtration
        assists in the regulation of body fluid
        and electrolytes
    C.  The kidneys rid the body of waste
        products via the process of urination
    D.  Approximately 1200 liters of blood enters
        the kidneys each day

## CORRECT ANSWER AND RATIONALE

D   The renal arteries deliver approximately 1200
    ml of blood to the kidneys each minute or 1700
    liters per day. (p. 814)

2.  Choose the one that doesn't belong in the group.

    A. Enuresis
    B. Micturation
    C. Urination
    D. Voiding

A   Options B, C, and D are all terms used to describe the process of emptying the bladder. Enuresis refers to involuntary urination during sleep. (p. 814)

3.  In order to accurately identify urinary elimination problems, the nurse should take which of the following into account?

    A. Physical and psychosocial factors affecting normal micturation
    B. Urine characteristics
    C. Results of urinary diagnostic tests
    D. All of the above

D   To identify problems in the urinary tract and take appropriate action, the nurse should first assess the person and take into account: Factors affecting micturation, characteristics of the urine, and the results of diagnostic tests. (p. 815)

4.  After which of the following meals would the nurse expect a person's urinary output to be lowest?

    A. Frankfurter with bun, prepared with sauerkraut, catsup, and mustard; potato chips, iced tea
    B. Canned tomato soup, smoked ham sandwich, salted crackers, and milk
    C. Bacon, two eggs, dry toast, and coffee
    D. Broiled chicken, fresh broccoli, fruit cocktail, and milk

B   All food items listed in option B are high in sodium content which could cause water retention and a reduced urinary output. Also, there are no foods listed that would have a diuretic effect. (p. 815)

5.  Urecholine, a cholinergic medication, has been ordered for an individual with post-operative urinary retention. The nurse knows that this medication will:

    A. Act as a diuretic and increase urine production
    B. Decrease the amount of urine being produced
    C. Stimulate contraction of the bladder, resulting in urination
    D. Suppress the central nervous system, further complicating the ability to void

C   Cholinergic medications stimulate contraction of the detrusor muscle, resulting in micturation. (p. 815)

6.  The timing of a 24-hour urine specimen collection should begin:

    A. After the procedure has been thoroughly explained to the individual
    B. Preferably during the early morning hours
    C. Right after the individual has emptied their bladder
    D. Whenever it is most convenient for the nurse and individual

C   To start a timed urinary specimen collection, the nurse should explain the procedure and then ask the person to void. Once the person has voided, the time is noted and the collection begun. (p. 817)

7.  The nurse should suspect a potential urinary elimination problem in the individual who:

    A. Has a 24-hour urine output of 400 ml
    B. Has a urine pH of 5.5
    C. Produces clear yellow, aromatic urine
    D. Voids approximately every 2 hours

A   The nurse should report urine outputs below 25 to 30 ml/hr (500 ml/day), which may indicate dehydration, kidney malfunction, or urinary tract obstruction. (p. 817)

8.  Several days after surgery, Mr. Allen voids
    300 cc of dark smoky urine.  The nurse knows
    that this may indicate:

    A.  Bleeding in the lower urinary tract
    B.  The presence of bacteria in the urine
    C.  That the urine is more concentrated
    D.  None of the above

D   Smoky or dark red urine indicates bleeding in
    the upper urinary tract.  (p. 818)

9.  When using a dipstick to test for glucose in
    the urine, the nurse should:

    A.  Compare dipstick color changes with
        appropriate charts
    B.  Document results of greater than 2% in
        the individual's chart
    C.  Obtain a double-voided specimen
    D.  Verify the results with another nurse

A   When testing for glucose in the urine via the
    dipstick method, the nurse should dip the stick
    into the urine, remove it, and tap it gently
    to remove excess urine.  Next, wait the speci-
    fied time and compare the color changes with
    the appropriate charts.  Usually, all results
    are recorded on the individual's chart.  A
    double-voided specimen is not necessary, nor
    verifying with another nurse in usual circum-
    stances.  (p. 818)

SITUATION:  Thirty-six year old Mrs. Barnes is
admitted to the hospital with a chief complaint of
burning with urination, urgency, and frequency.
Assessment reveals hematuria, fever, nausea and
vomiting, and flank pain.  After a thorough nursing assessment the following tentative nursing
diagnosis is made:  Alteration in urinary elimination due to urinary tract infection.  Questions 10
through 12 apply to this situation.

10. The physician will make a definitive UTI
    diagnosis based upon:

    A.  Individual's presenting signs and symptoms
    B.  Individual's past history of urinary
        tract infections
    C.  Results of clean-catch urine cultures
    D.  All of the above

C   Because the symptoms of a urinary tract
    infection vary greatly, it is necessary to
    perform cultures on clean-catch urine
    specimens to make a definitive diagnosis.
    (p. 824)

11. Which of the following individuals is least
    likely to develop a urinary tract infection?
    The person who has:

    A.  An indwelling urinary catheter
    B.  Had previous urinary tract infections
    C.  A urinary tract stone
    D.  Urinary incontinence

D   The person who is least likely to develop a
    UTI is the person with urinary incontinence.
    Other listed options are all at high risk for
    the development of a UTI.  (p. 824)

12. Nursing intervention for Mrs. Barnes would
    include all of the following except:

    A.  Altering urine pH (either alkanization or
        acidification depending on the infecting
        agent)
    B.  Encouraging her to void at least every
        two hours during the day
    C.  Encouraging her to take a shower instead
        of a bath
    D.  Increasing fluid intake, unless
        contraindicated

A   It would be useful to alter the pH of the
    urine with a special diet or an agent such as
    ascorbic acid to make it more acidic.  Acidic
    urine inhibits bacterial growth and increases
    the efficacy of certain urinary medications.
    Alkaline urine would enhance the growth of
    microorganisms.  (p. 824)

13. Mr. Caldwell recently underwent surgery for
    the formation of an ostomy that drains urine
    from the ureter into a surgically created
    ileal tissue pouch and out of the body onto
    the abdominal wall.  This is called a:

    A.  Cutaneous ureterostomy
    B.  Ileal conduit
    C.  Suprapubic cystostomy
    D.  Ureterosigmoidoscopy

B   An ileal conduit, connects the distal ureters
    to a dissected piece of the terminal ileum,
    which is brought out to open onto the
    abdominal wall, creating an ileostomy.
    (p. 825)

# 40

# MEETING BOWEL ELIMINATION NEEDS

## OBJECTIVES

1.0 Discuss normal anatomy and physiology of the lower gastrointestinal tract.

    1.1 Briefly describe the basic structure and function of the lower gastrointestinal tract. (p. 829)

2.0 Describe the act of defecation and factors that influence it.

    2.1 Identify ways in which an individual's toilet-training experience can influence future attitudes about bowel elimination. (p. 830)

    2.2 Explore the impact personal habits can have on an individual's bowel elimination pattern. (p. 831)

    2.3 Identify dietary factors that influence the bowel elimination process. (p. 831)

    2.4 Identify the relationship of fluid intake to normal bowel elimination. (p. 831)

    2.5 Discuss ways in which an individual's muscle tone influences the process of defecation. (p. 831)

    2.6 Give examples of medications that can alter an individual's bowel elimination pattern. (p. 831)

    2.7 Briefly discuss the impact of relaxation and privacy on bowel evacuation. (p. 835)

    2.8 Identify ways in which body position can influence the defecation process. (p. 835)

3.0 List data needed to assess an individual's bowel status.

    3.1 Identify essential data to be obtained in the nursing assessment of bowel elimination. (p. 830)

## TEACHING/LECTURE STRATEGIES

### Lecture/Discussion

Facilitate a discussion on the normal body processes of stool formation and excretion.

Ask students to review the normal anatomy and physiology of the lower gastrointestinal tract.

### Lecture/Discussion

Ask students to identify and briefly discuss the variables that can influence the normal defecation process.

### Lecture/Discussion

Assist students in describing the characteristics of stool that are used to assess the adequacy of GI functioning: Frequency, consistency, amount, and color. Ask students to differentiate between the characteristics that are normal and abnormal.

3.2 Identify normal and abnormal character-
    istics of stool that should be considered
    when assessing an individual's bowel
    status: Frequency, amount, color, con-
    sistency, shape, and odor. (p. 832)

## Clinical Laboratory Experience

Ask students to perform a bowel elimination
assessment on an assigned individual in the
clinical area. Assist them in formulating an
appropriate plan of care to assist the individual
with any identified bowel elimination disturbances.

4.0 Explain how to collect fecal specimens.

4.1 Outline essential information the nurse
    should be aware of when collecting stool
    specimens for assessment of an indi-
    vidual's bowel status. (p. 832)

## Lecture/Discussion

Ask students to describe the procedure for
collecting various types of stool specimens.

## Written Exercise

Have students list the data that should be
included in the assessment of an individual's
bowel elimination status.

5.0 Describe how to perform selected diagnostic
    tests on feces.

5.1 Briefly discuss the purpose of diag-
    nostic tests used to assess lower
    gastrointestinal functioning: Flat
    plate of abdomen, lower GI, proctoscopy,
    sigmoidoscopy, and colonoscopy. (p. 833)

5.2 Identify appropriate nursing measures
    that should be employed when preparing
    individuals for lower gastrointestinal
    diagnostic tests. (p. 833)

5.3 Identify factors responsible for the
    changes in bowel elimination that are
    often experienced after a surgical
    procedure or diagnostic test. (p. 831)

## Lecture/Discussion

Discuss the role of the nurse in assisting an
individual who is to have a diagnostic procedure
performed to evaluate functioning of the lower
gastrointestinal system.

## Clinical Laboratory Experience

Have several students perform guiac tests on
available stool specimens.

Arrange for students to accompany individuals to
the radiology department who are to undergo bowel
elimination studies.

6.0 Discuss nursing interventions to aid individ-
    uals in maintaining normal bowel elimination.

6.1 Briefly describe ways in which health
    teaching can be used to assist an indi-
    vidual to maintain normal bowel elimina-
    tion. (p. 834)

6.2 Discuss the importance of adequate
    dietary fiber in prevention of bowel
    elimination problems. (p. 834)

6.3 Describe the influence fluid intake can
    have on normal bowel functioning.
    (p. 834)

6.4 Discuss the role exercise plays in the
    maintenance of normal bowel elimination
    patterns. (p. 835)

6.5 Describe nursing interventions and
    attitudes related to bowel elimination
    habits. (p. 835)

## Lecture/Discussion

Ask students to list psychosocial factors that
affect their own bowel elimination status.

## Class Activity

Encourage students to visit a local pharmacy to
survey the variety of products that are available
for the regulation and care of the intestinal
tract. Ask them to share their findings in class.

7.0 Identify psychosocial components of defecation that may contribute to problems in bowel
elimination.

7.1 Identify major psychologic factors that
influence the process of normal defecation. (p. 830)

7.2 Identify cultural factors that have an
influence on the normal defecation
process. (p. 830)

8.0 Describe the following nursing diagnoses and
their management: alterations in bowel elimination due to (a) constipation, (b) fecal
impaction, (c) diarrhea, (d) flatulence, (e)
hemorrhoids, (f) fecal incontinence, and (g)
fecal diversion.

8.1 Identify common problems and selected
nursing diagnoses for individuals with
alterations in bowel elimination.
(p. 828)

8.2 Identify appropriate nursing goals for
an individual experiencing problems
related to bowel elimination. (p. 828)

8.3 Discuss criteria used to evaluate nursing care for individuals with bowel
elimination problems. (p. 828)

8.4 Describe the changes in bowel function
that may result from exposure to irritants within the GI tract. (p. 831)

8.5 Outline common bowel elimination changes
that occur as a result of the following: Age, motor and sensory disturbances, and intestinal pathology.
(p. 832)

8.6 Outline guidelines for assisting an
individual who has undergone hip surgery
with the process of defecation. (p. 836)

8.7 Identify and describe common causes of
constipation. (p. 836)

8.8 Identify individuals for whom constipation can be hazardous. (p. 836)

8.9 Summarize independent and dependent
nursing measures to assist individuals
experiencing constipation. (p. 837)

8.10 Identify five categories of laxatives
and describe the characteristics of
each. (p. 837)

8.11 Identify three purposes of enema
administration. (p. 838)

8.12 Explain the intent of administering
retention and return flow enemas.
(p. 838)

## Lecture/Discussion

Briefly describe common bowel elimination problems:
Fecal impaction, diarrhea, flatulence, hemorrhoids,
and fecal incontinence. Ask students to identify
factors that contribute to the development of each.

## Group Activity

Divide students into small groups. Ask each group
to develop a plan of care for individuals with one
of the common bowel elimination problems: Fecal
impaction, diarrhea, flatulence, hemorrhoids, and
fecal incontinence. Allow them to briefly present
their plan in class.

## Guest Speaker

Invite the ostomy nurse in each clinical facility
to a post-conference period to discuss their role
in the management of individuals with alterations
in bowel elimination due to fecal diversion:
Ileostomy and colostomy.

## Campus Laboratory Experience

Demonstrate the procedure for administering a
normal saline enema. Allow students to practice
the skill in a simulated laboratory situation.
Have students identify variations in the procedure
needed when performing other types of enemas.

## Clinical Laboratory Experience

Ask students to identify individuals in the
clinical area that display a high risk for the
development of bowel elimination problems. Have
them describe nursing measures that could be used
to prevent the occurrence of problems in each
identified individual.

Review the form that is used by the clinical
facility to record bowel elimination processes.

Have students identify the various appliances that
are used by individuals with alterations in bowel
elimination due to fecal diversion.

Upon demonstration of competency, have students
administer enemas to individuals in the clinical
area with supervision.

8.13 Summarize the relationship between the process of osmosis and enema administration. (p. 838)

8.14 Briefly describe the mechanisms by which various types of enema solutions promote bowel evacuation: Hypotonic, isotonic, and hypertonic solutions. (p. 838)

8.15 State the definition and describe the purposes of saline enema administration. (p. 839)

8.16 Discuss major contraindications and cautions the nurse should be aware of before administering a saline enema. (p. 839)

8.17 Identify basic teaching/learning needs of an individual who is to receive a saline enema. (p. 839)

8.18 Briefly discuss essential data the nurse should obtain before administering a saline enema. (p. 840)

8.19 List nursing actions that should be carried out in preparation for administering a saline enema. (p. 840)

8.20 Describe basic equipment that should be gathered by the nurse who is to administer a saline enema. (p. 840)

8.21 Outline steps the nurse should take to administer a saline enema. (p. 840)

8.22 Identify essential measures the nurse should perform upon completion of a saline enema administration. (p. 844)

8.23 Discuss assessment data that should be gathered by the nurse upon completion of a saline enema. (p. 844)

8.24 Describe the aftercare of basic equipment used to administer an enema. (p. 845)

8.25 Describe basic steps the nurse should take to administer other types of enemas: Hypertonic and retention. (p. 844)

8.26 Briefly describe complications that may occur as a result of enema administration: Fluid imbalance, electrolyte imbalance, tissue trauma, vagal nerve stimulation, and dependence. (p. 845)

8.27 Discuss measures the nurse can take to prevent or minimize complications due to enema administration. (p. 845)

8.28 Describe the development of a fecal impaction. (p. 845)

8.29 Identify clinical symptoms indicative of a fecal impaction. (p. 845)

8.30 Identify the major goal of treatment for individuals with altered bowel elimination due to fecal impactions.  (p. 846)

8.31 Discuss basic nursing measures that are utilized to assist an individual who has altered bowel elimination due to a fecal impaction.  (p. 846)

8.32 Briefly describe the meaning of diarrhea.  (p. 846)

8.33 Identify common causes of diarrhea.  (p. 846)

8.34 Identify symptoms that may accompany diarrhea.  (p. 846)

8.35 Identify data that should be obtained from a person experiencing alterations in bowel elimination due to diarrhea.  (p. 846)

8.36 Describe basic nursing intervention that will assist a person who is experiencing alterations in bowel elimination due to diarrhea.  (p. 846)

8.37 Discuss nursing measures that can be instituted to treat the accompanying symptoms of diarrhea.  (p. 847)

8.38 Describe the meaning of the term flatulence.  (p. 847)

8.39 Identify factors influencing the development of flatulence.  (p. 847)

8.40 Identify nursing goals and interventions for care of individuals with alterations in bowel elimination due to flatulence.  (p. 847)

8.41 Describe and state the possible causes of hemorrhoids.  (p. 847)

8.42 Describe basic treatment measures useful in assisting an individual experiencing alterations in bowel elimination due to hemorrhoids.  (p. 848)

8.43 Describe and identify possible causes of fecal incontinence.  (p. 848)

8.44 Identify basic nursing intervention for individuals with alterations in bowel elimination due to fecal incontinence.  (p. 848)

8.45 Describe basic purposes for the creation of two fecal diversion stomas:  Ileostomy and colostomy.  (p. 849)

8.46 Briefly discuss the psychological impact an ostomy may have on an individual.  (p. 849)

8.47 Identify ways in which the nurse can
offer psychological support to an individual with alterations in bowel elimination due to fecal diversion. (p. 849)

8.48 Outline guidelines for care of a person
with an ileostomy. (p. 849)

8.49 Discuss the basic care of an individual
with a colostomy. (p. 850)

---

MULTIPLE CHOICE QUESTIONS

CORRECT ANSWER AND RATIONALE

1. Which of the following statements is
   incorrect?

   A. Absorption of nutrients from digested
      material occurs in the small intestines
   B. Most of the water in digested material is
      absorbed in the large intestines
   C. The gastrocolic and duodenocolic reflexes
      are strongest when a person eats after
      fasting
   D. The rectum controls the process of
      defecation

   D   Although the defecation reflex begins in the
       rectum, the process is controlled by the
       internal and external sphincters of the anus.
       (p. 829)

2. Which of the following individuals is least
   likely to develop a problem with bowel
   elimination? The individual who:

   A. Consumes a low-fiber, high carbohydrate
      diet
   B. Has been on antibiotic therapy for two
      weeks
   C. Is experiencing a state of dehydration
   D. Takes morphine sulfate once a day for pain

   D   Individuals listed in options A, B, and C are
       all at high risk for the development of bowel
       elimination problems. Although morphine is a
       potent constipator, the person who takes it
       once a day is less likely to develop problems
       than the other individuals listed. (p. 831)

3. The nurse should be especially alert for the
   development of a paralytic ileus in a person
   who has:

   A. Delivered a child vaginally
   B. Had a lower gastrointestinal x-ray series
   C. Not had a bowel movement in several days
   D. Recently undergone abdominal surgery

   D   The person who has undergone abdominal surgery
       would be at greatest risk for the development
       of a paralytic ileus. The direct handling of
       the bowel itself causes a temporary stoppage
       of peristalsis called paralytic ileus.
       (p. 831)

4. An accurate stool analysis could be obtained
   from which of the following specimens? A
   stool specimen:

   A. For ova and parasites that has been left
      standing at room temperature for one hour
   B. For occult blood that has been
      refrigerated
   C. Obtained immediately after administering
      an oil retention enema
   D. That has been produced while voiding

   B   The nurse could accurately assess a stool
       specimen for occult blood after it has been
       refrigerated. Specimens contaminated with
       urine, oil, bismuth, or barium should not be
       used. It is necessary to maintain a specimen
       for ova and parasites at body temperature;
       therefore, they should be transported to the
       lab within 30 minutes of the defecation
       process. (p. 832)

5. Following a colonoscopy, the nurse should monitor Mr. Franklin for:

   A. Abdominal pain and distention
   B. Alterations in vital sign status
   C. Rectal bleeding
   D. All of the above

D  After direct visualization of the bowel, the nurse should continue to monitor vital signs and inspect frequently for fresh anal bleeding or abdominal pain and distention, which may indicate continued oozing at a biopsy site or bowel perforation. (p. 834)

6. When teaching an individual with cardio-vascular disease measures to improve their bowel elimination status, the nurse should encourage all of the following except:

   A. Avoid foods that cause a disruption in their bowel status
   B. Consume 1200 to 1500 cc of fluid daily, unless contraindicated
   C. Establish a daily bowel routine
   D. Perform abdominal isometric exercises

D  Isometric exercises are sometimes contraindi-cated in the individual with cardiac disease because they raise blood pressure and may cause coronary ischemia. Therefore, the nurse should consult the physician about the individual's health status before instituting an exercise program. (p. 835)

SITUATION: Mrs. Simmons, an 82-year-old individual, is admitted to the hospital with complaints of anorexia, headache, lethargy, and the continued passage of dry, hard stools. After a thorough assessment, you formulate the following nursing diagnosis: Alteration in bowel elimina-tion related to constipation. Questions 7 through 10 apply to this situation.

7. You know that Mrs. Simmons's constipation is most likely to result from:

   A. A diet low in dietary fiber
   B. Decreased peristalsis
   C. Lack of privacy in the nursing home
   D. The aging process

B  Constipation occurs when there is a decreased movement of feces through the large intestines, allowing more time for water absorption. Other factors listed would simply contribute to this problem. (p. 836)

8. Independent nursing measures to promote effective bowel elimination in Mrs. Simmons would include all of the following except:

   A. Administering oil retention enemas daily
   B. Encouraging increased fluid intake
   C. Giving six ounces of prune juice daily
   D. Providing ambulation activities three times daily

A  A physician's order would be required to administer an oil retention enema. All other listed measures would be independent nursing functions. (p. 837)

9. You have been asked to administer an oil retention enema for Mrs. Simmons. You know that the oil retention enema is given primarily to:

   A. Expel flatus
   B. Promote bowel regularity
   C. Soften the feces
   D. Stimulate the defecation process

C  A retention enema is retained in the bowel over a long period of time. It is usually administered to lubricate or soften a hard fecal mass, thus facilitating its expulsion through the anus. (p. 838)

10. In addition to the oil retention enema, the physician orders MOM 30 cc to be administered each evening at bedtime. MOM is an example of which type of laxative?

    A. Bulk-forming agent
    B. Emollient
    C. Osmotic agent
    D. Stimulant

C  MOM is an example of an osmotic agent. Osmotic agents promote bowel elimination by drawing water into the intestine to increase bulk and lubricate feces. (p. 837)

11. To prevent abrasions or perforations of the anterior rectal wall when administering an enema the nurse should:

   A. Administer the enema solution slowly
   B. Gently insert the enema tip 6-8 inches
   C. Inert the enema tip while the individual is in a Fowler's position
   D. All of the above

A  Abrasions or perforations of the anterior rectal wall can occur if the rectal tip is inserted too deeply; if fluid is inserted under excessively high pressure; or if the enema tip is inserted while the person is in a sitting position. (p. 839)

12. The nurse should be especially alert for the development of fluid and electrolyte disturbances in the person who has received which type of enema?

   A. Castile soap
   B. Oil retention
   C. Tap water
   D. All of the above

C  Fluid and electrolyte imbalances usually occur because of the tonicity of the enema solution. Caution should be used when administering hypotonic solutions to a person who is susceptible to fluid imbalance. The tap water enema is an example of a hypotonic solution. These enemas allow body absorption of water, thus promoting disturbances. (p. 845)

13. When a fecal impaction occurs, which of the following symptoms usually occurs first?

   A. Abdominal distention and fullness
   B. Inability to pass a normal stool
   C. Passage of small dry stools
   D. Seepage of liquid feces

B  The first symptom of an impaction is the inability to pass a normal stool. However, probably the most definitive symptom is the seepage of liquid stool from the anus. (p. 846)

# 41

# MEETING RESPIRATION NEEDS

## OBJECTIVES

1.0 Describe the normal structure and function of the respiratory system.

    1.1 Discuss the normal structure and function of the respiratory system. (p. 854)

    1.2 Briefly describe protective defense mechanisms of the respiratory tract. (p. 855)

2.0 Differentiate between acute and chronic respiratory dysfunction.

    2.1 Identify factors that may influence the development of upper airway dysfunctions. (p. 855)

    2.2 Identify specific forms of upper airway obstruction. (p. 855)

    2.3 Outline clinical signs indicative of upper airway distress. (p. 855)

    2.4 Identify conditions that affect the lower portion of the respiratory airway. (p. 856)

    2.5 Briefly discuss the etiology of the most common form of lower airway dysfunction, bronchospasm. (p. 856)

    2.6 Describe other causes of acute respiratory dysfunction: High spinal cord injury, neurologic diseases, and smoke or chemical irritation. (p. 856)

    2.7 Briefly describe two major categories used to classify conditions associated with chronic respiratory dysfunction. (p. 857)

    2.8 Identify specific diseases associated with obstructive lung disease. (p. 857)

    2.9 Identify basic causative factors for COPD and asthma. (p. 857)

    2.10 Discuss the clinical manifestations of the two basic types of asthma, extrinsic and intrinsic. (p. 857)

    2.11 Describe three types of restrictive lung diseases: Extrapulmonary disorders, disorders of the thoracic cage and diaphragm, and disorders of the lung parenchyma and pleura. (p. 857)

## TEACHING/LEARNING STRATEGIES

### Lecture/Discussion

Review the terminology listed on page 853 in the text.

Review the basic anatomy and physiology of the respiratory system.

### Lecture/Discussion

Briefly discuss the impact of immobility on a person's respiratory system functioning. Have students identify nursing management measures to prevent the respiratory complications caused by immobility.

Briefly discuss the etiology of the various chronic respiratory system disorders: Obstructive lung disease; restrictive lung disease; extrapulmonary disorders; disorders of the thoracic cage and diaphragm; and disorders of the lung parenchyma and pleura.

Have students differentiate between chronic and acute respiratory disorders.

### Clinical Laboratory Experience

Assist students in identifying individuals in the clinical area that are more prone to the development of alterations in respiratory functioning.

2.12 Describe the major effects obstructive
or restrictive respiratory disease may
have on the individual. (p. 858)

2.13 Outline physical body changes that are
commonly associated with COPD. (p. 858)

3.0 List causes of respiratory failure.

3.1 Define terminology used to describe the
process of respiratory failure: Hypercapnia, hypoxemia, ventilation, and
hypoventilation. (p. 859)

3.2 List the major causes of respiratory
failure. (p. 859)

3.3 Identify respiratory, cerebral, and
cardiovascular signs and symptoms
indicative of respiratory failure.
(p. 859)

3.4 Identify criteria used to determine the
presence of hypoxemia. (p. 868)

3.5 Identify manifestations and factors
contributing to the development of
cyanosis. (p. 868)

3.6 List factors that may alter or inhibit
clinical recognition of cyanosis.
(p. 868)

3.7 List five basic causes of inadequate
oxygenation. Give an example of each.
(p. 868)

3.8 Identify symptoms that are character-
istically associated with the three
levels of hypoxemia: Moderate, severe,
and grave. (p. 868)

4.0 Perform respiratory assessment under supervision.

4.1 Define terminology used to describe lung
volume and capacity: Tidal volume,
inspiratory reserve volume, expiratory
reserve volume, residual volume, total
lung capacity, vital capacity, inspiratory capacity, and functional residual
capacity. (p. 855)

4.2 Identify criteria used to assess people
with respiratory problems. (p. 859)

4.3 Describe various physical assessment
techniques that are employed in the
examination of people with respiratory
problems: Percussion, auscultation,
palpation of the chest, and inspection.
(p. 859)

4.4 Describe sounds that can be heard by
percussing the chest wall: Flat, dull,
resonant, tympany, and hyperresonant
sounds. (p. 861)

### Lecture/Discussion

Briefly discuss the causes of inadequate oxygenation: Inadequate oxygen in the inspired air,
hypoventilation, impaired diffusion, impaired
perfusion and transport of oxygen, and altered
uptake of oxygen by the tissues. Provide clinical
examples of each.

Ask students to identify assessment data useful in
determining the presence of hypoxemia.

Ask students to differentiate between the levels
of hypoxemia: Moderate, severe, and grave.

### Clinical Laboratory Experience

Assist students in identifying individuals who are
more prone to the development of respiratory failure. Have them identify the signs and symptoms of
impending respiratory failure: Respiratory, cerebral, and cardiac.

### Lecture/Discussion

Discuss the criteria used to evaluate the presence
of dyspnea. Point out common individual complaints
that may indicate the presence of dyspnea.

Provide a taped demonstration of normal and
abnormal breath sounds.

Ask students to identify and discuss terms that
are used to describe lung volumes and capacities.

### Written Exercise

Have students outline the data that is necessary
to assess a person's respiratory status. Ask them
to use this data to assess another classmate's
respiratory system functioning.

### Campus Laboratory

Demonstrate the procedures for auscultation,
percussion, inspection, and palpation. Allow
students to practice these techniques with another
classmate in the campus laboratory setting.

4.5 Describe basic observations the nurse
should make when conducting the inspection portion of a respiratory assessment.
(p. 861)

4.6 Discuss basic information the nurse
should gather when using palpation to
examine the respiratory system. (p. 861)

4.7 Identify criteria used to objectively
evaluate the effectiveness of oxygen
therapy. (p. 874)

4.8 Discuss the importance of continued
oxygen administration during exercise
for individuals with COPD and other
chronic respiratory disorders. (p. 875)

4.9 Briefly describe three methods of oxygen
administration devices available for
home use: Liquid portable oxygen systems, portable cylinders of gaseous
oxygen, and oxygen concentrators.
(p. 875)

4.10 Identify possible reasons for home
oxygen use. (p. 875)

4.11 Identify the purpose of medication
administration via the respiratory
tract. (p. 876)

4.12 Discuss methods used to delivery medication into the respiratory system.
(p. 876)

4.13 Describe the technique for using metered
dose inhalers to deliver medication into
the respiratory system. (p. 876)

4.14 Describe four categories of medications
that may be administered by aerosolization: Bronchodilators, mucolytics,
anti-inflammatory/anti-allergenic, and
antibiotics. (p. 877)

4.15 Explain the purpose of positive pressure
breathing. (p. 877)

4.16 Enumerate the undesirable effects that
may be caused by intermittent positive
pressure breathing. (p. 877)

4.17 Identify precautions the nurse should be
aware of when administering oxygen
therapy. (p. 880)

4.18 Discuss the teaching/learning needs of
individuals receiving oxygen therapy.
(p. 880)

4.19 Outline activities the nurse should take
in preparation for administration of
oxygen therapy. (p. 880)

4.20 Identify equipment the nurse should
gather in order to administer oxygen.
(p. 880)

## Clinical Laboratory Experience

Ask students to auscultate the lungs of an
assigned individual in the clinical area. Ask
them to share this experience in a post-conference
period.

4.21 List the sequence of steps the nurse should follow to administer oxygen therapy. (p. 880)

4.22 List the basic steps that a person should be taught to ensure effective incentive therapy. (p. 878)

4.23 Identify indications for instituting inspiratory muscle exercises. (p. 878)

4.24 Identify the common goals for breathing retraining techniques. (p. 878)

4.25 Discuss the purpose of rehabilitation programs for individuals with chronic respiratory disease. (p. 878)

4.26 List the major components of rehabilitation programs for people with chronic respiratory disease. (p. 878)

4.27 State the definition and describe the purposes of oxygen administration. (p. 880)

4.28 Discuss the nurse's responsibilities after beginning oxygen therapy; After-care of equipment, client assessment, aftercare of equipment, and documentation. (p. 882)

5.0 Interpret, with supervision, data collected from respiratory assessment.

5.1 Summarize normal laboratory arterial blood gas values; pH, $paCO_2$, $paO_2$, $HCO_3$, and $SaO_2$. Briefly discuss what these normal values indicate. (p. 859)

5.2 Describe normal breath sounds that are produced by the movement of air in and out of the lungs; Bronchial, bronchovesicular, and vesicular. State the anatomic location for each. (p. 860)

5.3 Describe abnormal lung sounds, their anatomic location, and whether they are heard on inspiration or expiration: Rales, rhonchi, pleural friction rub, increased breath sounds, and decreased breath sounds. (p. 860)

5.4 Describe the concept of dyspnea. (p. 861)

5.5 Identify terminology frequently used by an individual to describe dyspnea. (p. 861)

5.6 Briefly discuss the pathological manifestations caused by dyspnea. (p. 862)

5.7 Outline information that should be documented in the clinical record of an individual who is experiencing dyspnea. (p. 862)

## Lecture/Discussion

Focus discussion on the normal arterial blood gas values. Have students identify what each value indicates if within the normal range.

6.0 Present a learning/teaching session about smoking and its danger.

    6.1 Briefly discuss the hazards of cigarette smoking. (p. 862)

    6.2 Enumerate the effects of cigarette smoking on the respiratory system. (p. 862)

    6.3 Discuss the benefits obtained by a person who successfully completes a smoking cessation program. (p. 863)

7.0 Plan nursing care for people requiring various respiratory therapeutic measures.

    7.1 Identify common nursing diagnoses used to describe individuals with respiration needs. (p. 852)

    7.2 Identify common nursing goals related to care of the person with respiration needs. (p. 853)

    7.3 State outcome criteria essential for evaluating the nursing care of individuals with respiration needs. (p. 853)

    7.4 Discuss the overall purposes of various therapeutic respiratory treatment measures: Mobilization maneuvers, hydration, chest physical therapy, oxygen administration, medication, positive pressure breathing, respiratory exercises, and rehabilitation. (p. 863)

    7.5 Identify the benefits of various mobilization maneuvers, used to aid in the treatment of respiratory dysfunction: Turning, deep breathing, coughing, ambulation, and position changes. (p. 863)

    7.6 Describe the effects immobility can have on the respiratory system. (p. 863)

    7.7 Describe the anatomy of an effective cough. (p. 864)

    7.8 Identify hazards that are associated with coughing. (p. 864)

    7.9 Discuss the influence body position can have on the ability to cough effectively. (p. 865)

    7.10 Identify information that should be included in a teaching/learning session for effective coughing. (p. 865)

    7.11 Briefly discuss hydration methods used in the treatment of individuals with respiratory needs: Oral, parenteral, and topical. (p. 865)

### Lecture/Discussion

Ask students to discuss the effects of cigarette smoking on a person's respiratory system. Have them identify other body disorders that are commonly associated with cigarette smoking.

### Guest Speaker

Invite a representative from a local chapter of the American Lung Association to class to discuss the various smoking cessation clinics that are available within the community.

### Lecture/Discussion

Help students to understand differences in the basic oxygen delivery systems. Have them observe the use of each system in the clinical area.

Impress upon students the hazards associated with oxygen administration.

### Campus Laboratory Experiences

Demonstrate the procedure for assisting a person with effective coughing.

Demonstrate the technique that should be used when assisting individuals with the use of metered dose inhalers.

Demonstrate the technique used to assure effective incentive therapy.

Provide a demonstration of the techniques used in preparing and administering oxygen therapy. Allow students to practice the techniques in the campus laboratory facility.

### Clinical Laboratory Experience

Encourage students to observe the various types of respiratory equipment available in their clinical facility to assist a person with respiratory functioning.

Arrange for students to observe a respiratory therapist performing chest physical therapy maneuvers.

### Guest Speaker

Invite a respiratory therapist in each clinical facility to a post-conference period to discuss the various treatments performed on individuals with respiratory disorders.

7.12 Describe methods of topical hydration used in the treatment of respiratory problems: Humidifiers, aerosolization, and nebulization. (p. 866)

7.13 Discuss hazards associated with the use of respiratory hydration methods: Contamination, bronchospasm, shortness of breath, and overhydration. (p. 866)

7.14 Briefly describe chest physical therapy techniques that are commonly used for individuals with respiration needs: Postural drainage, chest percussion, and vibration. (p. 867)

7.15 Identify individuals for whom chest physical therapy would be inappropriate. (p. 867)

7.16 State the goal of oxygen therapy. (p. 868)

7.17 Outline major benefits of oxygen administration. (p. 869)

7.18 Briefly discuss favorable changes occurring in commonly observed symptoms of hypoxemia after the administration of oxygen. (p. 869)

7.19 Identify situations that would warrant continuous administration of oxygen. (p. 869)

7.20 List circumstances in which intermittent oxygen therapy should be used. (p. 869)

7.21 Discuss factors that should be considered when selecting the dosage of oxygen that is to be administered to an individual. (p. 869)

7.22 Identify information that should be included in a prescription for oxygen therapy. (p. 869)

7.23 Discuss factors that determine the amount of oxygen delivered by oxygen delivery systems. (p. 869)

7.24 State three measures that may be used to monitor the clinical effectiveness of a prescribed dosage of oxygen. (p. 870)

7.25 List important safety factors the nurse should keep in mind when administering oxygen therapy. (p. 870)

7.26 Identify nursing intervention that can be instituted to ensure the safety of an individual receiving oxygen therapy. (p. 870)

7.27 Describe the purpose of oxygen humidification. (p. 870)

7.28 Describe two basic categories of oxygen delivery systems; High flow oxygen systems and low flow oxygen systems. (p. 871)

7.29 Describe the basic characteristics of various low flow oxygen delivery systems: Nasal cannula; standard mask; and oxygen mask with reservoir bag, non-rebreathing. (p. 872)

7.30 Discuss the basic characteristics of various high flow oxygen delivery systems: Venturi mask and volume ventilator. (p. 872)

7.31 Discuss undesirable effects caused by oxygen therapy: oxygen-induced hypoventilation, oxygen toxicity, retrolental fibroplasia, and atelectasis. (p. 873)

---

## MULTIPLE CHOICE QUESTIONS

## CORRECT ANSWER AND RATIONALE

1. The nurse would expect to find rales most often when auscultating the lungs of an individual with:

   A. Alveolar fluid
   B. Asthma
   C. Cyanosis
   D. COPD

D  Rales are described as crackling sounds heard upon inspiration. They occur because of fluid passing through moisture. They are classified as wet (as in pulmonary edema) or dry (as associated with the pulmonary fibrosis of COPD). (p. 860)

2. The lung parenchyma:

   A. Includes the pleura and the thorax
   B. Is a membranous covering of the lung and thorax
   C. Provides the mechanism of gas exchange
   D. All of the above

C  The lung parenchyma (functional elements of the lung) consists of respiratory bronchioles, alveolar ducts, and alveolar sacs. The exchange of oxygen and carbon dioxide occurs primarily at the alveolar level. Gas exchange takes place by diffusion of oxygen and carbon dioxide across the alveolar capillary membrane. (p. 854)

3. When assessing a person with alterations in respiratory functioning, the nurse should understand that the vital capacity is equal to the:

   A. Inspiratory capacity plus ERV
   B. Tidal volume plus the RFC
   C. Tidal volume plus the RV
   D. Total lung capacity

A  The vital capacity of the lungs is the maximum amount of air that can be expelled from the lungs by a forceful effort, following a maximal inhalation. (p. 855)

4. Mr. Johnson has recently undergone thoracic surgery. The most likely etiology of his acute respiratory dysfunction after surgery would be:

   A. Pneumonia from prolonged bedrest
   B. A pneumothorax requiring a chest tube
   C. Residual tumor for which the surgery was performed
   D. Stridor with upper airway obstruction

B  Although an acute respiratory dysfunction can occur as a result of all the listed options, Mr. Johnson is most likely to develop problems because of a pneumothorax after surgery, which is a collapse of the lungs from air, blood, or other fluids that have collected in the pleural spaces. (p. 856)

5. Mr. Perry, a 52-year-old male, is admitted to the respiratory unit for extrinsic asthma. The nurse knows that extrinsic asthma is:

   A. A restrictive lung disease
   B. Caused by non-allergenic factors
   C. More common in the young
   D. Usually associated with inspiratory obstruction

C   Extrinsic asthma is caused by allergens. It is more common in children and young adults. Intrinsic asthma is caused by nonallergenic factors and is more common in middle-aged and older adults. (p. 857)

6. Which of the following blood gas values indicates respiratory failure?

   A. $paO_2$ 78, $paCO_2$ 42, pH 7.38
   B. $paO_2$ 78, $paCO_2$ 46, pH 7.40
   C. $paO_2$ 80, $paCO_2$ 42, pH 7.52
   D. $paO_2$ 78, $paCO_2$ 46, pH 7.32

D   Respiratory failure produces elevated $paO_2$, in combination with a decreased pH of the blood. (p. 858)

7. The nurse is aware that normal expiratory breath sounds include:

   A. Dry rales in the bases
   B. Scattered rhonchi
   C. Vesicular breath sounds peripherally
   D. All of the above

C   Vesicular breath sounds can be normally hear in the periphery. Other listed options are abnormal breath sounds. For a complete listing of normal and abnormal breath sounds, see page 860 in text. (p. 860)

8. As a nurse, you should know that dyspnea:

   A. And CO retention are often related
   B. Is abnormal if associated with activity
   C. Is rapid in occurrence in almost all cases
   D. Is objectively described to include retractions and stridor

A   Statements B, C, and D are all incorrect. Dyspnea and CO retention are, however, often related. (p. 861)

9. Cigarette smoking is a significant historical fact in predicting a person's risk for:

   A. Asthma
   B. Cancer of the stomach
   C. Premature spontaneous abortion
   D. All of the above

D   Cigarette smoking has been associated with all of the listed options. (p. 862)

SITUATION: Carrie, a 79-year-old nursing home individual, is admitted to the hospital with pneumonia. After a thorough history and physical, the physician orders the following: Turn, cough, and deep breathing exercises every two hours; use of a room humidifier; chest physical therapy three times a day; and oxygen at 5L/min per nasal cannula. Questions 10 through 12 apply to this situation.

10. In order to facilitate effective coughing for Carrie, the nurse should:

    A. Administer analgesics prior to coughing exercises
    B. Encourage the consumption of at least one quart of fluid daily
    C. Position Carrie in a semi-Fowler's position
    D. None of the above.

D   All responses are incorrect. The nurse would be unable to administer an analgesic without a physician's order; at least two to four quarts of fluid should be encouraged daily, unless contraindicated; and the person should be placed in a sitting position. (p. 864)

11. The nurse knows that chest physical therapy:

    A. Can be performed by almost anyone
    B. Is used primarily to prevent the collection of secretions in the upper airway passages
    C. Promotes tracheobronchial drainage and prevents pooling of secretions
    D. Should be performed immediately after mealtime

C   Goals of chest physical therapy include the promotion of tracheobronchial drainage, the prevention of secretion pooling, and an overall improvement in ventilation. It should never be performed immediately after a meal because nausea, vomiting, and aspiration of stomach contents can occur. Because of the complexity of techniques involved in chest physical therapy, it should only be performed by specially trained people. (p. 867)

12. When preparing Carrie's oxygen administration
set, the nurse should know that the nasal
cannula:

A. Delivers between 40 and 65 per cent of
oxygen
B. Has a liter flow rate of 4 to 10 LPM
C. Requires patent nasal passages to be
therapeutic
D. May promote feelings of confinement and
claustrophobia

C  The nasal cannula delivers from 1 to 6 liters
of oxygen per minute with a percentage of 22
to 40 per cent. To be effective, the
individual must have patent nasal passages.
Feelings of confinement and claustrophobia are
often associated with use of the standard
oxygen mask. (p. 871)


13. To effectively use an incentive spirometer,
the nurse should encourage a person to
initially:

A. Exhale to a point of minimal discomfort
B. Take a slow, deep inhalation
C. Place the mouthpiece between the teeth
and lips
D. None of the above

D  The first basic step for effective incentive
therapy is to exhale to a point of comfort.
Seven basic steps are listed on page 878 of
the text. (p. 878)

# PROVIDING IMMEDIATE LIFE SUPPORT

OBJECTIVES

1.0 Describe the pathophysiology of cardiopulmonary arrest.

    1.1 Review the structure and function of the
normal cardiovascular system. (p. 887)

    1.2 Describe the clinical characteristics of
acute and chronic failure of the respiratory system. (p. 887)

    1.3 Identify the systemic effects of hypox-
emia on the body. (p. 888)

    1.4 Discuss the clinical characteristics of
cardiovascular system failure. (p. 888)

    1.5 Summarize events that frequently lead to
a cardiopulmonary arrest. (p. 888)

    1.6 Identify the most frequent cause of
cardiac arrest. (p. 889)

    1.7 Briefly discuss the etiology of angina
pectoris. (p. 889)

    1.8 Identify secondary signs of cardiopul-
monary arrest. (p. 889)

2.0 Differentiate between respiratory and cardiac
arrest.

3.0 Differentiate between clinical and biologic
death.

4.0 Assess a person to identify cardiopulmonary
arrest.

    4.1 List the steps that should be taken to
determine a cardiopulmonary arrest.
(p. 890)

    4.2 Summarize the indications of impending
cardiopulmonary arrest. (p. 890)

    4.3 Discuss criteria that influence a
rescuer to begin cardiac compressions in
an unconscious person. (p. 894)

TEACHING/LEARNING STRATEGIES

**Lecture/Discussion**

Review the normal anatomy of the cardiovascular
system.

Summarize the changes that occur in the cardiopulmonary system as a result of an arrest.

**Lecture/Discussion**

Focus discussion on the etiology of acute or
chronic respiratory system failures and sudden
cardiac arrest.

**Written Exercise**

Ask students to outline the manifestations of
clinical and biologic death.

**Written Exercise**

Ask students to list the primary and secondary
signs of cardiopulmonary arrest.

**Clinical Laboratory Experience**

Arrange for students to visit the coronary care
department in their clinical facility for viewing
of the basic cardiac monitoring equipment.

5.0 Describe the accepted sequence of actions for basic life support.

5.1 Correctly utilize terminology related to immediate life support. (p. 886)

5.2 Briefly discuss historical perspectives influencing the development of current life support measures. (p. 886)

5.3 State the reason for administering a precordial thump to an individual who has experienced a cardiopulmonary arrest. (p. 891)

5.4 Outline the steps in the cardiopulmonary resuscitation process for an adult. (p. 891)

5.5 Briefly describe the reason it is necessary to open the airway of a person who has experienced a cardiopulmonary arrest. (p. 891)

5.6 Describe three methods that can be used by the nurse to establish an open airway in a person requiring CPR: Head tilt-chin lift, head tilt-neck lift, and jaw thrust method. (p. 891)

5.7 Describe the technique of mouth-to-mouth resuscitation for an adult. (p. 891)

5.8 Briefly describe the techniques involved in other rescue breathing methods: Mouth-to-nose, mouth-to-stoma, mouth-to-tracheostomy, and the jaw thrust without head tilt technique. (p. 891)

5.9 Describe factors that influence the rate and size of breaths needed to sustain an individual receiving CPR. (p. 893)

5.10 Identify the ratio for rate of breaths delivered to the number of cardiac compressions in basic CPR rescue techniques. (p. 894)

5.11 Explain the physiological changes that occur in a person receiving closed chest compressions. (p. 894)

5.12 List the steps that must be followed by a person to administer closed chest compressions. (p. 894)

5.13 Describe correct hand and finger placement in an individual delivering closed cardiac compressions. (p. 895)

5.14 Describe the rate of cardiac compressions that must be delivered for an adult during one-person and two-person CPR. (p. 895)

5.15 Summarize the CPR cardiac compression to ventilation ratio for one-rescuer and two-rescuer CPR. (p. 895)

## Lecture/Discussion

Ask students to explore their role in the event of a witnessed cardiovascular or respiratory arrest.

Ask students to identify agencies in the community who provide basic life support services in emergency situations.

5.16 Describe methods of evaluating the
effectiveness of CPR during two-person
CPR. (p. 896)

5.17 Outline the correct sequence of steps in
two-person CPR rescue attempts. (p. 896)

5.18 List the procedure for changing rescuer
roles during two-person CPR. (p. 897)

5.19 List factors that influence the decision
to terminate basic life support measures.
(p. 902)

5.20 Describe the major components of advanced
life support. (p. 903)

5.21 Discuss preliminary activities that
should be completed by the nurse before
beginning CPR. (p. 909)

5.22 List the steps involved in the CPR procedure for unwitnessed cardiopulmonary
arrest. (p. 910)

5.23 Enumerate the steps involved in the CPR
procedure for a witnessed cardiac
arrest. (p. 913)

5.24 Identify information that should be
documented in the clinical record of an
individual who has received CPR.
(p. 914)

6.0 Undertake regular, ongoing, supervised
instruction and practice for competency in
cardiopulmonary resuscitation (CPR).

**Lecture/Discussion**

Encourage students to obtain basic CPR certification yearly.

7.0 Perform cardiopulmonary resuscitation com-
petently for adults, children, and infants,
both within health care facilities and in the
community.

**Lecture/Discussion**

Ask students to review the policy at their
clinical facility regarding "Do not resuscitate"
orders.

Demonstrate the procedure for one- and two-person
CPR on an adult mannequin. Observe students as
they practice each technique.

Demonstrate the procedure for giving an infant
CPR. Observe students as they practice the
technique.

**Guest Speaker**

Invite a critical care nurse in the clinical
facility to speak in a post-conference period on
their role in witnessed cardiovascular or respiratory arrests.

8.0 Describe complications that can occur with
cardiopulmonary resuscitation.

8.1 Summarize major complications of CPR.
(p. 899)

**Lecture/Discussion**

Discuss the etiology of the various complications
associated with CPR: Spinal cord injuries, gastric
distention, aspiration, mechanical blockage of the
upper or lower airways, aspiration pnuemonia, rib
and xiphoid fractures, and myocardial contusion.

9.0 Describe and prevent errors in the performance of cardiopulmonary resuscitation.

    9.1 Briefly summarize performance errors and
        problems that may be encountered during
        CPR. (p. 897)

    9.2 Describe the consequences of improper
        hand placement by a rescuer during CPR.
        (p. 895)

10.0 Describe the differences between cardiopulmonary resuscitation for adults, children,
and infants.

**Lecture/Discussion**

Ask students to compare and contrast differences
in the techniques used to administer CPR to an
infant and an adult.

    10.1 Identify reasons for administering CPR
        to a newborn. (p. 897)

    10.2 Discuss other factors that can affect
        infant ventilation and create a need for
        resuscitation at birth. (p. 897)

    10.3 Identify common causes of respiratory
        arrests in infants and children.
        (p. 899)

    10.4 Discuss the proper sequence of steps
        involved in administering CPR to infants
        and children. (p. 899)

    10.5 Identify four signs of successful
        ventilation during CPR for infants and
        children. (p. 899)

    10.6 Compare the CPR technique required for
        infants with those required for children.
        (p. 902)

11.0 Offer psychosocial support for the significant others of individuals experiencing
cardiopulmonary arrest.

**Lecture/Discussion**

Have students explore the role of the nurse in
assisting the significant others of an individual
needing basic life support.

    11.1 Discuss the care of an individual's
        significant other when basic or advanced
        life support is necessary. (p. 903)

12.0 Offer psychological support to individuals
who recover from cardiopulmonary arrest.

**Lecture/Discussion**

Discuss the emotional reactions that may be displayed by the individual who has survived cardiopulmonary death: Denial, isolation of affect,
displacement, projection, hallucinatory or delusional behavior, and violent dreams.

    12.1 Describe the common reactions of an
        individual who has survived cardio-
        pulmonary death. (p. 903)

    12.2 Outline basic nursing intervention
        during the postcardiopulmonary arrest
        period. (p. 903)

13.0 Perform appropriate emergency intervention
for adults, children, and infants with
foreign body airway obstruction.

**Lecture/Discussion**

Ask students to give examples of individuals who
are prone to the development of a foreign airway
obstruction.

    13.1 Identify common causes of foreign body
        airway obstruction. (p. 904)

Have students identify the criteria used to
identify individuals with a foreign body airway
obstruction.

    13.2 Describe the sequence of steps involved
        in the Heimlich maneuver. (p. 904)

13.3 Identify Instances when the Heimlich
maneuver would be unsafe or Ineffective.
(p. 904)

13.4 Outline teaching/learning measures to
prevent foreign material airway obstruction. (p. 904)

13.5 Identify criteria that may be used to
assist in the recognition of a partial
or complete foreign body airway
obstruction. (p. 904)

13.6 Briefly discuss three techniques that
can be used to relieve foreign airway
obstruction: Back blows, manual
thrusts, and finger sweeps. (p. 905)

13.7 Summarize the prolonged effects a person
may experience as a result of hypoxia.
(p. 907)

13.8 Describe nursing activities that may be
necessary after removing an airway
obstruction. (p. 907)

13.9 Outline the action steps that should be
taken by the nurse for a complete airway
obstruction. (p. 908)

13.10 Discuss the proper management of foreign
body airway obstruction in Infants and
children. (p. 908)

## Campus Laboratory Experience

Provide a demonstration of the procedures used to
remove foreign airway obstructions:  Back blows,
manual thrusts, combined back blows and manual
thrusts, and finger sweeps.  Allow students to
practice the techniques on a mannequin in the
campus laboratory facility.

---

## MULTIPLE CHOICE QUESTIONS

## CORRECT ANSWER AND RATIONALE

1.  When making routine nursing rounds, you find
    Mrs. Still unconscious on the floor by her
    bed.  Immediate nursing intervention for Mrs.
    Still should include all of the following
    except:

    A.  Administering a sharp blow to the back
    B.  Performing abdominal or chest thrusts
    C.  Probing the mouth with a sweep of the
        finger
    D.  Transporting Mrs. Still back to bed

D   Options B, C, and D would be effective in
    removing an airway obstruction, if present.
    The individual should not be transported back
    to bed if found unconscious, but rather rescue
    techniques should be begun.  (p. 891)

2.  You open an individual's airway by tilting
    the head back and lifting the neck with one
    hand, while pushing down on the forehead with
    the other hand.  Which method are you using
    to open the airway?

    A.  Head tilt - jaw thrust method
    B.  Head tilt - neck lift method
    C.  Head tilt - chin lift method
    D.  Jaw thrust method

B   The situation describes the head tilt - neck
    lift method for opening an airway.  (p. 891)

3.  When performing two-person CPR rescue, the
    correct compression ratio is:

    A.  5:1
    B.  5:2
    C.  15:1
    D.  15:2

D   The correct compression ratio for two-person
    CPR rescue is 5:1.  When performing one-person
    CPR, the nurse should deliver a 15:2 ratio of
    compressions to ventilations.  (p. 895)

4. Which of the following findings is not commonly associated with acute respiratory failure?

   A. Acidemia
   B. Decreased arterial oxygen
   C. Increased arterial $CO_2$
   D. Increased blood pH

D   Acute failure of the respiratory system is marked by hypoxemia (a sudden fall in arterial oxygen) and hypercarbia (a rise in arterial $CO_2$). This results in respiratory acidosis, causing a fall in blood pH and acidemia. (p. 887)

5. Which of the following is not a cause of cardiopulmonary arrest due to an impaired circulatory system?

   A. Air embolism
   B. Electrolyte balance
   C. Hemorrhage
   D. Thrombus formation

B   Options A, C, and D are all examples of impaired circulatory events that lead to cardiopulmonary arrest. An electrolyte balance is an example of an altered state of homeostasis causing cardiopulmonary arrest. (p. 888)

6. The nurse can administer a precordial thump to a person who:

   A. Has a witnessed cardiopulmonary arrest
   B. Has ventricular fibrillation or tachycardia
   C. Is on a cardiac monitor
   D. All of the above

B   A precordial thump is done only when ventricular tachycardia or fibrillation is witnessed and monitored. (p. 890)

7. All of the following assessment data could be used to evaluate the effectiveness of ventilation in an infant receiving CPR except:

   A. Bilateral expansion of the chest
   B. Bilateral breath sounds upon auscultation
   C. Increased heart rate to 80 beats/minute
   D. Improvement of skin color and peripheral pulses

C   Options A, B, and D could be used to evaluate the effectiveness of ventilation efforts. The pulse rate should, however, increase to a regular rate of 100 beats per minute or more. (p. 899)

8. In order to provide effective aid to a choking victim, the nurse should administer:

   A. Abdominal thrusts to an obese individual
   B. Abdominal thrusts to a child, if back blows are ineffective
   C. Chest thrusts to a pregnant female
   D. All of the above

C   Thrusts to the lower chest are used when the individual's abdominal girth is too great to allow the rescuer to wrap their hands around the abdomen to perform abdominal thrusts. (p. 905)

# 43

# CARING FOR PEOPLE REQUIRING AIRWAY MANAGEMENT

## OBJECTIVES

1.0 Identify causes of airway obstruction.

   1.1 Understand terminology used in the care of people requiring airway management. (p. 917)

   1.2 List factors that may influence the potency of a person's airway. (p. 917)

   1.3 Identify the sites and causes of upper airway obstruction. (p. 917)

   1.4 Identify clinical data indicative of a nonpatent airway (p. 918)

   1.5 Identify nursing measures useful in the prevention of airway obstruction. (p. 918)

   1.6 Identify the physiological manifestations that might be observed in individuals with lower airway obstruction. (p. 919)

   1.7 Identify individuals who have a greater risk for the development, of lower airway obstructions. (p. 919)

2.0 Describe the method of inserting oropharyngeal and nasopharyngeal airways.

   2.1 Describe basic nursing intervention for a person with a suspected nonpatent airway. (p. 918)

   2.2 Briefly describe the purpose of oropharyngeal airway placement. (p. 919)

   2.3 Identify individuals in whom an oropharyngeal airway would be appropriate. (p. 919)

   2.4 Discuss the nursing care of an individual with an oropharyngeal airway. (p. 919)

   2.5 Describe the procedure for insertion of an oral airway. (p. 919)

   2.6 Briefly describe two types of respiratory airways: Oropharyngeal and nasopharyngeal. (p. 919)

   2.7 Outline the sequence of steps for the insertion of a nasopharyngeal airway. (p. 920)

## TEACHING/LEARNING STRATEGIES

### Lecture/Discussion

Have students list the clinical signs indicative of upper and lower airway obstructions.

Ask students to compare and contrast the factors that cause upper and lower airway obstructions.

### Clinical Laboratory Experience

Assist students in identifying individuals in the clinical facility who are more prone to the development of upper and lower airway obstructions.

### Lecture/Discussion

Demonstrate the procedure for insertion of an oropharyngeal airway and a nasopharyngeal airway. Allow students to practice the procedures on a mannequin in the campus laboratory facility.

3.0 List methods of promoting tracheobronchial hydration.

    3.1 Discuss the reason for humidification of artificial airways. (p. 922)

    3.2 Describe various devices used to provide humidification and oxygenation to people requiring artificial airways. (p. 922)

    3.3 List three methods by which tracheobronchial secretions can be hydrated. (p. 923)

### Campus Laboratory Experience

Describe the devices used to provide humidification and oxygenation to people requiring artificial airways. Arrange for students to view these devices in the clinical laboratory setting.

4.0 Discuss tracheobronchial suctioning, including side effects and precautions.

    4.1 Identify factors that influence the route chosen for suctioning of an airway. (p. 923)

    4.2 Outline the steps involved in airway suctioning: Oropharyngeal and nasopharyngeal. (p. 923)

    4.3 Identify general factors the nurse should take into consideration when performing airway suctioning techniques. (p. 923)

    4.4 Identify criteria used to select the type of catheter necessary for various respiratory suctioning maneuvers. (p. 924)

    4.5 Briefly describe the function of a coude-tip suction catheter. (p. 925)

    4.6 Identify side effects that may occur as a result of respiratory suctioning. (p. 926)

    4.7 Identify the major purpose of tracheobronchial tree suctioning. (p. 926)

    4.8 Identify contraindications and precautions the nurse should be aware of when performing tracheobronchial tree suctioning. (p. 926)

### Lecture/Discussion

Discuss the side effects that can occur as a result of respiratory suctioning procedures. Ask students to identify appropriate nursing intervention that can be used to prevent each side effect.

### Campus Laboratory Experience

Demonstrate the procedures used to perform nasopharyngeal and tracheal suctioning. Allow students to practice each technique on a mannequin in the campus laboratory facility.

### Clinical Laboratory Experience

Arrange for students to observe a nurse or respiratory therapist performing respiratory suctioning procedures.

5.0 Perform safe tracheobronchial suctioning under supervision.

    5.1 Summarize assessment data that can be utilized to determine the need for respiratory suctioning. (p. 926)

    5.2 Describe preliminary nursing activities that should be performed in preparation for tracheobronchial tree suctioning. (p. 928)

    5.3 List the equipment needed to perform tracheobronchial tree suctioning. (p. 928)

    5.4 Describe the steps involved in the suctioning of the tracheobronchial tree via various routes: Oral, nasal, and artificial airways. (p. 928)

### Lecture/Discussion

Ask students to identify the criteria that can be used to assess a person's need for respiratory suctioning.

### Clinical Laboratory Experience

After demonstrating proficiency, allow students to perform respiratory suctioning techniques on assigned persons in the clinical area with supervision.

5.5 Explain nursing responsibilities upon completion of tracheobronchial tree suctioning. (p. 930)

5.6 Describe data that should be documented in the clinical record of a person who has received tracheobronchial tree suctioning. (p. 930)

6.0 List types of artificial airways and their purposes.

6.1 Define the term "artificial airway." (p. 920)

6.2 Identify situations that necessitate the insertion of an artificial airway. (p. 920)

6.3 Describe the purpose and function of two types of artificial airways: Endotracheal and tracheostomy tubes. (p. 920)

6.4 Compare the routes of placement for endotracheal and tracheostomy airway devices. (p. 922)

6.5 Discuss major differences in cuffed and uncuffed artificial airways. (p. 922)

**Lecture/Discussion**

Compare and contrast cuffed and uncuffed artificial airways.

Bring examples to class of oropharyngeal airways, nasopharyngeal airways, endotracheal tubes, and tracheostomy tubes to class for student viewing.

**Clinical Laboratory Experience**

Arrange for students to briefly observe a person using a continuous mechanical ventilator.

7.0 Describe safety precautions important in caring for people using artificial airways.

7.1 Discuss problems associated with the use of artificial airways. (p. 921)

7.2 Describe techniques the nurse can utilize to intervene effectively in problems associated with the use of artificial airways. (p. 921)

7.3 Briefly discuss the risks associated with placing and maintaining artificial airways. (p. 923)

7.4 Describe basic vacuum pressures used to aspirate respiratory secretions. (p. 924)

7.5 Describe the proper care of the inner and outer cannula of a tracheostomy tube. (p. 930)

7.6 Describe the technique that should be used by the nurse to secure tracheostomy ties. (p. 930)

7.7 Discuss nursing measures that should be performed to care for tracheostomy dressings. (p. 931)

7.8 Identify techniques that should be used to prevent infection in the tracheostomy person. (p. 931)

7.9 Identify individuals requiring the use of continuous mechanical ventilation. (p. 931)

**Lecture/Discussion**

Focus discussion on the problems that are commonly associated with the use of artificial airway devices. Discuss appropriate nursing intervention for the management of each problem.

Discuss the care and safety concepts involved in the care of individuals requiring tracheostomy care.

1. The nurse is aware that stridor:

   A. Is more common in adults than children
   B. Is a serious indicator of lower airway obstruction
   C. May indicate airway obstruction at the level of the larynx
   D. All of the above

C  Stridor, a high-pitched respiratory crowing sound, is a serious indicator of upper airway obstruction, usually at the level of the larynx or epiglottis. It occurs more commonly in children than adults. (p. 918)

2. A complete or prolonged partial airway obstruction can lead to:

   A. Decreased paO levels
   B. Increased paCO levels
   C. Respiratory arrest
   D. All of the above

D  Complete or prolonged airway obstruction may lead to hypoxemia, hypercapnia, and even apnea. (p. 918)

3. Which of the following individuals is least likely to develop an airway obstruction? A person who has:

   A. Been overmedicated with an analgesic
   B. Recently received spinal anesthesia
   C. Severe chronic obstructive pulmonary disease
   D. Suffered a cerebrovascular accident or "stroke"

B  Individuals likely to develop nonpatent airways include the elderly; neurologically impaired people; those who are overmedicated; and people who are weak or debilitated from chronic disease. (p. 919)

4. When inserting an oropharyngeal airway, which of the following measures would be contra-indicated?

   A. Initially hyperextending the person's neck
   B. Inserting the airway in a "normal" position
   C. Sliding the tip of the airway back over the person's tongue upside down
   D. Using a tongue blade to facilitate insertion

B  The tongue can inadvertently be pushed backward causing further airway obstruction if the airway is inserted in a "normal" position. (p. 919)

5. The physician may decide to insert an endotracheal tube in the person who:

   A. Has an immovable obstruction blocking the upper airway
   B. Has respiratory stridor
   C. Needs tracheal suctioning
   D. Requires long-term airway management

C  An endotracheal tube is sometimes inserted to allow tracheal suctioning. A tracheostomy tube would normally be inserted in situations such as those described in options A, B, and D. (p. 920)

6. Which of the following statements related to cuffed artificial airways is incorrect?

   A. Can increase the risk of infection if improperly used
   B. Causes less trauma to the tracheal mucosa than an uncuffed tube
   C. Prevents the escape of ventilated air into the upper airway
   D. Prevents oral secretions from passing into the lower airway

B  Options A, C, and D are all true statements. Long-term use of a cuffed artificial airway can promote pressure damage to the tracheal mucosa. (p. 922)

7. When performing airway suctioning techniques, all of the following are appropriate except:

   A. Placing an unconscious person in a semi-Fowler's position
   B. Suctioning only after complete insertion of the catheter
   C. Twisting the catheter while withdrawing it
   D. Using normal saline to flush the catheter after removal

A   An unconscious person should be placed in a lateral position for airway suctioning. (p. 923)

8. When using a portable suction unit for airway suctioning, the nurse knows that the safe range for vacuum pressure is:

   A. 80 to 100 mmHg
   B. 80 to 120 mmHg
   C. 80 to 140 mmHg
   D. Any of the above

B   The safe range for vacuum pressure in adult respiratory suctioning is 80 to 120 mmHg. (p. 924)

9. In performing routine tracheostomy care, the nurse should:

   A. Remove the outer cannula every eight hours for cleansing
   B. Secure the tracheostomy ties with a square knot
   C. Use cut gauze for tracheostomy dressings
   D. Use gloves during the entire procedure

B   Before providing tracheostomy care, the nurse should understand that: The outer cannula always remains in place to maintain the airway; cut gauze should never be used because filaments can work their way loose into the stoma; and sterile gloves are always used to decrease the risk of infection. (p. 931)

# 44

# CARING FOR PEOPLE WITH WOUNDS

1.0 Identify appropriate goals of nursing for people experiencing wounds.

    1.1 Identify nursing goals of care for individuals with wounds and other alterations in skin integrity. (p. 934)

2.0 Discuss the psychosocial impact of being wounded and plan appropriate care.

    2.1 Summarize typical psychosocial responses a person might have to injury. (p. 934)

    2.2 Identify factors that influence a person's psychosocial response to injury. (p. 934)

    2.3 Identify data that should be included in the nursing assessment of psychosocial responses to injury. (p. 934)

    2.4 Describe basic nursing intervention for psychosocial problems that may occur as a result of injury. (p. 935)

3.0 Describe a clear classification of the various types of wounds.

    3.1 Understand terminology used in the care of people with wounds. (p. 933)

    3.2 Discuss the meaning of "wound." (p. 933)

    3.3 Briefly describe various classifications used to describe a wound: Closed and open; intentional and accidental, incisions and lacerations, abrasions and contusions, penetrating, perforating, and puncture wounds; and clean, contaminated, and infected wounds. (p. 937)

    3.4 Describe the systems used to classify burns: Depth and rule of nines. (p. 938)

    3.5 Describe the procedure for calculating the percentage of body surface burns. (p. 939)

    3.6 Describe wound situations that warrant the use of surgical clips or staples. (p. 948)

    3.7 List specific wound uses for adhesive skin closures. (p. 949)

## TEACHING/LEARNING STRATEGIES

### Lecture/Discussion

Focus discussion on the general goals of wound care.

### Lecture/Discussion

Explore the psychosocial factors that influence a person's reaction to injury. Ask students to identify data useful in assessing a person's psychosocial response to injury.

### Written Exercise

Have students outline appropriate nursing intervention to deal with the fears and concerns of an injured person.

### Lecture/Discussion

Ask students to review the terminology listed on page 993 in the text.

Discuss the various ways in which wounds can be classified: Closed and open; intentional and accidental; incisions/lacerations; abrasions/contusions; penetrating/perforating/puncturing; and clean/contaminated/infected.

### Written Exercise

Ask students to use the rule of nines to calculate the total percentage of body surface burns for a hypothetical individual.

4.0  Describe in your own words the process of
     wound healing.

     4.1  Identify terms used to describe the
          wound healing process. (p. 938)

     4.2  List the three stages of the wound heal-
          ing process. (p. 938)

     4.3  Discuss the physiological changes that
          occur during the wound healing and
          inflammation phase of the healing
          process. (p. 940)

     4.4  Briefly explain the physiological
          changes occurring in the fibroplasia
          phase of the healing process. (p. 940)

     4.5  Discuss physiological changes that occur
          in the final stage of the healing pro-
          cess. (p. 940)

5.0  Identify factors influencing wound healing
     along with specific nursing intervention to
     support each factor.

     5.1  Identify and briefly discuss factors
          influencing the wound healing process.
          (p. 941)

     5.2  List four purposes for suturing wounds.
          (p. 947)

     5.3  Identify four techniques used to achieve
          wound closure. (p. 947)

     5.4  Identify factors that influence the
          selection of wound closure methods for a
          wound. (p. 947)

     5.5  Describe characteristics of various
          types of sutures: Natural, synthetic,
          absorbable, nonabsorbable, monofilament,
          and braided. (p. 947)

     5.6  Identify and briefly describe two types
          of adhesive skin devices used for wound
          closure. (p. 949)

     5.7  Discuss the major uses of wound drains.
          (p. 959)

     5.8  Identify two ways for assessing the
          amount of fluid lost from a wound
          drain. (p. 959)

     5.9  Identify major types of wound drains and
          their specific purposes. (p. 960)

     5.10 Discuss the important role nutrition
          plays in the wound healing process.
          (p. 960)

     5.11 Discuss the therapeutic and prophylactic
          uses of anti-microbial agents in wound
          care. (p. 961)

     5.12 Briefly describe the routes by which
          antimicrobial agents may be administered.
          (p. 961)

Lecture/Discussion

Ask students to briefly summarize the stages of
wound healing: Wound and inflammation phase,
fibroplasia phase, and scar maturation phase.

Lecture/Discussion

Discuss the general principles of wound healing
and ask students to give examples of nursing
measures that apply to each.

Facilitate a discussion on the various factors
that have an influence on the wound healing
process.

Compare and contrast the different methods used to
facilitate wound closure: Suturing, surgical
clips and staples, and adhesive skin closures.

Discuss the common types and purposes of wound
drains. Arrange for students to observe persons
in the clinical area with each type of drain:
Penrose, red rubber, T-tube, intracath/pediatric
feeding tube, and Gauze wick/NuGauze/iodoform
gauze.

5.13 Describe three groups of antimicrobial agents: Antibacterial agents, anti-fungal agents, and antiviral agents. (p. 961)

6.0 Assess wounds for signs of healthy healing or the presence of complications.

6.1 Discuss important factors to consider when caring for individuals with injuries caused by burns. (p. 938)

6.2 Identify data the nurse should include when assessing factors that influence a person's process of healing. (p. 941)

6.3 Briefly describe indices used to assess wound healing: Pain, wound drainage hemorrhage, inflammatory response, abscess formation, extension of infec-tion, necrosis, and wound dehiscence. (p. 942)

6.4 Identify indices used to assess wound drainage. (p. 942)

6.5 Identify techniques the nurse can use to accurately determine the amount of blood or drainage lost from a wound site. (p. 942)

6.6 Summarize baseline data that should be included in an initial assessment of a wound. (p. 943)

6.7 Summarize factors that should be in-cluded in an ongoing wound assessment. (p. 943)

6.8 Identify assessment data that should be gathered by the nurse when encountering an individual with an accidental wound. (p. 944)

6.9 Identify data required to assess a sutured wound. (p. 947)

7.0 Apply the nursing process to support healthy processes of wound healing.

7.1 Discuss supportive measures useful in aiding with the wound healing process. (p. 944)

7.2 Outline guidelines that should be utilized when providing first aid care of accidental wounds. (p. 944)

7.3 Understand basic scientific principles relevant to the care of people with wounds. (p. 945)

7.4 Identify factors that influence the technique of cleansing chosen for a wound. (p. 946)

7.5 Describe the procedure for cleansing wounds that have previously been sutured or closed with adhesive strips. (p. 946)

## Lecture/Discussion

Have students identify data that should be used to assess an individual's progress in wound healing.

Discuss the systematic approach the nurse should use to assess and manage persons who have sus-tained accidental wounds.

## Clinical Laboratory Experience

Arrange for students to view several different types of wounds in the clinical area. Ask them to assess the wounds for signs of healthy healing or the presence of complications.

## Lecture/Discussion

Ask students to identify data required to assess a person with sutures or surgical clips and staples.

Ask students to review the scientific principles and their related nursing interventions relevant to the care of wounds that is provided on page 945 in the text.

## Campus Laboratory Experience

Demonstrate the procedures for irrigating fresh accidental and surgical wounds. Allow students to practice the techniques in a simulated laboratory setting.

## Clinical Laboratory Experience

Upon demonstrating proficiency, allow students to perform cleansing and irrigating techniques on assigned persons in the clinical area.

7.6 List the steps that the nurse should take to cleanse a fresh accidental wound. (p. 946)

7.7 Discuss variations in the cleaning procedure that are necessary for other wounds, such as: surgical wounds and pressure sores. (p. 946)

7.8 Outline appropriate nursing measures for individuals who have a sutured wound. (p. 947)

7.9 Identify essential guidelines the nurse can utilize for infection control during wound care. (p. 961)

7.10 Discuss specific aspects of environmental control when caring for individuals with wounds. (p. 962)

Upon demonstrating proficiency, allow students to perform sterile wet and dry dressing changes on assigned persons in the clinical area with supervision.

8.0 Apply the nursing process to reduce undesirable responses to wound healing and complications.

8.1 Identify wounds that require advanced intervention measures. (p. 936)

8.2 Outline clinical signs of infection: Local and generalized. (p. 942)

8.3 Discuss the significance of increased pain at a wound site. (p. 942)

8.4 Discuss the impact abscess formation can have on the wound healing process. (p. 942)

8.5 Briefly discuss data indicative of an extension of an infectious process. (p. 942)

### Written Exercise

Ask students to outline a plan of care for the individual requiring wound management.

9.0 Initiate emergency care for wound dehiscence or evisceration.

9.1 Identify factors that promote the occurrence of: Necrosis and wound dehiscence. (p. 943)

9.2 Describe the steps that take place in the wound dehiscence process. (p. 943)

9.3 Outline basic nursing intervention for care of an individual with a wound dehiscence. (p. 943)

### Lecture/Discussion

Ask students to identify the clinical signs of wound dehiscence and eviceration. Focus discussion on the emergency care of each.

10.0 Carry out appropriate skills that aid wound healing.

10.1 Describe the steps that should be taken for suture removal. (p. 948)

10.2 Identify key points the nurse should keep in mind when applying adhesive strips. (p. 949)

10.3 Describe purposes for the application of a wound dressing. (p. 949)

### Guest Speaker

Invite the infection control nurse in each clinical facility to a post-conference period to discuss the individual's role in the care of individuals with wounds.

10.4 Briefly describe three wound dressing categories: Dry sterile, wet sterile, and clean. (p. 950)

10.5 Identify the purpose for dry sterile dressing changes. (p. 450)

10.6 Discuss contraindications and precautions the nurse should be aware of when applying dry sterile dressings (p. 950)

10.7 List equipment needed to apply a dry sterile dressing. (p. 950)

10.8 Describe preliminary activities that should be completed by the nurse prior to applying a dry sterile dressing. (p. 950)

10.9 Describe the steps that should be taken by the nurse in order to apply a dry sterile dressing. (p. 951)

10.10 Describe basic nursing responsibilities upon completion of a dry sterile dressing change. (p. 952)

10.11 Describe the proper technique for cleansing a linear and a circular wound. (p. 952)

10.12 Describe the purpose of wet sterile dressing changes. (p. 952)

10.13 List precautions the nurse should take into consideration when applying wet sterile dressings. (p. 952)

10.14 Describe the preliminary activities that must be performed by the nurse when planning to apply a wet sterile dressing. (p. 953)

10.15 Outline the steps that should be followed for a wet sterile dressing change. (p. 953)

10.16 Identify differences in the application of sterile and clean dressings. (p. 953)

10.17 Describe the three component layers of a dressing: Contact layer, intermediate layer, and the outer layer. (p. 954)

10.18 Discuss the specific uses and indications for different dressing types: Silk, fine mesh gauze, coarse mesh gauze, fluffs, abdominal pads, and burn dressings. (p. 954)

10.19 Discuss specific uses of hydrophobic or hydrophilic dressings: Petroleum gauze, adaptic, scarlet red ointment, furacin, xeroform, film wound dressings, and chemical sealants. (p. 954)

## Campus Laboratory Experience

Demonstrate the procedure for applying adhesive skin closures. Allow students to practice the technique on assigned individuals in the clinical area under supervision.

Provide a demonstration of the procedures for applying wet and dry sterile dressings. Allow students to practice the techniques in a simulated laboratory experience.

Discuss the general principles of bandage application. Afterwards, demonstrate the procedure for applying roller bandages. Allow students to practice the techniques on another classmate.

## Clinical Laboratory Experience

Upon demonstration of proficiency, allow students to apply bandages to assigned persons in the clinical area with supervision.

10.20 Identify common wound situations that require the application of wound packing. (p. 955)

10.21 Identify risks involved with the use of wound packing materials. (p. 955)

10.22 Identify two types of devices that are used to secure dressings. (p. 955)

10.23 Outline the major features of different types of adhesive tape: Heavy, cotton-backed adhesive tape; paper, plastic, and acetate taffeta, and foam adhesive. (p. 955)

10.24 Identify the key points the nurse should remember when applying or removing adhesive tape. (p. 955)

10.25 Briefly describe adverse reactions that may be caused by adhesive tape. (p. 955)

10.26 Identify situations that warrant the use of montgomery straps. (p. 956)

10.27 Describe the procedure for securing a dressing with montgomery straps. (p. 956)

10.28 Discuss the difference in a dressing and a bandage. (p. 956)

10.29 Describe the major purpose of bandage application. (p. 956)

10.30 List materials commonly used for bandages. (p. 956)

10.31 Describe the application of a bandage. (p. 956)

10.32 Describe a roller bandage. (p. 957)

10.33 Outline the steps involved in the procedure for application of a roller bandage. (p. 957)

10.34 Discuss different types of turns used to apply roller bandages: Circular, spiral, spiral reverse, figure-of-eight, spica, and recurrent. (p. 957)

10.35 Describe two major types of roller bandages: Cotton gauze and elasticized or rubberized. (p. 958)

10.36 Describe the value of using tubular bandages: Elasticized net and stockinettes/tube-gauze. (p. 958)

10.37 Briefly describe the purpose for applying a Jones dressing. (p. 959)

10.38 Identify the teaching and learning needs of a person who has had a Jones dressing applied. (p. 959)

10.39 Describe the various features of different wound drainage/suction systems: Hemovac suction, TLS surgical drainage system, TLS bulb drainage system, Vac-U-Care system, and Vac-U-Care bulb. (p. 960)

10.40 Identify instances in which it would be necessary to use an electrical pump (Gumco) for wound suction/drainage. (p. 960)

10.41 Describe methods that may be used to immobilize a wound. (p. 962)

10.42 Describe the functions of therapeutic heat and cold in the wound healing process. (p. 962)

10.43 Identify measures the nurse can utilize to control wound odor. (p. 962)

11.0 Develop and implement a learning/teaching plan for a wounded individual and significant others.

11.1 Identify educational needs of a person who has a sutured wound. (p. 948)

11.2 Outline the educational needs of a person who is having a dry sterile dressing applied. (p. 950)

12.0 Evaluate the nursing process as it is applied to the care of wounded people.

12.1 Discuss behavioral outcomes that may be used to evaluate the care of an individual with a wound. (p. 963)

13.0 Document wound assessment and management.

13.1 List information that should be included in the clinical record of a person with a sutured wound. (p. 948)

13.2 List data that should be documented in the clinical record of a person after the application of a wet sterile dressing. (p. 952)

### Lecture/Discussion

Ask students to identify the educational needs of a wounded individual and their significant others.

### Lecture/Discussion

Ask students to identify the criteria used to evaluate the wound healing process.

### Clinical Laboratory Experience

After viewing a wound in the clinical area, assist students in writing a sample nursing record describing the wound.

---

## MULTIPLE CHOICE QUESTIONS

1. The nurse is aware that the vasovagal response occurs as a result of all of the following except:

   A. Decreased blood flow to brain
   B. Failure of the vasomotor system
   C. Intense emotional experiences
   D. Vagal stimulation of the heart

## CORRECT ANSWER AND RATIONALE

B  The vasovagal response or "emotional" fainting is a "pathophysiologic" response due to large amounts of psychologic input, not intense vasomotor failure. Intense vagal heart stimulation causes a decrease in blood pressure, which is followed by a severe decline in heart rate. This reduced heart rate elicits unconsciousness by decreasing blood flow to the brain. (p. 934)

2. When attempting to get out of bed alone, Mr. Gilbert falls and receives a sharp blow to the back of his head. Your nursing assessment reveals no break in skin, a large ecchymotic area, and a developing hematoma. This type of injury is correctly labeled as a:

A. Accidental wound
B. Closed wound
C. Contusion
D. All of the above

D Any of the listed options can be used to describe the wound received by Mr. Gilbert. (p. 935)

SITUATION: Nineteen-year-old John is involved in an automobile accident, which resulted in a fire. He is admitted to the emergency room with burns covering both the legs and arms, and the entire front side of the body. There is no injury to the head, back, or genital regions. Questions 3 and 4 relate to this situation.

3. Using the rule of nines, calculate the percentage of total body surface that has been burned.

A. 45%
B. 54%
C. 72%
D. 80%

C The total body surface burned can be calculated according to the rule of nines as follows: Arms-18%, legs-36%, and the front side of the body-18%, for a total of 72%. (p. 939)

4. The burns on John's lower extremities appear white in color. The skin surface is elevated, soft, and pliable. The depth of these burns can be classified as:

A. Second degree burns
B. Deep partial thickness burns
C. Full thickness burns
D. Partial thickness burns

B The burns described are an example of a deep partial thickness burn. For a complete listing of assessment data used to clinically diagnose the depth of a burn injury, see page 939 in the text. (p. 939)

5. A wound that has been sutured closed usually heals by:

A. Delayed closure
B. Primary union
C. Secondary union
D. Third intention

B A wound that heals without infection or separation of the wound edges, heals by first intention or primary union. A good example is a wound whose edges have been approximated or closed via the use of sutures. (p. 938)

6. Arrange the steps of the wound healing process in order:

A. Inflammation, fibroplasia, remodeling
B. Inflammation, remodeling, fibroplasia
C. Inflammation, remodeling, proliferation
D. Proliferation, inflammation, remodeling

A The wound healing process occurs in the following order: Wounding and inflammation, fibroplasia (proliferation) phase, and the scar maturation (remodeling) phase. (p. 940)

7. Which of the following factors would be least likely to interfere with the wound healing process?

A. Cortisone therapy
B. Hematoma formation
C. Liver disease
D. Presence of granulation tissue

D Granulation tissue forms as a result of the normal healing process. (p. 941)

8.  When examining a person with a local wound
    infection, the nurse would expect to find:

    A.  Anesthesia, redness, loss of functioning
    B.  General malaise, increase in TPR, and pain
    C.  Pallor, warmth, edema
    D.  Redness, heat, changes in vital signs

D   Signs of local infection may include any of
    the following: Redness, pain, heat, swelling,
    decreased or loss of functioning, and changes
    in vital signs.  General malaise is a sign of
    a general body infection.  (p. 942)

9.  During an intense coughing episode, Mr.
    Fuller's surgical abdominal wound eviscerates.
    The nurse's initial reaction should be to:

    A.  Attempt to replace the affected tissues
    B.  Cover the area with a large sterile
        dressing
    C.  Notify the physician
    D.  Promote a calm, supportive environment

D   Because of the frightening nature of this
    situation, the nurse should initially attempt
    to maintain a calm, supportive environment.
    The area should then be redressed with a
    sterile dressing and the physician notified.
    (p. 943)

10. Which of the following actions would be
    appropriate when cleansing a fresh,
    accidental wound?

    A.  Cleaning the area around the wound with
        an antiseptic solution
    B.  Irrigating the wound with hydrogen
        peroxide
    C.  Using a hypodermic syringe and needle to
        irrigate the wound
    D.  Using 50 cc's of solution to irrigate a
        wound one inch long and one inch deep

A   The nurse can clean the area around a wound
    with an antibacterial soap solution, allowing
    no solution to enter the fresh wound.  Options
    B, C, and D are all incorrect.  (p. 946)

11. In cleansing a linear wound, where should the
    nurse's first cleansing stroke be?

    A.  Down the center of the wound
    B.  On the distal side of the wound
    C.  On the proximal side of the wound
    D.  Sequence doesn't matter

A   The nurse's first cleansing stroke should be
    down the center of the wound.  This prevents
    contamination of the wound from microorganisms
    on the skin surface adjacent to the wound.
    (p. 952)

12. The nurse should use a figure-of-eight turn
    when applying a roller bandage to:

    A.  An amputation site
    B.  Circumferential areas that increase in
        size
    C.  Cylindrical body parts
    D.  Immobilize joints

D   A figure-of-eight turn is used when applying a
    roller bandage to immobilize a joint.  (p. 957)

13. Which of the following is the most accurate
    method for documenting the amount of fluid
    lost via a wound drain:

    A.  Describing the amount of drainage present
        on the dressing
    B.  Recording the number and size of dress-
        ings changed
    C.  Recording the weight difference between
        the new and old dressing
    D.  Any of the above

D   Option C is the most effective way the nurse
    can communicate the amount of fluid produced
    from a wound drain.  To be accurate, options A
    and B would have to be used together.  (p. 959)

# CARING FOR PEOPLE REQUIRING HEAT
# AND COLD APPLICATIONS

## OBJECTIVES

1.0 Describe the anatomic and physiologic bases for the application of heat and cold.

   1.1 Understand the meaning of terminology used in the care of people who require the application of heat, and cold. (p. 966)

   1.2 Summarize the basic structure and function of body receptors for heat and cold. (p. 967)

   1.3 Identify factors that influence the sensation of heat and cold by the body. (p. 967)

   1.4 Briefly describe, using an example, the process of thermal receptor adaptation. (p. 967)

   1.5 Explain the physiological changes that result from neural transmission of thermal signals. (p. 967)

   1.6 Describe the process by which cutaneous circulation aids in the body in maintaining homeostatis. (p. 967)

   1.7 Explain the phenomenon of consensual response as it applies to the application of heat and cold. (p. 968)

   1.8 Summarize the physiological effects of heat and cold application. (p. 968)

   1.9 Identify the effects of heat and cold application on: Cellular metabolism, circulatory response, inflammatory response, connective tissue, synovial fluid, nerve conduction, muscle, and pain. (pp. 968-969)

2.0 Compare and contrast the therapeutic uses of heat and cold.

   2.1 Identify situations in which the application of heat would be therapeutic. (p. 969)

   2.2 Identify situations in which the application of cold would be therapeutic. (p. 969)

## TEACHING/LECTURE STRATEGIES

### Lecture/Discussion

Review the role of the hypothalamus in body thermoregulation.

Discuss the mechanism of thermal receptor adaptation.

Ask students to describe the process that occurs in neural transmission of thermal signals.

Discuss the role of skin circulation in the thermoregulatory process.

### Lecture/Discussion

Ask students to compare and contrast the physiological effects of heat and cold.

Assist students in understanding the physiologic bases and therapeutic indications for the application of heat and cold.

Describe the therapeutic ranges of temperature for the application of heat and cold.

2.3 Summarize the physiologic bases for applying heat to the person who is experiencing: Pain, inflammation, muscle spasm, contractures, or stiffness. (p. 970)

2.4 Describe the therapeutic action of heat in the following conditions: Pain, inflammation, muscle spasm, contractures, and stiffness. (p. 970)

2.5 Identify the physiologic basis for the therapeutic application of cold for a person experiencing: Traumatic injury, pain, inflammation, muscle spasm, contractures, and muscle spasticity. (p. 970)

2.6 Describe therapeutic temperature ranges for heat treatments. (p. 971)

2.7 Identify common terms used to describe temperature. (p. 970)

2.8 Identify the usual temperature range for terminology used to describe temperature: Very hot, hot, warm, tepid, cool, cold, and very cold. (p. 971)

3.0 Name variables affecting heat and cold therapies.

3.1 Identify criteria essential for assessing a person who is receiving heat or cold applications. (p. 979)

3.2 Summarize important guidelines the nurse should be aware of when caring for individuals receiving heat or cold applications. (p. 980)

4.0 List contraindications of heat and cold therapies.

5.0 Describe complications that may result from improper applications of heat and cold.

5.1 Briefly discuss the adverse effects that may occur as a result of heat application. (p. 970)

6.0 Describe the important precautions to observe during application of heat and cold.

6.1 Identify precaution and contraindications the nurse should take into consideration before applying heat. (p. 971)

6.2 Summarize the precautions and contraindications associated with applications of cold. (p. 972)

## Written Exercise

Ask students to list situations in which heat/cold applications would be appropriate.

## Clinical Laboratory Experience

Assist students in identifying individuals in the clinical area for which heat and cold applications would be contraindicated.

## Lecture/Discussion

Focus discussion on the precautions and contraindications the nurse should be aware of when applying heat or cold.

6.3 List essential components that must be included in a physician's order for heat or cold applications. (p. 979)

7.0 Describe commonly used heat and cold modalities.

7.1 Briefly describe methods of heat application: Superficial or deep, mild or vigorous, and dry or moist. (p. 972)

7.2 Describe the administration of dry heat via the following methods: Hot water bottles, disposable chemical packs, electric heating pads, Aqua K pads, heat cradles, incandescent lamps, paraffin wax, hydrocollator packs, irritants and counterirritants, and diathermy. (p. 973)

7.3 Summarize indirect and direct methods of cold application (p. 977)

7.4 Identify major factors influencing the application of cold. (p. 977)

8.0 Apply the nursing process to application of heat and cold.

8.1 Outline appropriate nursing measures for the application of heat via a hot water bottle. (p. 973)

8.2 Identify the responsibilities of a nurse who is using an electric heating pad to apply heat. (p. 973)

8.3 Discuss the nurse's responsibility with regard to the use of Aqua K pads. (p. 973)

8.4 List nursing actions that should be carried out when caring for persons with heat cradles. (p. 975)

8.5 Articulate the nurse's responsibility with regard to the use of infrared or gooseneck lamps. (p. 975)

8.6 Identify guidelines for the application of heat with chemical counterirritants. (p. 975)

8.7 List and discuss important factors in caring for persons receiving diathermy therapy. (p. 976)

8.8 Identify the methods for administering moist heat. (p. 976)

8.9 Identify basic steps involved in the application of hot compresses. (p. 976)

8.10 Briefly describe methods used to apply paraffin wax. (p. 976)

## Lecture/Discussion

Discuss the modes for therapeutic application of moist heat; Compresses, paraffin wax, tub bath/soaks, sitz bath, and contrast bath.

Discuss the modes for therapeutic application of dry heat: Hot water bottle, chemical pack, electric heating pad, Aqua K pad, Baker heat cradle, Gooseneck lamps, hydrocollator packs, and irritants/counterirritants.

## Clinical Laboratory Experience

Arrange for students to view equipment used to apply therapeutic heat and cold applications.

## Written Exercise

Ask students to summarize in writing the information that should be included in the nursing assessment of a person requiring heat and cold applications.

Have students formulate criteria to be used to evaluate a person's response to heat and cold applications.

## Clinical Laboratory Experience

Allow students to participate in the care of an individual who is receiving heat or cold applications.

8.11 Identify essential aspects of care for the person receiving a therapeutic bath. (p. 976)

8.12 Identify specific concepts and principles related to the sitz bath. (p. 976)

8.13 Describe the steps taken to administer a contrast bath. (p. 977)

8.14 Outline appropriate nursing measures for the application of cold packs and cold compresses. (p. 978)

8.15 Identify essential responsibilities of the nurse when caring for individuals with hypothermia blankets. (p. 978)

8.16 Identify ways in which the nurse can apply a tepid sponge. (p. 979)

8.17 Identify the special needs of a person who is receiving a tepid sponge bath. (p. 979)

8.18 Summarize the responsibilities of the nurse in the application of cold via the ice application, ice immersion, and evaporation methods. (p. 979)

8.19 Discuss criteria used to evaluate the care of individuals receiving heat or cold applications. (p. 981)

9.0 Respond to a person's psychosocial needs concerning the application of heat and cold.

9.1 Identify the steps the nurse should follow to apply heat with a disposable chemical pack. (p. 973)

10.0 Provide appropriate learning/teaching opportunities for people and their significant others regarding applications of heat and cold.

10.1 Identify educational needs of the person who is to receive a cold/heat application. (pp. 973-977)

**Lecture/Discussion**

Ask students to identify the educational needs of an individual receiving a heat or cold application.

---

| MULTIPLE CHOICE QUESTIONS | CORRECT ANSWER AND RATIONALE |
|---|---|
| 1. Which of the following statements is **incorrect**? <br><br> A. Cold sensations are more easily identified than heat sensations <br> B. The body has more warm receptors than cold receptors <br> C. The sensations produced by heat and cold are very similar <br> D. Thermosensitive pain responses are elicited only in response to extreme heat or cold | B   Options A, C, and D are all correct. The body generally has more cold receptors than warm receptors. (p. 967) |

2. The nurse should understand that the physiologic effects of heat include all of the
   following <u>except</u>:

   A. Decreased distention of connective tissue
   B. Increased need for oxygen
   C. Increased nerve conduction velocity
   D. Increased pain threshold

A  The application of local heat increases the
   distention of connective tissue. All other
   responses are correct. For a complete summary
   of the physiological responses to heat see
   page 968 in the text. (p. 968)

3. Direct heat application would be contraindicated in all of the following situations
   <u>except</u>:

   A. For a person with appendicitis
   B. For a recently sprained joint
   C. In a person with a suspected malignancy
   D. In a person with an edematous extremity

D  Direct heat application would be contraindicated in the individuals listed in options A,
   B, and C. It could produce increased pain and
   inflammation in the person with appendicitis;
   increased pain and swelling in the recently
   sprained joint; and increased malignant cell
   growth in the person with a neoplasm. (p. 969)

4. Which of the following <u>is not</u> an effect of
   local cold application?

   A. Anesthetization of body parts
   B. Decreased bleeding
   C. Reduction of inflammation
   D. Decreased fluid accumulation

D  The local application of cold at the site of
   accumulated fluid would cause vasoconstriction, thereby having no reducing effect. It
   can be used to initially prevent the accumulation of fluid in injured body tissues.
   (p. 970)

5. Mrs. Irwin has been admitted to the hospital
   with thrombophlebitis of the left lower
   extremity. If the physician requests application of moist heat to this extremity, which
   of the following equipment could be used?

   A. Aqua K pad
   B. Electric heating pad
   C. Hydrocollator pack
   D. Hot water bottle

A  The equipment listed in options B, C, and D
   produce dry heat. The Aqua K pad can deliver
   both dry and moist heat. (p. 973)

6. In preparing an Aqua K pad for use, the nurse
   demonstrates correct technique by performing
   all of the following <u>except</u>:

   A. Placing the unit at a level slightly
      below the body part being treated
   B. Setting the temperature at 105 degrees F
   C. Removing air bubbles from the unit
   D. Taking measures to avoid kinking or
      tangling of the tubing

A  The Aqua K unit will function better when
   placed at a level equal to, or slightly above,
   the body part being treated. This prevents
   the motor from having to push water against
   gravity. (p. 973)

7. A person is to receive a sitz bath to promote
   circulation to the perineal area. The nurse
   is aware that a sitz bath is generally
   administered for:

   A. 15 to 20 minutes
   B. 20 to 25 minutes
   C. 30 to 45 minutes
   D. One hour

B  Sitz baths are generally prescribed for 20 to
   25 minutes. (p. 977)

8. Which of the following individuals is <u>most</u>
   likely to sustain a burn injury when
   receiving heat therapy? The person who:

   A. Has a large gooseneck lamp positioned 18
      inches away from the body
   B. Receives moist heat to an extremity
   C. Receives no instruction prior to the
      application of an electric heating pad
   D. Uses a hot water bottle for 20 to 30
      minutes

A  The individual in option A is at greatest risk
   because the large gooseneck lamp should be
   positioned approximately 24 to 30 inches away
   from the body to prevent burns. The individual
   in option C would also be a risk if they chose
   to self-regulate the electric heating pad.
   (p. 973)

# 46
# CARING FOR PEOPLE WITH URINARY CATHETERS

OBJECTIVES

1.0 List the purposes of urinary catheterization.

    1.1 Review terminology used in the care of individuals with urinary catheters. (p. 982)

    1.2 Review the normal structure and function of the urinary system. (p. 983)

    1.3 Identify common reasons for urinary catheterization. (p. 984)

    1.4 Enumerate the various factors that must be considered in the assessment of a person's need for urinary catheterization. (p. 984)

2.0 Describe the variety of catheters available and state uses for each.

    2.1 Define catheter and catheterization. (p. 985)

    2.2 Identify different types of urinary catheters according to configuration, material, size, and purpose. (pp. 985-987)

    2.3 List three routes that may be used for urinary catheterization. (p. 987)

    2.4 Briefly describe the three routes of urinary catheterization: Ureteral, suprapubic, and urethral. (p. 987)

3.0 Describe the following interventions: male and female catheterization, irrigation of a urinary catheter, obtaining a specimen from a catheter, and removal of a urethral catheter.

    3.1 Discuss the importance of maintaining sterility when inserting urinary catheters. (p. 987)

    3.2 Briefly discuss contraindications and precautions the nurse should be aware of when inserting urethral urinary catheters. (p. 988)

    3.3 Identify essential data the nurse should obtain before performing urethral urinary catheterization. (p. 988)

    3.4 List nursing actions that should be carried out in preparation for urethral catheterization. (p. 988)

TEACHING/LEARNING STRATEGIES

Lecture/Discussion

Ask students to review the normal structure and function of the urinary system.

Provide clinical examples of individuals requiring urinary catheterization.

Lecture/Discussion

Assist students in understanding the situations in which different types of catheters would be appropriate.

Campus Laboratory Experience

Obtain examples of the various types of catheters that are available. Place in the campus laboratory for student viewing.

Lecture/Discussion

Ask students to compare and contrast the techniques used for male and female urinary catheterization.

Compare and contrast the various techniques used in irrigation of the bladder: internal and external procedures.

Campus Laboratory Experience

Demonstrate the procedure for male and female urinary catheterization. Have students practice each technique on a mannequin in the campus laboratory facility.

3.5 List the equipment needed to perform a urethral catheterization. (p. 988)

3.6 Describe the draping procedures for males and females receiving urethral catheters. (p. 989)

3.7 Identify basic steps in the procedure for urethral catheterization. (p. 980)

3.8 Describe nursing responsibilities upon the completion of the procedure for urethral catheterization. (p. 993)

3.9 Describe an alternate position that may be used when performing female urethral catheterizations. (p. 993)

3.10 Identify measures the physician can perform to remove a catheter with an uninflated balloon. (p. 995)

3.11 Outline nursing responsibilities following catheter removal. (p. 995)

3.12 Describe basic nursing intervention useful in assisting a person with bladder training. (p. 995)

3.13 Identify equipment the nurse should gather to remove an indwelling catheter. (p. 995)

3.14 List the sequence of steps for removal of indwelling urinary catheters. (p. 995)

3.15 Identify criteria used to determine the need for catheter removal. (p. 995)

3.16 List criteria that can be used to determine the need for irrigation of a urinary catheter. (p. 997)

3.17 Briefly describe methods used to irrigate urinary catheters. (p. 997)

3.18 Describe reasons for clamping a urinary catheter. (p. 998)

3.19 Describe the correct method for taping a urinary catheter in the male and female person. (p. 999)

3.20 Discuss the procedure for collecting sterile urine specimens in catheterized individuals. (p. 1001)

4.0 Discuss the techniques and advantages of intermittent self-catheterization.

4.1 Identify factors that influence the success of intermittent catheterization. (p. 994)

4.2 Identify the reasons for intermittent urinary catheterization. (p. 994)

Demonstrate the procedure for removing a foley catheter. Allow time for students to practice this procedure.

Demonstrate the procedures for internal and external urinary catheter irrigation. Ask students to practice each technique in a simulated campus laboratory experience.

## Clinical Laboratory Experience

Upon demonstration of proficiency, allow students to perform male and female urinary catheterizations on persons in the clinical area with supervision.

Assist students in the selection of appropriate equipment when preparing to perform a urinary catheterization.

Assist students in performing internal and external urinary catheter irrigations for assigned persons in the clinical facility.

## Lecture/Discussion

Have students compare and contrast the techniques used for normal urinary catheterization with those used for intermittent self-catheterization.

Enumerate the advantages and disadvantages of intermittent urinary catheterization. (p. 994)

5.0 Discuss the physical and psychologic hazards of catheterization, and how they can be prevented.

    5.1 Identify specific complications associated with the use of urinary catheters. (p. 984)

    5.2 Identify the educational needs of individuals undergoing urethral urinary catheterization. (p. 988)

    5.3 Discuss the etiology of autonomic dysreflexia or hyperreflexia. (p. 996)

    5.4 Identify clinical indications of autonomic dysreflexia or hyperreflexia. (p. 996)

    5.5 Describe the treatment for autonomic dysreflexia and hyperreflexia. (p. 996)

    5.6 Describe actions the nurse might take to relieve bladder spasms in a catheterized individual. (p. 999)

    5.7 Identify factors that increase the bladder's resistance to infection. (p. 999)

    5.8 Identify the most common organisms infecting the bladder. (p. 999)

    5.9 Identify common sources of contamination for the person with a urinary catheter. (p. 999)

    5.10 Identify the physiological manifestations of a urinary tract infection. (p. 999)

    5.11 Identify factors that influence loss of tissue integrity in catheterized individuals. (p. 1001)

    5.12 Outline guidelines for maintaining psychologic comfort in a person with a urinary catheter. (p. 1002)

6.0 Discuss nursing intervention for a person with an indwelling catheter.

    6.1 Identify information that should be documented in the clinical record of a person who has undergone a urethral catheterization. (p. 993)

    6.2 Summarize nursing intervention for people with indwelling urethral catheters. (p. 996)

    6.3 Identify clinical signs indicating an obstructed urinary catheter. (p. 996)

    6.4 Outline guidelines for the prevention of urinary catheter obstruction. (p. 996)

    6.5 Outline teaching/learning guidelines to facilitate comfort and safety in a person with a urinary catheter. (p. 998)

## Lecture/Discussion

Emphasize the hazards and benefits of urinary catheterization.

Have students list the common ways in which contamination occurs during urinary catheterization.

Ask students to state some of the usual concerns a person might have regarding urinary catheterization. Ask them to address these concerns when performing urinary catheterization on people in the clinical area.

## Group Activity

Divide students into small groups. Ask each group to formulate a plan of care to assist catheterized persons with the maintenance of one of the following: Catheter patency, comfort and safety, bladder sterility/prevention of infection, tissue integrity, and psychologic comfort. Ask each group to present their plan in class.

## Written Exercise

Ask students to list the information that should be recorded in the clinical record after performing a urinary catheterization. Ask them to write a sample recording that includes all the information they listed.

Ask students to outline the educational needs of a person who is going home with a urinary catheter.

## Clinical Laboratory Experience

Assist students in formulating an appropriate plan of care for catheterized persons they are caring for in the clinical facility.

6.6 Identify intervention strategies useful
in the prevention of urinary tract
infections in catheterized individuals.
(p. 999)

6.7 Discuss nursing intervention methods
used to prevent altered tissue integrity
in a catheterized person. (p. 1002)

7.0 Discuss the physical, psychosocial, sexual,
and learning needs of people going home with
an indwelling catheter.

7.1 Identify the basic steps a person should
be taught when planning to insert a
urinary catheter by the clean technique
method. (p. 994)

7.2 Describe the basic educational needs of
individuals going home with a urinary
catheter. (p. 1002)

8.0 Describe nursing intervention to help people
who suffer embarrassment and loss of independence because of their need for catheterization.

---

| MULTIPLE CHOICE QUESTIONS | CORRECT ANSWER AND RATIONALE |
|---|---|

**MULTIPLE CHOICE QUESTIONS**

1. The nurse knows that urinary catheterization
should be performed for all of the following
reasons except:

    A. Facilitate bladder decompression prior to
    surgery
    B. Obtain a sterile urine specimen
    C. Prevent skin breakdown in the incontinent
    individual
    D. Relieve lower urinary tract obstructions

2. If asked to assess a person for residual
urine volume, which type of catheter should
the nurse use?

    A. Indwelling catheter
    B. Macelot catheter
    C. Retention catheter
    D. Straight catheter

3. Which statement related to urinary
catheterization is true?

    A. A catheter should be inserted 7 to 8
    inches in the male.
    B. A female person should always be cathe-
    terized in a dorsorecumbent position.
    C. If the catheter fails to enter the
    urinary meatus on the first attempt, the
    catheter should be removed and another
    attempt made.
    D. Urethral catheterization is always a
    sterile procedure.

**CORRECT ANSWER AND RATIONALE**

B    Because urinary catheterization is a
potentially hazardous procedure, it is
generally considered more acceptable to
obtain a sterile urine specimen via the
mid-stream or "clean-catch" method. (p. 984)

D    A straight, single lumen catheter is used to
check a person for residual urine. Other
types of catheters would be used if the
physician requested for the catheter to be
left in place for a certain residual volume.
(p. 986)

A    Option A is the only true statement. Other
options are incorrect for the following
reasons: Clean technique may be used for
intermittent self-catheterization; an alternative lateral position may be used for
female catheterization; and the nurse should
obtain a new, sterile catheter if the first
insertion attempt fails. (pp. 987; 991-993)

4. The nurse lubricates the catheter tip prior to insertion primarily to:

A. Decrease the person's discomfort during insertion
B. Facilitate insertion of the catheter through the meatus
C. Relax the external sphincter
D. All of the above

B   The catheter tip should be lubricated prior to insertion to reduce friction, thereby facilitating catheter insertion. (p. 990)

5. When performing routine catheter care according to hospital policy, the nurse would document all of the following except:

A. Cleansing agent used
B. Character of the urine
C. Condition of the urethral meatus
D. Time of the catheter care

A   It would not be necessary to document the cleansing agent used if following a stated hospital policy for catheter care. (p. 1000)

6. Which of the following nursing measures are appropriate when removing a urinary catheter?

A. Explaining to the person that the catheter is to be removed
B. Instructing the person to maintain a good fluid intake after removal
C. Monitoring the person's fluid intake and output for at least 24 hours
D. All of the above

D   All statements are correct. (p. 995)

7. In preparing for bladder irrigation, the nurse knows that all of the following are correct except:

A. A closed bladder irrigating system reduces the risk of urinary tract infection
B. If blood is present, the irrigation flow rate may be increased to keep the system patent
C. It is always necessary to disconnect the catheter from the tubing to irrigate a triple lumen tube
D. Room temperature sterile solutions are usually used for irrigation

C   A triple lumen system does not have to be broken when irrigating because it has a special lumen for that purpose. Open irrigation of a continuous irrigation set should only be performed when there is an obstruction. (p. 997)

8. Which of the following nursing measures would not be effective in reducing the risk of infection in a catheterized individual?

A. Cleansing the perineal area at least once daily
B. Emptying the collection bag at least three times a day
C. Encouraging fluid intake between 2000-2500 ml/day
D. Keeping the tubing and collection bag below the level of the bladder

B   Option B is incorrect because it does not indicate the time intervals between each emptying. The collection bag should be emptied at least every eight hours, and more frequently if urine output is high. Urine left sitting in the collection bag for long periods of time is an excellent medium for bacterial growth. (p. 1000)

# CARING FOR PEOPLE REQUIRING GASTROINTESTINAL TUBES

OBJECTIVES

1.0 Describe the anatomy and physiology of the gastrointestinal (GI) tract.

   1.1 Summarize the structure and function of the gastrointestinal tract. (p. 1006)

2.0 Discuss the reasons for GI intubation.

   2.1 Identify individuals requiring the insertion of gastrointestinal tubes. (p. 1006)

   2.2 Identify factors that influence the type of gastrointestinal tube inserted. (p. 1009)

   2.3 Describe the purpose for inserting a nasogastric or nasoenteric tube. (p. 1016)

3.0 Explain the principles and methods of applying GI suction.

   3.1 Discuss the purposes of gastrointestinal intubation: Decompression, compression, gavage, lavage, and gastric analysis. (p. 1009)

   3.2 Describe factors that affect the drainage and movement of fluids in gastrointestinal tubes: Pressure differences, viscosity, diameter of the tube, length of the tube, and suction. (p. 1014)

   3.3 Enumerate the various reasons suction is used in conjunction with gastrointestinal tubes. (p. 1015)

   3.4 Outline the nurse's responsibility with regard to suction equipment used in conjunction with gastrointestinal tubes. (p. 1015)

   3.5 Describe the essential steps to be followed when emptying drainage containers and recording output. (p. 1024)

4.0 Recognize and explain the uses of different types of gastric and intestinal tubes.

   4.1 Identify and briefly describe the various routes used for gastrointestinal intubation. (p. 1008)

TEACHING/LEARNING STRATEGIES

Lecture/Discussion

Ask students to review the terminology listed on page 1006 in the text.

Review the structure and function of the gastrointestinal tract.

Lecture/Discussion

Discuss the purposes for gastrointestinal intubation: Decompression, compression, gavage, lavage, and gastric analysis. Provide clinical examples of each.

Clinical Laboratory Experience

Assist students in identifying individuals in the clinical area who may need enteral nutrition.

Lecture/Discussion

Help students to understand the physics of tube drainage: Pressure difference, viscosity, diameter of the tube, length of the tube, and suction.

Clinical Laboratory Experience

Demonstrate the procedure for emptying gastrointestinal drainage containers. Review the forms used in each clinical facility for recording GI drainage.

Lecture/Discussion

Ask students to differentiate between the different routes of gastrointestinal tubes: Nasogastric, orogastric, intestinal, esophogastrostomy, gastrostomy, and jejunostomy.

4.2 Identify the basic features of gastric and intestinal tubes. (p. 1009)

4.3 Summarize significant facts and characteristics of gastric and GI tubes: Levin, salem sump, vivonex, Sengstaken-Blakemore, Minnesota, Ewald, Cantor, Miller-Abbott, Baker, pediatric feeding, gastrostomy feeding, and weighted feeding tubes. (p. 1010)

4.4 Describe two major differences between gastric and intestinal tubes. (p. 1013)

4.5 Briefly describe the value of specialized feeding tubes. (p. 1014)

5.0 Understand the methods and be prepared to practice the techniques of gastric and enteric intubation and irrigation.

5.1 Summarize the contraindications and precautions the nurse should be aware of when inserting a nasogastric or nasoenteric tube. (p. 1016)

5.2 Outline the preliminary responsibilities of the nurse inserting a nasogastric or nasoenteric tube. (p. 1017)

5.3 List equipment needed to insert a nasogastric or nasoenteric tube. (p. 1017)

5.4 Identify the steps necessary for insertion of a nasogastric or nasoenteric tube. (p. 1017)

5.5 Describe the technique for inserting an intubation tube with a stylet. (p. 1020)

5.6 Describe the steps that should be taken to insert an orogastric tube. (p. 1021)

5.7 Briefly discuss the definition and purpose for the irrigation of gastrointestinal tubes. (p. 1022)

5.8 Explain the precautions and contraindications that the nurse should keep in mind when irrigating a gastrointestinal tube. (p. 1022)

5.9 Outline the nursing preliminary responsibilities when preparing to irrigate a gastrointestinal tube. (p. 1022)

5.10 Identify the equipment the nurse should gather to perform the procedure for irrigation of a gastrointestinal tube. (p. 1022)

5.11 Using the nursing process, describe the steps that should be taken to irrigate a gastrointestinal tube. (p. 1022)

Describe the different types of tubes used for gastrointestinal intubation. Provide examples of each for student viewing.

## Campus Laboratory Experience

Arrange for students to view the various equipment used to provide gastrointestinal suction.

## Lecture/Discussion

Focus discussion on the role of the nurse in insertion of each type of gastrointestinal tube.

Ask students to compare and contrast the procedures for inserting a nasogastric and orogastric tube.

Discuss the nurse's role and responsibilities in the insertion of intestinal tubes for decompression purposes.

## Campus Laboratory Experience

Demonstrate the procedure for insertion of a nasogastric or nasoenteric tube. Have students practice the insertion procedures for each in the campus laboratory facility.

Provide a demonstration of the technique used to irrigate a gastrointestinal tube. Allow students to practice the technique in simulated campus laboratory experience.

## Clinical Laboratory Experience

Upon demonstration of proficiency, allow students to insert nasogastric and nasoenteric tubes for assigned individuals in the clinical area with supervision.

5.12 Identify data that should be documented in the clinical record of an individual after irrigation of a gastrointestinal tube. (p. 1024)

6.0 Administer medications via GI tubes.

6.1 Describe the nurse's responsibility with regard to the instillation of medication into gastrointestinal tubes. (p. 1026)

6.2 Identify the equipment needed to administer a medication via a gastrointestinal tube. (p. 1026)

6.3 List the sequence of steps that should be followed by the nurse to administer a medication via a gastrointestinal tube. (p. 1026)

7.0 Apply the nursing process in planning care for individuals requiring intubation.

7.1 Discuss nursing measures that can be utilized to psychologically prepare an individual for gastrointestinal intubation. (p. 1016)

7.2 Identify the assessment data that should be obtained by the nurse after inserting a nasogastric or nasoenteric tube. (p. 1020)

7.3 Briefly describe information that should be documented in the clinical record of an individual after the insertion of a nasogastric or nasoenteric tube. (p. 1020)

7.4 List nursing actions that should be carried out for an individual who has had an intestinal tube inserted for decompression purposes. (p. 1021)

7.5 Describe the nursing intervention strategies effective in meeting the physical and psychological needs of individuals with gastrointestinal tubes. (p. 1021)

7.6 Outline a general nursing plan of care for individuals with nasogastric/enteric tubes. (p. 1025)

8.0 Discuss the psychologic implications of gastric and intestinal intubation.

## Clinical Laboratory Experience

Demonstrate the procedure for administering medications via gastrointestinal tubes. Allow students to practice this technique in the clinical setting with close supervision.

## Lecture/Discussion

Ask students to review the material on page 1025 in the text related to common nursing diagnoses and nursing interventions for individuals with nasogastric/enteric tubes.

## Lecture/Discussion

Ask students to explore ways in which they can psychologically prepare an individual for the insertion of a gastrointestinal tube.

Ask students to describe ways of promoting independence and a positive self-concept in an individual who has a gastrointestinal tube.

9.0 Teach people and their significant others about GI tubes.

    9.1 Discuss the educational needs of an individual who is having a nasogastric or nasoenteric tube inserted. (p. 1016)

    9.2 Identify the educational needs of an individual requiring irrigation of a gastrointestinal tube. (p. 1022)

10.0 Apply the nursing process in planning care for individuals on enteral feeding programs.

    10.1 Briefly describe the meaning of enteral hyperalimentation or enteral nutrition. (p. 1027)

    10.2 Identify individuals who would benefit from enteral hyperalimentation or enteral nutrition. (p. 1027)

    10.3 Identify the routes and types of gastro-intestinal tubes that may be used to administer enteral hyperalimentation. (p. 1027)

    10.4 List the basic requirements that must be fulfilled in order for a tube feeding to provide adequate nourishment for an individual. (p. 1027)

    10.5 Identify special equipment that may be needed to administer enteral nutrition. (p. 1028)

    10.6 Identify specific nursing measures for care of individuals receiving enteral nutrition. (p. 1028)

11.0 Describe the different types of enteral feeding programs.

    11.1 Identify factors that influence the type of tube feeding that is chosen for an individual. (p. 1027)

    11.2 Describe the procedure for administering enteral nutrition by the continuous-drip and intermittent-drip methods. (p. 1027)

    11.3 Identify specific features of various commercially prepared enteral feeding formulas. (p. 1028)

    11.4 Discuss nursing intervention to facilitate the implementation of an enteral feeding program at home. (p. 1029)

    11.5 Discuss the teaching/learning needs of individuals who require enteral feedings at home. (p. 1032)

### Lecture/Discussion

Ask students to identify the educational needs of an individual and their significant others regarding GI tubes.

### Lecture/Discussion

Have students summarize the requirements that must be met if a tube feeding preparation is to adequately nourish an individual.

Focus discussion on appropriate nursing intervention measures for people receiving enteral nutrition.

### Clinical Laboratory Experience

Ask students to formulate a plan of care to meet the enteral nutrition needs for an assigned individual in the clinical area.

### Lecture/Discussion

Discuss the different types of commercially prepared enteral feeding formulas.

Compare and contrast the different methods for proving enteral feedings: Continuous-drip and intermittent-drip.

### Guest Speaker

Identify the individual in each clinical facility who is responsible for instituting home enteral feeding programs. Invite them to a post-conference period to discuss the different types of programs that are available.

12.0 Describe nursing interventions for problems associated with GI intubation.

    12.1 Identify conditions that predispose a gastrointestinal tube to becoming clogged. (p. 1022)

    12.2 Identify common problems and selected nursing diagnoses for people receiving enteral feedings. (p. 1030)

    12.3 Outline common interventions for the specific problems associated with individuals who are receiving enteral feedings. (p. 1031)

13.0 Assist with placement of balloon-tipped intestinal tubes.

## Lecture/Discussion

Discuss common problems associated with gastrointestinal tube use. Ask students to review appropriate nursing intervention for each problem as stated on pages 1030-1031 in the text.

## Clinical Laboratory Experience

Arrange for students to assist with the placement of balloon-tipped intestinal tubes. Afterwards, ask them to share their experience with other students.

---

## MULTIPLE CHOICE QUESTIONS

1. The nurse knows that an NG tube is most often ordered postoperatively to:

    A. Control bleeding within the GI system
    B. Increase peristaltic activity in the lower GI tract
    C. Provide fluid and nutrients
    D. Remove flatus and accumulated gases in the stomach

2. Which type of gastrointestinal tube can be used for both compression and decompression purposes?

    A. Levin
    B. Ewald
    C. Minnesota
    D. Baker

3. Nurses demonstrate the correct technique for inserting a nasogastric tube when they do all of the following except:

    A. Ask the person to flex their head for initial insertion of the tube
    B. Determine insertion depth by measuring from the tip of the nose to the xiphoid process
    C. Place the individual in a sitting position prior to insertion
    D. Stand on the right side of the bed, if right-handed

## CORRECT ANSWER AND RATIONALE

D    Decompression, or the removal of accumulated gas and fluids from the stomach, is commonly employed after surgery to help prevent vomiting and distention. (p. 1009)

C    The Sengstaken-Blakemore and Minnesota tubes are used for both compression and decompression in individuals with bleeding esophageal varices. (p. 1009)

B    The distance of tube insertion should be measured from the tip of the nose to the earlobe, plus the distance from the earlobe to the top of the xiphoid process. (p. 1017)

4. If excessive gasping, dyspnea, or cyanosis occurs while inserting a nasogastric tube, the nurse should:

   A. Ask the individual to inhale and exhale slowly through the mouth
   B. Immediately pull back on the tube
   C. Notify the physician
   D. Remove the tube and try insertion at a later time

B  The signs listed in this situation indicate respiratory distress. The nurse should immediately pull back on the tube; it may be in the trachea. (p. 1018)

5. Following the insertion of a Cantor tube through the nose and into the stomach, the nurse should:

   A. Ask the individual to slowly inhale and exhale
   B. Attach the tube to low intermittent suction
   C. Place the individual on their right side
   D. Tape the tube in place

C  The nurse should place the individual on their right side to facilitate passage of the tube through the pylorus into the small intestine. The tube should not be taped nor hooked to suction until it has reached the desired location. (p. 1021)

6. The nurse can promote a positive body image and independence in the individual with a gastrointestinal tube by:

   A. Encouraging frequent ambulation
   B. Encouraging verbalization of feelings about the tube
   C. Promoting self-care activities
   D. All of the above

D  All of the listed options would be useful in promoting a positive self-concept or body image. (pp. 1022, 1025)

7. Which of the following statements related to the administration of medications via a gastrointestinal tube is false?

   A. Allow the medication to flow through the tubing by gravity drainage
   B. Before instilling medication, check for tube placement
   C. Check the residual volume of feedings administered in the last hour
   D. Reconnect the individual to suction when the medication has completely cleared the tubing

D  The nurse should wait at least 15 minutes before reconnecting the tube to suction to allow the medication to be absorbed. (p. 1026)

# INTRODUCTION TO PRINCIPLES OF MEDICATION ADMINISTRATION

OBJECTIVES

1.0 Work accurately with metric, apothecaries and household measurement systems and be able to convert one to another.

    1.1 List and describe the three mathematical systems used to describe drug dosages. (p. 1044)

2.0 Define terms and abbreviations commonly used in prescribing and administering medications.

    2.1 Define common terms used when caring for the medication needs of an individual. (p. 1034)

    2.2 Define the meaning of the term "drug." (p. 1037)

    2.3 Identify and describe the three names by which a drug may be prescribed, administered, and sold. (p. 1037)

    2.4 Identify common abbreviations used for prescribing and administering medications. (p. 1043)

3.0 Identify and explain facts and principles that guide the nurse in the preparation and administration of medications, and apply them in the clinical setting.

4.0 Use dependable sources of information about medications.

5.0 Describe the roles and responsibilities of the nurse and other members of the health care team in medication administration.

    5.1 Discuss the role and responsibilities of the nurse in medication administration. (p. 1035)

TEACHING/LEARNING STRATEGIES

Class Activity

Ask students to perform drug calculations using the household, apothecary, and metric systems of measurement.

Lecture/Discussion

Review the terminology listed on page 1034 in the text.

Class Activity

Have students identify the generic, chemical, and proprietary names of ten medications.

Have students interpret the common abbreviations used for prescribing and administering medications.

Lecture/Discussion

Ask students to list the information a nurse should know before administering medications.

Written Exercise

Have students list the "five rights" for administering medications. Emphasize the importance of performing these checks each time a medication is administered.

Written Exercise

Have students demonstrate the use of a drug reference text by preparing medication reference cards on five medications. Ask them to use the form provided on page 1042 in the text as a guide.

Guest Speaker

Invite a pharmacist in each clinical facility to a post-conference period to discuss their role in medication administration.

5.2 Discuss the responsibilities that the physician must assume in relation to medication administration. (p. 1035)

5.3 Describe the pharmacist's role and responsibilities in medication administration. (p. 1035)

6.0 Discuss the rights and responsibilities of individuals receiving medications.

6.1 Outline the basic rights of an individual receiving medication. (p. 1036)

### Lecture/Discussion

Facilitate a discussion on the responsibilities and rights of individuals receiving medications.

### Communication Activity

Ask students to solicit information from individuals in the community regarding their perception of their rights and responsibilities when receiving medications. Allow time for students to share this information in class.

7.0 Discuss the historical, ethical, legal, and legislative aspects of medication administration.

7.1 Discuss historical factors that have influenced the current practice of medication administration. (p. 1036)

7.2 Briefly discuss the nurse's legal responsibilities and obligations associated with the preparation, administration, and evaluation of medications. (p. 1036)

7.3 Identify the legislative groups that regulate the control of drugs in the United States. (p. 1037)

7.4 Explore various ethical issues the nurse administering medications may encounter: Drug misuse, drug dependence, and the administration of experimental drugs. (p. 1037)

### Lecture/Discussion

Ask students to identify the legal aspects involved in medication administration.

### Values Clarification

Explore student feeling related to the ethical issues nurses must face when working with medications: Drug misuse, drug dependence, and the administration of experimental drugs.

8.0 List drug classifications and discuss the pharmacokinetics and effects of medications.

8.1 Describe the categories by which drugs are classified: Prescription and over-the-counter. (p. 1037)

8.2 List the criteria used to determine whether or not a medication should be available over-the-counter or by prescription only. (p. 1036)

8.3 Describe the states of drug metabolism: Absorption, distribution, biotransformation, and excretion. (p. 1038)

8.4 Explain the impact of pharmacokinetics on the action of a drug. (p. 1038)

### Lecture/Discussion

Encourage students to review the summary of general medication classifications and actions beginning on page 1039 in the text.

Facilitate a discussion on the desirable and undesirable effects of all medications.

Have students differentiate between the different effects medications can produce: Therapeutic, adverse, toxic, local, systemic, and synergistic.

8.5 Describe factors that influence the rate of a drug's absorption: Solubility, concentration, site of absorption, circulation, and the total surface area involved in the absorption. (p. 1038)

8.6 Explore factors that affect the distribution of a drug within the body. (p. 1038)

8.7 Understand the classifications and actions of general medications as outlined in Table 48-1 in the text. (p. 1040)

8.8 Identify the major body organ involved in the metabolism of a medication. (p. 1042)

8.9 Describe the mechanisms by which drugs are excreted from the body. (p. 1042)

8.10 Briefly discuss the therapeutic intent of medication administration. (p. 1042)

8.11 Differentiate between the adverse effects and toxic effects a drug may have on an individual. (p. 1042)

9.0 Describe the common systems of medication administration.

9.1 Describe the four major kinds of medication administration systems in current use: Stock supply system, individual cubicle system, unit dose system, and self-medication. (p. 1043)

10.0 List routes of medication administration.

10.1 Briefly describe the routes by which medications may be administered: Oral (sublingual and buccal); Topical (Optic, otic, nasal, vaginal, rectal, pulmonary); and Parenteral (Subcutaneous, intramuscular, intradermal, intravenous, intra-arterial, intracardiac, intraosseous, and intrathecal). (p. 1038)

11.0 Define the elements of a medication order and list the types of orders; discuss the importance of accurate medication computation; discuss the timing of medication administration; and describe safety measures pertinent to medication administration.

11.1 List the necessary elements that must be included in a medication order. (p. 1043)

11.2 Identify the nurse's responsibility in regard to written and verbal medication orders. (p. 1043)

Lecture/Discussion

Ask students to differentiate between the four major kinds of medication systems in use: Stock supply system, individual cubicle system, unit dose system, and self-medication system. Have them identify the technique that is being used in their clinical facility.

Lecture/Discussion

Discuss the different terms used to designate the frequency of medication administration: Single, standing, stat, and PRN. Give examples of each for student identification purposes.

Help students to understand the factors the nurse must consider when planning the times of medication administration.

Facilitate a discussion on the safety precautions pertinent to medication administration: Clear and verifiable communications, safeguarding medications, and safeguarding the individual.

11.3 Identify terminology used to designate the frequency of medication administration. (p. 1043)

11.4 Identify factors that affect the timing of medication administration. (p. 1047)

11.5 Outline guidelines the nurse should use to make decisions related to medication administration. (p. 1053)

## Written Exercise

Ask students to list the seven parts of a drug order.

12.0 Discuss the nursing process as it applies to medication administration.

12.1 Identify basic knowledge the nurse needs before giving any medication. (p. 1038)

12.2 Outline basic safety guidelines that should be followed when administering medications. (p. 1047)

## Clinical Laboratory Experience

Arrange for students to observe a nurse on their clinical unit as medications are administered.

13.0 Take an accurate and complete medication history.

13.1 List information that should be included in an individual's medication history. (p. 1049)

13.2 Identify the specific purpose and types of data that should be obtained when assessing the physiological factors affecting the pharmacokinetics of medications. (p. 1050)

## Clinical Laboratory Experience

Ask students to take a complete medication history on an assigned individual in the clinical facility.

14.0 Assess physical and psychosocial factors that affect choice of medication and route.

14.1 Identify and briefly describe the psychosocial factors that should be assessed when administering medications. (p. 1051)

14.2 Identify factors useful in assessing individuals with special medication administration needs. (p. 1052)

## Lecture/Discussion

Ask students to explain the concepts of absorption, distribution, biotransformation, and excretion.

Ask students to discuss how age, weight, sex, and the condition of the individual can influence physiological functioning of medications.

Ask students to identify psychosocial factors that can influence an individual's response to medication therapy.

15.0 Identify and assist individuals who are receiving medications and who have special needs, e.g. children, the elderly, and individuals with chronic pain.

15.1 Describe, using examples, three basic methods used to correctly calculate pediatric drug dosages. (p. 1046)

15.2 Identify individuals who may need special assistance when taking medications. (p. 1052)

15.3 Describe basic nursing intervention useful in assisting individuals with special medication administration needs. (p. 1052)

## Written Exercise

Have students calculate pediatric drug dosages using Clark's rule.

## Clinical Laboratory Experience

Assist students in identifying individuals in the clinical facility that might require special assistance when taking medications.

16.0 Describe the methods of teaching self-care to persons receiving medications.

    16.1 Outline the educational needs of individuals who are taking medications at home. (p. 1052)

    16.2 Identify factors that influence the occurrence of drug errors in individuals taking medication at home. (p. 1052)

## Clinical Laboratory Experience

Have students identify the educational needs of an individual in the clinical facility who will be self-administering medications upon discharge from the hospital. Ask them to develop a teaching/learning plan to meet the identified needs of the individual.

## MULTIPLE CHOICE QUESTIONS

1. The "five rights of medication administration" include:

    A. Generic name, action, drug, dose, time
    B. Person, drug, route, dose, and time
    C. Person, drug, dose, time, expiration date
    D. Person, room, drug, dose, time

B   The nurse can prevent medication errors by observing the "five rights of medication administration" which include: Right person, right drug, right route, right dose, and right time. (p. 1036)

2. The law regulating the use and sale of medications in the United States is the:

    A. Controlled Substance Act
    B. Federal Drug Act
    C. Food, Drug, and Cosmetic Act
    D. National Food and Drug Act

C   The Federal Food, Drug, and Cosmetic Act of 1938 is the major statute regulating drugs in the United States. (p. 1037)

3. Which of the following statements is incorrect?

    A. Adverse drug effects occur from overdoses of medication
    B. All medications have both desirable and undesirable effects
    C. A drug may increase or decrease the effect of another drug
    D. Toxic drug doses may result in death

A   Adverse effects of a medication pertain to those body responses that are unintended or harmful. They occur with normal doses, whereas toxic effects are adverse reactions resulting from overdoses or abnormal accumulation of the drug in the body. (p. 1042)

4. Which of the following associations is incorrect?

    A. ac - before meals
    B. ad lib - freely
    C. OD - left eye
    D. QID - four times a day

C   OD is the abbreviation for right eye (p. 1043)

5. Mrs. Parker is to receive Ampicillin 250 mg po BID. This means that she should receive the medication:

    A. After meals twice a day
    B. By mouth twice a day
    C. By mouth three times a day
    D. Twice a day when needed

B   The abbreviations po BID means by mouth twice a day. (p. 1043)

6. A physician order reads: Demerol 50 mg IM every 4 hr as needed for pain. This is an example of which type of medication order?

    A. One time order
    B. Routine order
    C. Single order
    D. PRN order

D   A PRN medication order, such as the one listed in the situation, can be administered at the nurse's discretion within the time limitations given. (p. 1044)

7. All of the following dosages are described according to the apothecary system of measurement except:

A. 15 g
B. 1 mg
C. 4 ounces
D. 1 pint

B  The apothecary system of measurement includes: Minums, dram, ounce, grain, pound, pint, quart, and gallon. A milligram is a unit of measurement used in the metric system of measurement. (p. 1046)

8. Which of the following associations is incorrect?

A. 2 tsp. = 10 cc
B. 2 pints = 1 liter
C. 1 quart = 1000 ml
D. 2 ounces = 50 cc

D  Options A, B, and C are correct. One ounce is equal to 30 cc, so 2 ounces is equal to 60 cc. (p. 1048)

9. As you prepare to administer an injection of penicillin, the individual asks you what the medication is and why he is receiving it. Your best response would be:

A. "It is a medication for your urinary tract infection."
B. "It is a medication that your physician prescribed for your urinary tract infection."
C. It is penicillin and it is for your urinary tract infection."
D. "You'll have to ask your physician. I can't give you that information."

C  People receiving medication have the right to know the medication name, actions, and side effects. This understanding and knowledge promotes adherence to the treatment plan. (p. 1052)

# 49

# ADMINISTERING ORAL AND TOPICAL MEDICATIONS

## OBJECTIVES

1.0 State the steps for preparing and administering an oral medication, and explain the rationale.

1.1 Understand terminology used in the administration of oral and topical medications. (p. 1055)

1.2 Discuss benefits and disadvantages of oral medication administration. (p. 1055)

1.3 Differentiate between various solid forms of oral medication: Tablets, capsules, powders, pills, and lozenges. (p. 1055)

1.4 Differentiate between various forms of oral liquid medication: Syrup, solution, suspension, emulsion, elixir, and tincture. (p. 1055)

1.5 Identify factors that influence the oral administration of medications. (p. 1056)

1.6 Identify significant environmental factors that can have an influence on the effect of medications administered orally. (p. 1056)

1.7 Identify dietary factors influencing oral medication administration. (p. 1056)

1.8 List possible reasons an individual may have difficulty ingesting oral medications. (p. 1056)

1.9 Identify oral medications that cannot be altered for the purpose of easier administration. (p. 1057)

1.10 Describe the basic purpose of oral medication administration. (p. 1056)

1.11 Identify the contraindications and precautions the nurse should take into consideration when administering oral medications. (p. 1057)

1.12 List the educational needs of an individual receiving oral medications. (p. 1058)

1.13 Identify essential assessment data that should be obtained prior to oral medication administration. (p. 1058)

## TEACHING/LEARNING STRATEGIES

### Lecture/Discussion

Ask students to review the terminology listed on page 1055 in the text.

Ask students to identify factors that could affect oral medication administration.

Ask students to identify essential data to be obtained in the nursing history of an individual receiving medications.

Have students discuss the variations in methods of medication administration required for infants, children, and elderly individuals.

### Written Exercise

Ask students to outline the essential steps that should be followed when administering medications.

### Clinical Laboratory Experience

Assist students in identifying examples of the different oral and topical forms of medication during a clinical experience.

Encourage students to review medication policies for their clinical facility.

2.0 Prepare and administer oral medications.

    2.1 List the equipment needed to administer oral medications. (p. 1058)

    2.2 Describe the steps the nurse should follow in order to administer oral medications. (p. 1058)

    2.3 Summarize the nurse's responsibilities after administering oral medications. (p. 1061)

    2.4 Describe data that should be documented in the clinical record of an individual who has received an oral medication. (p. 1061)

### Lecture/Discussion

Demonstrate the procedure for administering oral medications. Have students practice the procedure in a simulated campus laboratory experience.

### Clinical Laboratory Experience

Provide an example of the forms that are used to document medication administration in each clinical facility. Allow time for students to practice using the form for their clinical facility.

Upon demonstration of proficiency, allow students to administer oral medications to assigned individuals under supervision.

3.0 Alter oral medications in order to ease ingestion, e.g., crushing tablets, diluting medications.

    3.1 Outline guidelines the nurse can follow to facilitate oral medication ingestion in individuals who have difficulty swallowing. (p. 1057)

### Lecture/Discussion

Ask students to identify medications that should not be crushed or altered for administration purposes.

### Clinical Laboratory Experience

Have students identify individuals in the clinical facility that may experience problems when taking oral medications.

4.0 Describe the types of medications used for topical administration.

    4.1 Discuss the advantages and disadvantages of topical medication administration. (p. 1061)

    4.2 Briefly describe the various topical medication preparations: Lotions, creams, ointments, powders, gels, liquids, and aerosols. (p. 1061)

    4.3 Review the structure and function of the integumentary system. (p. 1062)

    4.4 Identify ways in which the skin can influence the absorption of a topical medication. (p. 1062)

    4.5 Identify the three most common sites for instillation and irrigation of medication. (p. 1065)

### Lecture/Discussion

Discuss the advantages and disadvantages of topical medication administration.

Ask students to identify the distinguishing characteristics of different types of topical medications: Lotions, creams, ointments, powders, gels, liquids, and aerosols.

Have students identify factors that enhance the absorption of topical medications.

5.0 Differentiate between sterile and nonsterile body cavities.

### Lecture/Discussion

Ask students to identify specific topical medication procedures that require sterile aseptic practice.

6.0 Describe methods of administering topical medications to the skin and mucous membranes, and the underlying rationale.

    6.1 List nursing actions that should be carried out when preparing to administer topical medications to the skin. (p. 1062)

### Lecture/Discussion

Have students differentiate between the positions used for instilling ear drops in adults and children.

6.2  Outline guidelines the nurse should
     follow when applying topical lotions,
     creams, ointments, or gels to the skin
     surface.  (p. 1063)

6.3  Identify the steps involved in the
     topical application of powders and
     aerosol medications to the skin
     surface.  (p. 1063)

6.4  Outline guidelines the nurse should
     follow when giving medicated baths or
     soaks, and when applying wet dressings.
     (p. 1063)

6.5  Identify types of medications that may
     be administered by the insertion method
     of administration.  (p. 1064)

6.6  Describe the essential steps that should
     be taken by the nurse to insert vaginal
     and rectal suppositories.  (p. 1064)

6.7  Briefly describe the most common methods
     of medication administration to mucous
     membranes:  Insertion, instillation/
     irrigation, and inhalation.  (p. 1064)

6.8  Identify essential steps and nursing
     responsibilities for instillation of
     nasal medications.  (p. 1065)

6.9  Outline the basic steps the nurse should
     follow when administering eye drops or
     ointment.  (p. 1065)

6.10 Describe the procedure for irrigation of
     the eyes.  (p. 1066)

6.11 Describe the sequence of steps that
     should be followed to place otic drops
     or perform irrigation of the external
     auditory canal.  (p. 1066)

6.12 Describe the anatomical differences
     between the auditory canal of an adult
     and that of an infant.  (p. 1066)

6.13 Outline nursing responsibilities with
     regard to irrigation of the vaginal
     canal.  (p. 1067)

6.14 Compare and contrast the techniques used
     in nose, eye, and ear instillations and
     irrigations.  (p. 1067)

6.15 Discuss the role of the nurse in the
     administration of medication by
     inhalation.  (p. 1067)

6.16 Briefly describe two groups of medicinal
     substances that are administered by the
     inhalation method:  Volatile and non-
     volatile.  (p. 1068)

7.0  Explain the precautions necessary for topical
     administration of medications.

## Campus Laboratory Experience

Demonstrate the procedure for administering
various forms of topical medications:  Insertion
of rectal or vaginal suppositories, instillation
and irrigation of nasal, eye, ear, and vaginal
medications, and inhalation of medication into the
lungs.  Have students practice each procedure in a
simulated campus laboratory experience.

## Lecture/Discussion

Ask students to describe the assessment data that
should be gathered before administering topical
medications.

8.0 Differentiate between local and systemic
effects of medications.

9.0 Safely administer topical medications to skin
and mucous membranes.

## Clinical Laboratory Experience

Upon demonstration of proficiency, allow students
to administer topical forms of medications under
supervision.

---

## MULTIPLE CHOICE QUESTIONS

1. Which of the following liquid medication
forms may be contraindicated in the diabetic
individual?

   A. Elixir
   B. Syrup
   C. Tincture
   D. All of the above

2. Mrs. Barker is to receive an enteric coated
form of aspirin three times daily. If she
has difficulty swallowing the medication, the
nurse should:

   A. Crush the medication and give it to her
      in juice
   B. Have her take the medication in an
      upright sitting position
   C. Mix the medication with soft foods
   D. Place the medication farther back on the
      tongue to facilitate swallowing

3. The nurse should plan to teach the individual
who is receiving medications about all of the
following except:

   A. Frequency of the medication and how it
      works
   B. Name of the medication and how it works
   C. Possible synergistic effects of the
      medication
   D. Way in which the medication is to be given

4. The most accurate method for identifying an
individual who is to receive medication is to:

   A. Read the name on the I.D. band
   B. Read the name at the door or bedside
   C. Ask the person to state their name
   D. Address the person by name

5. The nurse should document the administration
of a medication:

   A. When the medication is being prepared
   B. Before leaving for the day
   C. Immediately after administration
   D. Within one hour from the time it was
      administered

## CORRECT ANSWER AND RATIONALE

D   All listed options may contain sugar, so
    should be given cautiously to the diabetic
    individual. (p. 1056)

B   If a person has difficulty swallowing, the
    nurse should: Administer the medication with
    at least 60 to 100 cc of fluid, if appro-
    priate, and have the individual assume a
    standing or upright position. (p. 1057)

C   The individual should be given the information
    listed in options A, B, and D. (p. 1058)

A   The most accurate method of identification
    prior to any procedure is to check the name on
    the individual's I.D. band. If the individual
    is confused or the wrong label has been placed
    on the room or bed, the nurse may administer
    the medication to the wrong individual.
    (p. 1060)

C   The nurse should document drug administration
    immediately after leaving the individual's
    room. This reduces the possibility of the
    medication being repeated by another nurse.
    It should never be documented before
    administration because the individual may be
    unable to take the medication, may refuse it,
    or may not be present on the unit. (p. 1061)

6. The nurse should use sterile technique when administering which type of topical medication?

   A. Vaginal suppositories
   B. Opthalmic solutions
   C. Nasal medications
   D. Otic solutions

7. Mr. Lily is to have one drop of a 1% Epinephrine solution instilled OD b.i.d. The nurse demonstrates correct medication administration technique when doing all of the following except:

   A. Instills one drop of medication into the right eye
   B. Drops the medication onto the lower conjunctival sac
   C. Asks the individual to look straight ahead when instilling the medication
   D. Uses sterile technique to administer the medication twice daily

B  Sterile technique is advocated when instilling eye medications because of the sensitive nature of the tissue. Clean technique is generally used for the other listed options. However, the nurse should use sterile technique when instilling medication into the ears if it is suspected that the system is not intact. (pp. 1064-1067)

C  The nurse should ask the person to "look up" and then deposit the medication. This technique reduces stimulation of the corneal reflex, which could cause injury if the person startles or jerks away. (p. 1066)

# 50

# ADMINISTERING PARENTERAL MEDICATIONS

OBJECTIVES

1.0 Identify factors to consider in choosing a site for an injection.

    1.1 Define important terminology related to the administration of parenteral medications. (p. 1071)

    1.2 Identify and briefly describe major routes used by the nurse to administer parenteral medications. (p. 1071)

    1.3 Describe other parenteral routes for medication administration: Intra-arterial, intracardiac, intra-articular, intraperitoneal, intrapleural, and intrathecal. (p. 1071)

    1.4 Briefly discuss basic medication characteristics that influence the nurse's selection of route and site of injection in parenteral medications. (p. 1072)

    1.5 Describe data that should be collected to assess an individual's mental attitude toward injections. (p. 1073)

2.0 Describe the anatomy of the site selected.

    2.1 Identify criteria essential for assessing potential parenteral injection sites. (p. 1072)

    2.2 Identify the purpose and most common injection sites for intradermal medication administration. (p. 1080)

    2.3 Identify the various factors that must be considered in assessment of a site for intradermal administration of a medication. (p. 1080)

    2.4 Identify the purpose and most common sites for injection of subcutaneous medications. (p. 1081)

    2.5 Briefly describe the technique used to identify the various sites for intramuscular injection: Ventrogluteal, Quadriceps femoris, dorsogluteal, and mid-deltoid. (p. 1084)

TEACHING/LEARNING STRATEGIES

Lecture/Discussion

Ask students to review the terminology listed on page 1070 in the text.

Ask students to identify factors that can influence the administration of parenteral medications.

Lecture/Discussion

Discuss the technique for locating intramuscular injection sites: Ventrogluteal, quadraceps femoris, dorsogluteal, and mid-deltoid.

Campus Laboratory Experience

Demonstrate the procedure for locating intramuscular injection sites. Ask students to practice each method of location with another classmate.

Identify the sites used to administer intradermal and subcutaneous injections. Ask students to identify each of the sites on another classmate.

3.0 Select appropriate needle gauge and length to use in parenteral therapy, based on medication characteristics, route ordered, and physical size and condition of the individual.

    3.1 Compare and contrast the purpose, syringe type, needle length and gauge, and recommended injections volumes for the various parenteral routes: Intradermal, subcutaneous, Intramuscular, and intravenous. (p. 1076)

    3.2 Identify criteria the nurse should use to select the appropriate needle and syringe. (p. 1076)

4.0 Discuss techniques that reduce the discomfort associated with injections.

    4.1 Identify nursing intervention measures to reduce the discomfort and anxiety that often accompany parenteral medication administration. (p. 1074)

5.0 Identify hazards of parenteral therapy.

    5.1 Enumerate the advantages of administering medications via a parenteral route. (p. 1071)

    5.2 Discuss the disadvantages of administering medications via a parenteral route. (p. 1072)

    5.3 Enumerate the advantages and disadvantages of intravenous therapy. (p. 1090)

6.0 Apply aseptic principles to parenteral therapy.

    6.1 Describe the nurse's responsibilities related to the proper care and handling of syringes and needles. (p. 1078)

7.0 List indications and contraindications for parenteral routes.

    7.1 Identify common contraindications and precautions the nurse should consider when administering intradermal medications. (p. 1081)

## Class Activity

Ask students to list the criteria that should be used in choosing the appropriate needle and syringe. Give them specific clinical examples and ask them to identify appropriate syringes and needles to be used.

## Campus Laboratory Experience

Obtain examples of the different size needles and syringes used for administering injections. Allow students to view them in the campus laboratory facility.

## Lecture/Discussion

Focus discussion on the advantages and disadvantages of using parenteral routes for medication administration purposes.

Help students to understand the complications that can occur in conjunction with IV therapy. Emphasize methods the nurse can use to prevent the occurrence of each.

## Group Activity

Discuss appropriate nursing intervention for common IV complications: Infiltration of IV solution, Phlebitis, Infection of site, air embolism, hypersensitivity reaction, circulatory overload, hypoglycemia, and hyperglycemia.

## Lecture/Discussion

Ask students to identify appropriate aseptic practices that should be performed when administering parenteral medications.

Emphasize the importance of using good aseptic technique when administering parenteral medications.

## Lecture/Discussion

Ask students to discuss the advantages of using a heparin lock system instead of a continuous IV infusion system.

7.2  Identify contraindications and precautions the nurse should consider when administering any intramuscular medication. (p. 1086)

7.3  Identify major contraindications and precautions associated with percutaneous venipuncture. (p. 1092)

8.0  Identify individuals requiring special consideration during administration of parenteral medications.

8.1  Discuss assessment data indicative of individuals with problems of altered circulation, musculature and integument. (p. 1073)

8.2  Discuss the responsibilities of the nurse in assessing children who are to receive parenteral medications. (p. 1073)

8.3  Identify essential sources of data to obtain when assessing elderly individuals receiving parenteral medication. (p. 1074)

9.0  Prepare and administer medications by intradermal, subcutaneous, and intramuscular injections knowledgeably, skillfully, and safely.

9.1  Identify essential data that should be assessed prior to the administration of parenteral medications. (p. 1072)

9.2  Outline basic principles of parenteral drug administration that the nurse should understand before administering parenteral medications: Safety considerations and asepsis. (p. 1075)

9.3  Describe the procedure for cleansing the skin prior to venipuncture. (p. 1076)

9.4  Outline appropriate nursing measures for removing/administering parenteral medications stored in various types of containers: Ampules, vials, and prepackaged, prefilled cartridges and prefilled syringes. (p. 1078)

9.5  Identify assessment data indicative of an allergic reaction to a medication that has been administered intradermally. (p. 1080)

9.6  List nursing actions that should be carried out after the injection of an intradermal medication. (p. 1081)

9.7  Describe the practice of using rotating-site charts for individuals receiving subcutaneous injections over a prolonged period of time. (p. 1081)

## Lecture/Discussion

Ask students to discuss the physiological changes related to aging that influence the effectiveness of parenteral medication administration.

## Clinical Laboratory Experience

Assist students in identifying individuals in the clinical area that would require special consideration during the administration of parenteral medications.

## Lecture/Discussion

Have students describe the information that should be included when documenting injections.

Ask students to identify the appropriate angle at which the needle is inserted when giving intradermal, subcutaneous, and intramuscular injections.

## Written Exercise

Have students list the information that should be included in the nursing assessment of an individual receiving parenteral medications.

## Campus Laboratory Experience

Demonstrate the technique for removing medications from ampules and vials. Allow students to practice each technique in the campus laboratory setting.

Demonstrate the Z-track technique for administering intramuscular injections. Ask students to perform this procedure on a mannequin in the campus laboratory setting.

## Clinical Laboratory Experience

Upon demonstration of proficiency, allow students to administer intradermal, subcutaneous, and intramuscular injections to individuals in the clinical area under supervision.

Arrange for students to observe venipuncture procedures being performed on individuals in their clinical facility.

9.8 Identify the teaching/learning needs of individuals who are receiving intra-dermal medications. (p. 1081)

9.9 Identify assessment data that should be gathered by the nurse prior to adminis-tering an intradermal medication. (p. 1082)

9.10 List the equipment needed by the nurse to administer a medication intra-dermally. (p. 1082)

9.11 Describe the steps that the nurse should follow to properly administer an intra-dermal medication. (p. 1082)

9.12 Describe the responsibilities of the nurse upon completion of the adminis-tration of an intradermal medication. (p. 1082)

9.13 Identify data that should be documented in the clinical record after the ad-ministration of an intradermal medica-tion. (p. 1082)

9.14 Identify basic contraindications and precautions that should be remembered when administering subcutaneous medications. (p. 1083)

9.15 Briefly describe the educational needs of an individual receiving subcutaneous injections of medication. (p. 1083)

9.16 Identify data that should be gathered by the nurse when assessing a person prior to the injection of a subcutaneous medication. (p. 1083)

9.17 Identify equipment needed to administer a subcutaneous injection. (p. 1083)

9.18 Identify the steps that the nurse should follow to administer medication subcutaneously. (p. 1083)

9.19 Describe nursing responsibilities upon completion of a subcutaneous medication injection. (p. 1084)

9.20 List the data the nurse should document in an individual's clinical record after administering a subcutaneous injection. (p. 1084)

9.21 List items that should be included in a general assessment prior to administering an intramuscular medication. (p. 1085)

9.22 Outline guidelines for administering intramuscular medications via the Z-track method of administration. (p. 1085)

9.23 Briefly discuss reasons for utilizing the air-lock technique when adminis-tering an intramuscular medication. (p. 1085)

9.24 Identify the essential teaching needs of an individual receiving an intramuscular medication. (p. 1086)

9.25 Describe the preliminary planning and assessment and planning activities of the nurse administering an intramuscular injection of medication. (p. 1087)

9.26 Identify the equipment the nurse should gather to administer medication intramuscularly. (p. 1087)

9.27 Describe the steps involved in the administration of intramuscular injections. Include in this description, general considerations, the air-lock technique, and the Z-track method of administration. (p. 1087)

9.28 Discuss nursing actions that should be carried out after administering an intramuscular injection of medication. (p. 1090)

9.29 List data that should be documented in the clinical record after administering an intramuscular medication. (p. 1090)

9.30 Outline the teaching/learning needs of individuals receiving percutaneous venipuncture for peripheral IV therapy purposes. (p. 1092)

10.0 Perform a venipuncture for withdrawal of a blood sample or administration of an infusion.

10.1 Briefly describe equipment used to administer intravenous medications. (p. 1090)

10.2 Identify factors that influence the choice of equipment used in administering intravenous medications. (p. 1090)

10.3 Discuss the advantages of using a heparin lock system for intravenous therapy. (p. 1090)

10.4 Identify factors the nurse should consider when selecting a venipuncture site for peripheral IV therapy. (p. 1092)

10.5 Define and briefly describe the purpose of percutaneous venipuncture. (p. 1092)

10.6 Discuss preliminary assessment and planning activities that should be performed by the nurse prior to percutaneous venipuncture. (p. 1093)

10.7 Identify the equipment needed to perform a percutaneous venipuncture. (p. 1093)

10.8 Describe the steps that should be followed to perform percutaneous venipuncture. (p. 1093)

## Lecture/Discussion

Ask students to identify the information that should be included when documenting a venipuncture procedure. Have them write a sample nursing recording for venipuncture insertion for a hypothetical situation.

Ask students to outline the assessment data that should be included in the assessment of an individual receiving intravenous therapy.

## Campus Laboratory Experience

Demonstrate the technique for percutaneous venipuncture. Have students practice the technique on a mannequin in the campus laboratory setting.

Have students identify common venipuncture sites on another classmate.

## Clinical Laboratory Experience

Ask students to review the policy for IV insertion for their clinical facility.

10.9 Describe appropriate nursing measures
that should be performed by the nurse
after a percutaneous venipuncture.
(p. 1094)

10.10 Describe data to be included when
documenting a percutaneous venipuncture. (p. 1095)

10.11 Describe assessment data useful in
identifying individuals who may require
intravenous therapy. (p. 1095)

10.12 Identify data useful in assessing an
individual's response to IV therapy.
(p. 1095)

10.13 Identify common problems/complications
associated with IV therapy and venipuncture. (p. 1096)

10.14 Discuss possible nursing measures that
can be utilized to reduce complications
often encountered with IV therapy and
venipuncture. (p. 1096)

---

| MULTIPLE CHOICE QUESTIONS | CORRECT ANSWER AND RATIONALE |
|---|---|
| 1. You are to administer an intradermal medica-tion to Mr. Johnson for diagnostic purposes. All of the following injection sites would be appropriate except:<br><br>A. Lateral aspect of the upper arm<br>B. Lower ventral abdominal wall<br>C. Inner surface of the forearm<br>D. Anterior aspect of the upper chest | B Substances used for skin testing can be potent. Therefore, the less vasculary ID layer is used to retard absorption. The ventral mid-forearm and the scapulae are the most common ID injection sites. Other sites include the upper arm and upper chest. (p. 1080) |
| 2. When a subcutaneous medication ordered for an emaciated individual, the nurse should administer the medication with a:<br><br>A. 1/2 inch needle at a 45 degree angle<br>B. 3/8 inch needle at a 90 degree angle<br>C. 5/8 inch needle at a 45 degree angle<br>D. 5/8 inch needle at a 90 degree angle | C For a small child or an emaciated adult, the nurse should use a 5/8 inch needle at a 45 degree angle, or a 1/2 inch needle at a 90 degree angle. This technique decreases the possibility of the needle entering the muscular tissue. (p. 1083) |
| 3. An obese individual is to receive Diluadid 2 mg IM PRN. The nurse demonstrates correct administration technique when performing all of the following except:<br><br>A. Select a one inch, 22 gauge needle for administration<br>B. Maintains sterile technique throughout the procedure<br>C. Administers the medication at a 90 degree angle<br>D. Uses the air-lock technique when instilling the medication | A The nurse should select a longer needle when administering intramuscular medications to an obese individual to assure penetration of the needle into muscular tissue. (p. 1084) |

4.  Which intramuscular injection site is
    relatively free of major nerves and blood
    vessels?

    A.  Deltoid
    B.  Dorsogluteal
    C.  Ventrogluteal
    D.  Vastus lateralis

D   The nurse should use caution when selecting
    the IM sites listed in options A, B, and C to
    avoid major nerves, arteries, and veins.  The
    quadraceps femoris site (vastus lateralis and
    rectus femoris muscles) is relatively free of
    major nerves and blood vessels.  (p. 1088)

5.  Mrs. Sanford's IV site is swollen, red,
    painful, and cold to touch.  What does this
    indicate?

    A.  Infection at the site
    B.  Inflammation of the vein
    C.  Infiltration of IV solution
    D.  Hypersensitivity reaction

C   An IV site that appears edematous, blanched or
    red, painful and cold indicates an
    infiltration of IV solution.  (p. 1097)

6.  When an IV infiltration is suspected, the
    nurse should:

    A.  Discontinue the IV and restart it in
        another site
    B.  Ask another nurse to confirm the
        observations
    C.  Irrigate the IV and observe the reaction
        at the site
    D.  All of the above

A   The nurse should discontinue the IV and, if
    necessary, restart the infusion at an
    alternative site, preferably in another
    extremity.  (p. 1097)

NOTES

NOTES

NOTES

NOTES

NOTES